Personalized Mechanical Ventilation

Jorge Hidalgo • Robert C Hyzy
Ahmed Mohamed Reda Taha
Yasser Younis A. Tolba
Editors

Personalized Mechanical Ventilation

Improving Quality of Care

Springer

Editors
Jorge Hidalgo
Critical Care Division
Belize Healthcare Partners
Belize, Belize

Robert C Hyzy
Pulmonary and Critical Care
University of Michigan
Ann Arbor, MI, USA

Ahmed Mohamed Reda Taha
Critical Care Institute
Cleveland Clinic
Abu Dhabi, UAE

Yasser Younis A. Tolba
Critical Care
King Faisal Specialist Hospital & Research
Riyadh, Saudi Arabia

ISBN 978-3-031-14137-9 ISBN 978-3-031-14138-6 (eBook)
https://doi.org/10.1007/978-3-031-14138-6

This Springer imprint is published by the registered company Springer Nature Switzerland AG
The registered company address is: Gewerbestrasse 11, 6330 Cham, Switzerland

Preface

Much has been written in recent years about the emergence of "personalized medicine." Of course, medicine has always been tailored to individual circumstances, and in a sense, personalized medicine is not terribly new. However, advances in medical knowledge in terms of genetics, biomarkers, and other features, with subsequent acknowledgment of the heterogeneity of treatment effect (HTE) in clinical trials, have required clinicians to be evermore cognizant of the need to approach therapeutic endeavors by patient subgroups.

The last few decades have seen advances in patient outcomes and quality of care resulting from the initiation and use of various checklists and protocols. Yet, a one-size-fits-all approach to patients requiring mechanical ventilation is woefully insufficient to meet individual patient needs. While the use of lung-protective ventilation in ARDS has been implemented in a somewhat standardized fashion, there are multiple other circumstances intensivists confront, where the application of mechanical ventilation is far from standardized. Hence, the application of mechanical ventilation to patients also requires a personalized approach.

We are pleased then to offer this new book by Springer Incorporated entitled "Personalized Mechanical Ventilation." Over the course of 26 chapters, mechanical ventilation use in circumstances such as obesity, trauma, pregnancy, and shock, as well as many others, is addressed. Each chapter affords the intensivist a fresh perspective on how to utilize mechanical ventilation in each condition. We have secured contributions from an array of international experts to offer their perspective on a large array of clinical scenarios where mechanical ventilation is employed. We believe that busy intensivists will find this work useful as they attempt to treat their critically ill patients.

Abu Dhabi, UAE — Ahmed Mohamed Reda Taha
Ann Arbor, MI — Robert C Hyzy
Belize, Belize — Jorge Hidalgo
Riyadh, Saudi Arabia — Yasser Younis A. Tolba

Prologue

It is a real honor for me to be the bearer of some considerations in the prologue of this exquisite new scientific work, where authors from all over the world, mainly the Middle East, the United States, and Latin America, join together to offer their experiences about the management of mechanical ventilation focusing its use on a personalized, directed, and unique way according to the needs and problems that each group of patients deserves.

This new work makes a necessary and invaluable account of respiratory physiology and the findings found at the patient's bedside, covering in an orderly manner the elements that make up the anatomy of a ventilator, its circuits, and ventilatory modes, and which throughout history have been used for the benefit of the critically ill patient.

When talking about mechanical ventilation, it seems that everything has been said. However, it surprises us when trying to customize new methods. We find questions regarding how should patients with a unilateral lung injury be managed, postoperative ventilation, rapid extubation, when and how, and ventilation in patients with COVID 19, among others.

The authors also analyze the pros and cons of multiple ventilation with a single ventilator, almost in the style of an in-depth editorial, thus arriving at the state of the art of weaning from mechanical ventilation.

I can only congratulate the distinguished authors of this magnificent work in a very special way since it will surely give answers to many situations that arise in daily life with the use of this formidable tool considered by some as the right hand of critical medicine: "Personalized Mechanical Ventilation."

Punta Pacific Hospital/Johns Hopkins Medicine
Panama City, Panama

Jorge Sinclair Avila

Special Thanks

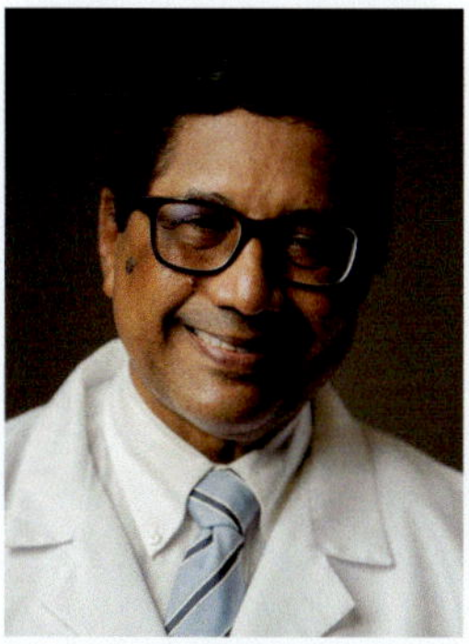

Jorge Sinclair, MD, FCCM, FACP, FCCP
Associate Dean for International and Global Education,
School of Medicine University of Panama.

We would like to express our deep gratitude to Professor Jorge Sinclair, for his academic contribution, enthusiastic encouragement, and useful and constructive recommendations on this project.

Contents

Respiratory Physiology and Mechanics at the Bedside

Ahmed Mohamed Reda Taha and Prashant Nasa

1 Introduction

Mechanical ventilators are sophisticated machines working on complex algorithms to deliver positive-pressure ventilation to patients. Mechanical ventilators are often handled by healthcare professionals with limited training in their different settings and functions. The mechanical ventilation strategy for a particular disease depends on the pathophysiology of the disease and the experience or familiarity of the intensive care unit (ICU) staff to a specific ventilator mode. Understanding of basic physiology of the respiratory system and physics of airflow dynamics is paramount to optimize mechanical ventilation settings. Lung-protective ventilation (LPV) for patients on invasive mechanical ventilation has consistently shown mortality benefit. The core principle of the LPV strategy is to reduce the harm of positive-pressure ventilation, also called ventilator-induced lung injury (VILI). ICU management is progressing towards precision-based medicine, defined as treatment tailored to the pathophysiology of the disease instead of based on averages. Respiratory mechanics are a surrogate representation of lung function using pressure, volume, or flows. Understanding respiratory physiology and mechanics represents the first step towards a personalized approach to ventilator management in the ICU. This chapter reviews the applied physiology of the respiratory system, equation of motion, dynamic and static respiratory mechanics, and their implication in the management of invasive or noninvasive mechanical ventilation.

The original version of the chapter has been revised. A correction to this chapter can be found at https://doi.org/10.1007/978-3-031-14138-6_27

A. Mohamed Reda Taha (✉)
Critical Care Institute, Cleveland Clinic, Abu Dhabi, UAE

P. Nasa
NMC Specialty, Dubai, UAE

J. Hidalgo et al. (eds.), *Personalized Mechanical Ventilation*,
https://doi.org/10.1007/978-3-031-14138-6_1

2 Lung Volumes and Capacity

Understanding lung volume and capacity helps to diagnose an obstructive versus restrictive condition, response to therapeutics, prognosis, and assessment of weaning or tracheal extubation (Fig. 1). Functional residual capacity (FRC) is the volume of gas remaining in the lung after normal passive expiration. FRC can be represented mathematically as the sum of expiratory reserve volume and residual volume (Fig. 1). End-expiratory lung volume (EELV) is defined as the addition of positive end-expiratory pressure (PEEP) to the FRC of patients on mechanical ventilation. EELV is simply the volume present in the lungs before the start of the next tidal volume breath. EELV represents the balance of opposing forces and elastic recoil of lungs and chest wall, along with PEEP. The gas exchange in the lung is primarily dependent on the EELV, and mechanical ventilation settings should target optimizing the EELV, thereby reducing the risk of VILI [1]. The decrease in EELV is observed with alveolar collapse, alveolar flooding seen in pulmonary edema or severe pneumonia, and decreased thoracic compliance in obesity or abdominal surgery.

The distribution of tidal volume in a reduced EELV characterized by smaller aerated lung volume may cause VILI in the form of barotrauma or volutrauma. The PEEP titration may avoid end-expiratory alveolar collapse and hence reduction of EELV. The recruitment maneuvers are also targeted to increase the aerated portion of the lung and EELV. The personalized approach to invasive mechanical ventilation, thus, requires measurement of EELV. Unfortunately, the EELV measurement

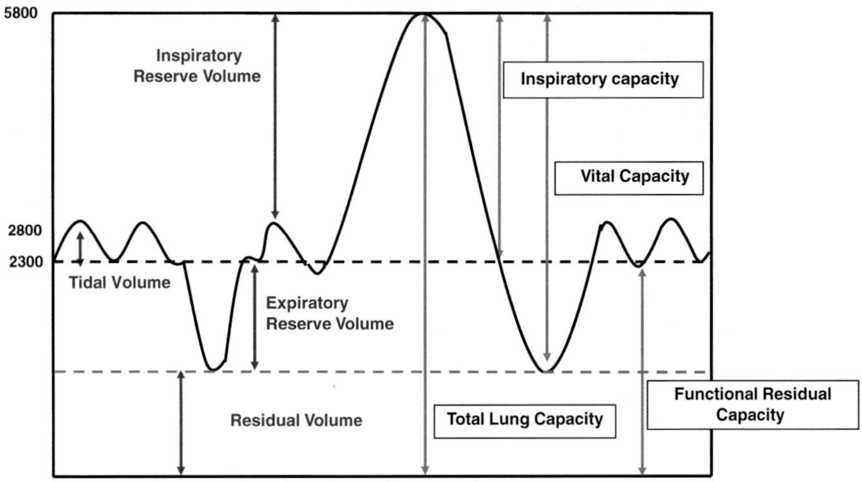

Fig. 1 Lung volumes and capacity. In approximate values: tidal volume (500 mL), expiratory reserve volume (1100 mL), residual volume (1100 mL), inspiratory reserve volume (3000 mL), total lung capacity (5800 mL), vital capacity (4600 mL), functional residual capacity (2300 mL), inspiratory capacity (3500 mL)

is laborious and impractical at the bedside because residual volume calculation needs techniques based on the dilution of trace gases. However, the newer commercial ventilators, using the alteration of a fraction of inspired oxygen, started calculating EELV during controlled ventilation modes.

3 Equation of Motion

The equation of motion is a fundamental concept that describes the overall forces required to drive gases across the respiratory system. The mathematical representation of the equation of motion helps in understanding respiratory mechanics during invasive mechanical ventilation. The equation states that the pressure required to (both inspiratory muscles and the ventilator) drive the gases into the lungs is equal and opposite to the force offered by the patient's respiratory system. The force of the respiratory system has three components: an elastic component (distension of the lung parenchyma), a resistive component (airway resistance till respiratory bronchiole), and an inertial component (changes in the lung parenchyma caused by volume acceleration). At usual respiratory frequencies of under 1 Hz (60 rpm), the inertial component is negligible and can be excluded for calculation.

Equation of motion:

$$\mathbf{P_{MUS} + P_{VENT} = Resistive\ component + Distention\ component + Inertial\ component}$$

$\mathbf{P_{MUS}}$: Pressure generated by the inspiratory muscles. In case of complete paralysis without any inspiratory muscle effort, $\mathbf{P_{MUS}}$ will become zero. $\mathbf{P_{VENT}}$: Pressure generated at the ventilator end and reflects airway pressure (Paw) or Pao (pressure at airway opening). Resistance component: Resistance of the respiratory system, which equals to flow ($\dot{V}$) X resistance (**R**). Distension component: Respiratory system elastance (inverse of respiratory system compliance) X change in volume (**ΔV**).

$$\mathbf{P_{MUS} + P_{VENT} = \left(\dot{V} \times R\right) + \left(\Delta V / compliance\right) + PEEP + inertance}$$

PEEP is the total PEEP, which includes set PEEP on the ventilator and intrinsic PEEP.

Inertance is the component contributed by system inertia, which is generally insignificant for calculation purpose and can be ignored.

4 Alveolar Pressure (P_{alv})

Alveolar pressure, defined as the pressure in the alveoli at the end of inflation, is a surrogate of alveolar distension during inspiration. Due to the resistance component, pressure at airway opening (Pao) is always greater than Palv. The end-inspiratory breath hold of 0.5–2 s equilibrates the system pressure, stopping the flow and reducing the resistance component to zero (Fig. 2). The measured Pao at static flow is called plateau pressure (Pplat), and once the equilibrium is achieved in the airway, it is the surrogate of alveolar pressure. Pplat is dependent on two variables, tidal volume and compliance:

$$\mathbf{P_{plat} = Vt / C_{rs}}$$

Vt: Tidal volume. C_{rs}: Compliance

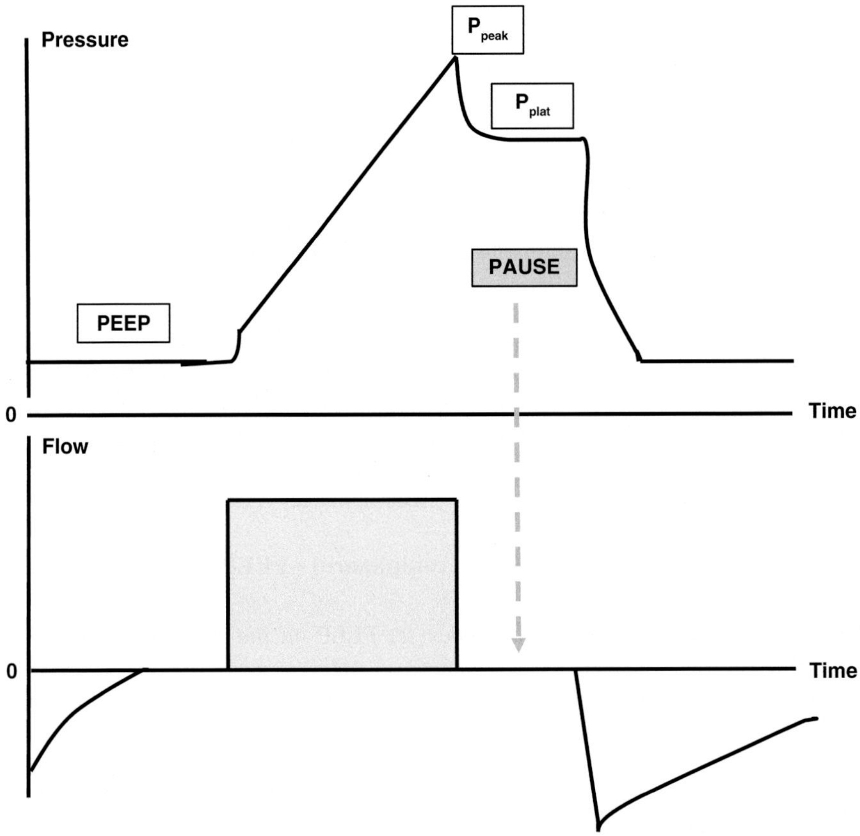

Fig. 2 Pressure-time and flow-time waveforms during volume control ventilation, illustrating the effect of an end-inspiratory pause (breath hold). In the period of no flow, the pressure equilibrates to the alveolar pressure or plateau pressure (P_{plat}). *Pplat* plateau pressure, *PEEP* positive end-expiratory pressure, *PIP* peak inspiratory pressure

The end-inspiratory pause of ≥3 s provides the most accurate P_{plat} in both diseased and healthy lung. Shorter pauses of 0.5 s may overestimate P_{plat} acute respiratory distress syndrome (ARDS) and chronic obstructive pulmonary disease (COPD) [2].

The high P_{plat} indicates alveolar overdistension and risk of VILI. The P_{plat} should be less than 30 cmH_2O to reduce VILI, and some evidence supports even lower P_{plat} targets (<25 cmH2O) in patients with ARDS [3, 4].

The newer generation ventilators can provide Pplat without the need for inspiratory breath hold. The real-time determination method of P_{plat} uses the expiratory time constant (τ_E), estimated from the expiratory flow curve:

$$\mathbf{P_{plat} = \left(Vt \times P_{insp}\right) - \left(Vt \times PEEP\right) / \, Vt + \tau_E \times \dot{V}insp}$$

Pinsp: inspiratory peak pressure, $\dot{V}$ insp: inspiratory flow.

5 Driving Pressure

Driving pressure is the pressure generated in the alveoli above PEEP while delivering the tidal volume. The driving pressure can be calculated by the difference between P_{plat} and PEEP and correlates to global lung strain:

$$\textbf{Driving pressure} = \mathbf{P_{plat} - PEEP}$$

PEEP includes total PEEP, including set PEEP and intrinsic PEEP.

There is growing evidence supporting the monitoring of driving pressure during LPV strategy on invasive mechanical ventilation. The studies in intensive care and perioperative settings found driving pressure compared to tidal volume to be a better predictor of clinical outcomes [5–7]. The driving pressure greater than 15 cm of H_2O was associated with increased mortality [relative risk (RR) 1.41]; even with conventional targets of LPV, Pplat [<30 cmH_2O] and Vt [<7 mL/kg/ideal body weight (IBW)] are in target ranges for protective ventilation [6]. In a meta-analysis, during general anesthesia in the operation theatre, the driving pressure [odds ratio (OR) 1.16] was the only ventilatory parameter associated with increased risk of postoperative pulmonary complications [7].

6 Transpulmonary Pressure

The transpulmonary pressure (P_L) is the pressure required to drive the air into the lungs; it includes pressure to move the air through the airways (airway opening—alveolar pressure) and to overcome the elastic recoil of the lungs (calculated as alveolar pressure—pleural pressure):

$$\textbf{Transpulmonary pressure } (P_L) = \textbf{airway opening pressure} - \textbf{pleural pressure}.$$

In static flow conditions (at either end inspiration or end expiration), transpulmonary pressure approximates elastic recoil pressure and surrogates to lung stress during ventilation [8].

The pleural pressure can be calculated through an esophageal manometry with a special balloon and is not always feasible. Hence, P_{plat} pressure or driving pressure is taken as a surrogate of lung stress or VILI and approximates P_L in most situations except where chest or abdominal wall compliance is altered. The divergence of driving pressure and P_L is seen during conditions of raised intra-abdominal pressure (e.g., laparoscopic insufflation, obesity, ascites, supine position) [9–13].

7 Intrinsic PEEP

The positive pressure produced by the trapped gas in the alveoli at the end of expiration is called intrinsic PEEP, auto-PEEP, or occult PEEP. Intrinsic PEEP can be calculated by end-expiratory breath hold when the flow stops and pressure equilibrates (Fig. 3). The total PEEP includes the set PEEP on the ventilator and any intrinsic PEEP:

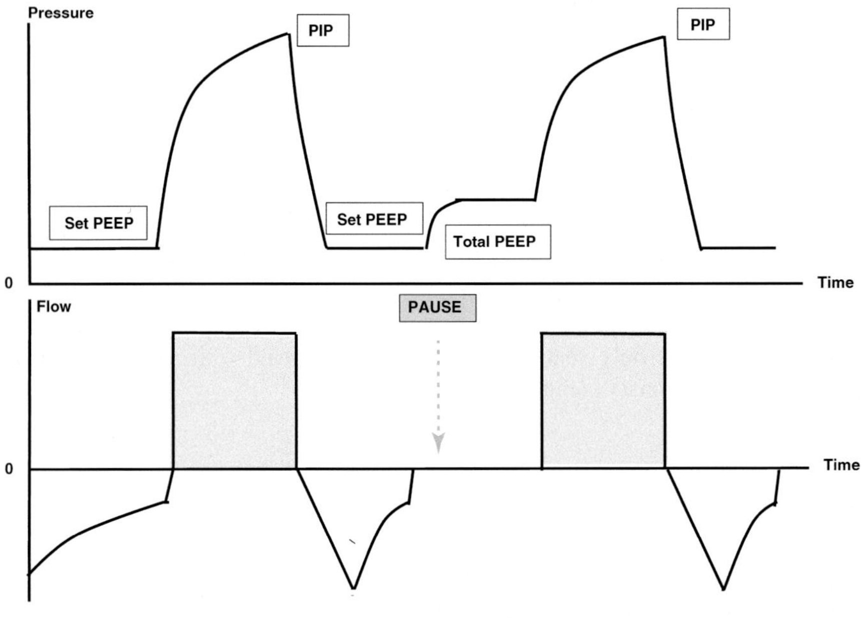

Fig. 3 Pressure-time and flow-time waveforms during volume control ventilation, illustrating the effect of an end-expiratory pause (breath hold). In the period of no flow, the pressure equilibrates to the alveolar pressure and reflects total PEEP. The difference between the total PEEP and set PEEP provides intrinsic PEEP. *PEEP* positive end-expiratory pressure, *PIP* peak inspiratory pressure

$$\textbf{Intrinsic PEEP} = \textbf{Total PEEP}\left(\textbf{end-expiratory pause}\right) - \textbf{set PEEP}$$

The pressure calculation should be done in the absence of any active expiratory effort, which may generate a positive pressure due to chest retraction at the end of expiration that can be misinterpreted as intrinsic PEEP. Intrinsic PEEP may cause dynamic hyperinflation by progressive increasing in end-expiratory lung volumes.

8 Respiratory System Compliance

Compliance (C_{rs}) is the distensibility of the lungs and is defined as the change in lung volumes per unit pressure change. C_{rs} is the inverse of the elastance and can be static or dynamic. The normal value of C_{rs} is 60–100 mL/cmH_2O. The static compliance (with no flow) reflects the elastic recoil pressures of the lungs and can be measured using the following formula:

$$\textbf{Static } \mathbf{C_{rs}} = \mathbf{Vt}/\left(\mathbf{P_{plat}} - \mathbf{PEEP}\right)$$

As the name suggests, dynamic compliance is a continuous measurement, dependent on the elastic and airway resistance. The dynamic compliance can be calculated using a pressure-volume curve. The pressure-volume curves are different for inspiration and expiration due to hysteresis, as the pressure required for lung inflation is higher than deflation (Fig. 4). However, the curves meet at two points, end

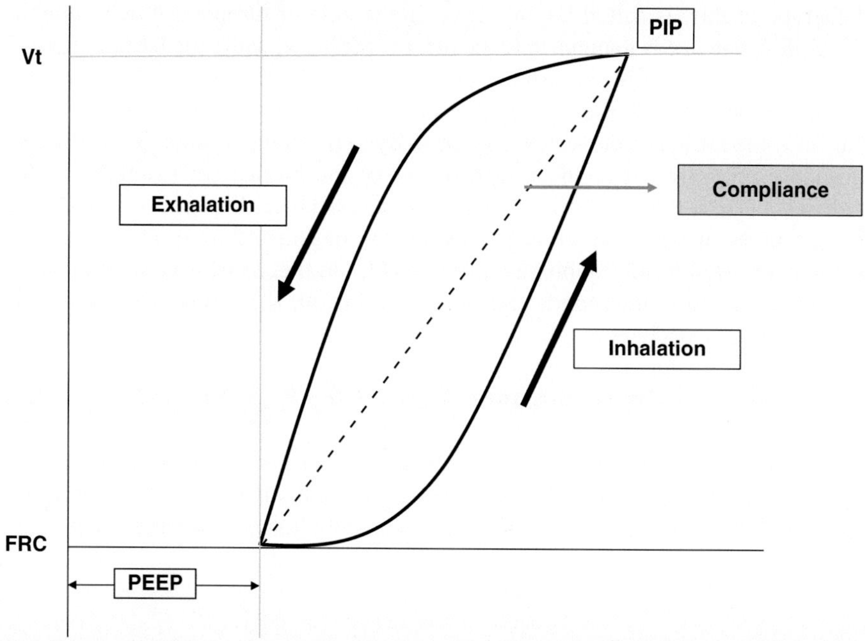

Fig. 4 Pressure-volume curve. *PIP* pressure inspiratory pressure, *PEEP* pressure end-expiratory pressure, *Vt* tidal volume, *FRC* functional residual capacity

inspiration and end expiration. The line connecting the two points provides the dynamic compliance of the lungs [14].

The ventilators may display dynamic C_{rs} (during pressure-controlled ventilation) based on the calculation:

$$\textbf{Dynamic } \mathbf{C_{rs}} = \mathbf{Vt/(PIP - PEEP)}$$

PIP is the peak inspiratory pressure.

A shorter inspiration time, increased airway resistance (R_{aw}), intrinsic PEEP, or active inspiratory effort can create a divergence between the static and dynamic C_{rs} [15].

9 Resistance

Resistance is the opposing friction to airflow during respiration. Resistance of the respiratory system is contributed by airway resistance (R_{aw}), viscoelastic properties of lung or chest wall, and lung parenchyma (due to unequal time constant of different regions). The normal value of resistance is 0.5–2.5 cmH_2O/L/s. R_{aw} depends on the air viscosity and density, and length and radius of airways, and increases with either changes in the flow (higher flow rates on the ventilator) or narrowing of the airways (bronchospasm). In large airways, the flow is described as turbulent when it is at a low velocity, while through narrow tubes, it tends to be more orderly and streamlined and flows in a straight line. This type of flow is called laminar flow. in the case of turbulent flow to double the airflow one needs to quadruple the driving pressure, while the laminar flow is directly proportional to the driving pressure, such that to double the flow rate, one needs only double the driving pressure (Poiseuille's Law). In case of laminar flow, the radius of the airway is a primary dependent variable. Resistance is inversely proportional to the fourth power of the radius; for example, if the radius is halved, there is a 16-fold increase in resistance. Resistance of the lung is a property of volume and decreases during lung insufflation on inspiration, while expiration has an oppositive effect [16]. On mechanical ventilation with assist volume-controlled mode and square waveform, R_{aw} can be measured with end-inspiratory occlusion:

$$\textbf{Airway resistance } \mathbf{(R_{aw}) = (PIP - P_{plat})/Vt}$$

However, during the pressure-controlled mode, inspiratory resistance is difficult to measure, as peak and plateau pressure are usually the same. The ventilators can calculate and display airway resistance and compliance using the equation of motion through the linear least-squares fitting. The software digitizes the variables pressure, volume, and $\dot{V}$ at high speed (100 Hz) and provides real-time compliance and resistance. Though the least-squares fitting method can be applied during the whole breathing cycle, it is recommended to apply it during the inspiratory phase to overcome expiratory flow limitation seen in chronic obstructive pulmonary disease (COPD) [17]. There is an important assumption made (P_{MUS} is zero), and thus, the calculation is valid only in patients without any spontaneous effort [18].

The elastic component of the lung parenchyma also contributes to resistance. Resistance due to elastic component would be high in cases of increased lung and/or chest wall elastance (e.g., ARDS, idiopathic pulmonary fibrosis (IPF)).

10 Expiratory Time Constant

The time constant (TC) is defined as the time (in seconds) required to inflate (inspiratory time constant) and deflate (expiratory time constant) the lungs to a certain percentage of tidal volume. The expiratory TC (TC_{exp}) is a product of resistance and compliance, providing a real-time dynamic assessment of the respiratory mechanics.

One TC_{exp} is the time required by the alveoli to deflate 63% of its volume, while in three TC_{exp}, alveoli will be empty by 95%.

The TC_{exp} can diagnose various lung pathologies, assess the severity of the disease, monitor the effect of prone positioning, optimize settings on the ventilator, and troubleshoot respiratory events on mechanical ventilation. TC_{exp} is reliable even in patients who are spontaneously breathing and on NIV (assuming that expiration is passive and there are no unintentional leaks):

$$\mathbf{TC}_{\mathrm{exp}} = \mathbf{R}_{\mathbf{aw}} \times \mathbf{C}_{\mathbf{rs}}$$

11 Diagnosis of the Lung Conditions

The normal value of TC_{exp} in patients on invasive mechanical ventilation is between 0.5 and 0.7 s. However, pseudo-normal expiratory TC_{exp} can be seen with decreased compliance and increased resistance.

TC_{exp} less than 0.5 s implies decreased compliance in patients of lung fibrosis, kyphoscoliosis (decreased chest wall compliance), or severe ARDS [19]. TC_{exp} of longer than 0.7 s indicates increased resistance, e.g., COPD, right mainstem bronchus intubation, or kinking of the endotracheal tube (Fig. 5).

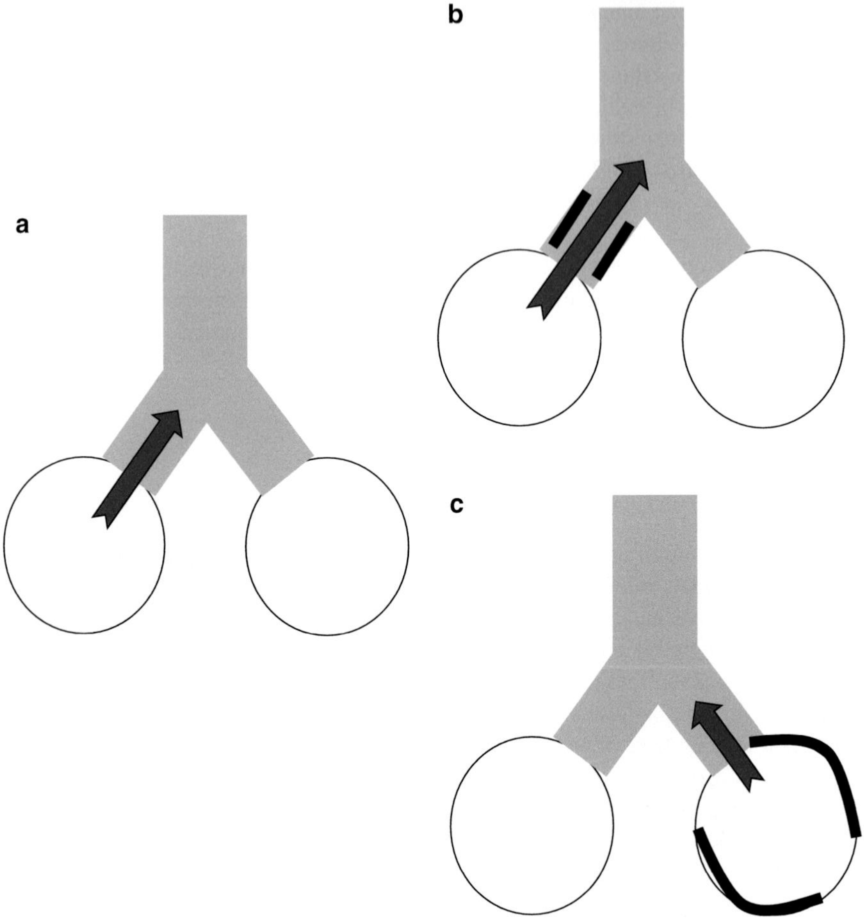

Fig. 5 Expiratory time constant. (**a**) Normal lungs with expiratory time constant (arrow). (**b**) Obstructive airway disease with longer time constant (arrow). (**c**) Restrictive airway disease with shorter time constant (arrow)

12 Optimization of Ventilatory Settings

Patients with a shorter TC_{exp} are at risk of VILI and should be closely monitored for targets of LPV (i.e., tidal volume, driving pressure, and plateau pressure). In contrast, patients with a longer expiratory TC are at risk of dynamic hyperinflammation and should be monitored periodically for the auto-PEEP.

13 Monitoring of Prone Position

During prone positioning of the intubated patient, the TC_{exp} can be used to assess the respiratory mechanics. The increase in TC_{exp} and compliance with prone positioning are markers of lung recruitment, while no increase in lung compliance but increased TC_{exp} is caused by kinking or mispositioned endotracheal tube.

14 Troubleshooting of Respiratory Events

The sudden drop in oxygen saturation or increase in airway pressure needs a rapid and correct diagnosis. The trends of TC_{exp} can help to understand respiratory mechanics in these events. An increase in TC_{exp} usually indicates an obstruction caused by one of the following: an endotracheal tube kinking, blockade or mispositioning, a patient biting the endotracheal tube, an excess of tracheal secretions, or bronchospasm. Conversely, a decrease in expiratory TC indicates a drop in compliance, e.g., pneumothorax, pleural effusion, or atelectasis. Without a change in expiratory TC, sudden desaturation indicates a drop in cardiac output or a massive pulmonary embolism.

15 Dead Space/Dead Space Fraction

The inspired gas that does not take part in gas exchange is termed dead space (Vd). It determines the fraction of wasted ventilation.

Total (or physiological) dead space includes anatomical and alveolar dead space. In a healthy adult, the alveolar dead space is negligible. Anatomical dead space represents the air that fills the conducting passages starting from the upper airway to the lower respiratory tract (up to respiratory bronchioles). This volume constitutes up to one-third of the normal tidal volume. The respiratory zone that takes part in actual gas exchanges comprises respiratory bronchioles, alveolar duct, alveolar sac, and alveoli. The abnormality of the alveolocapillary membrane or ventilation/perfusion mismatch causes the physiologic dead space to exceed above anatomical dead space.

The normal dead space-to-tidal volume (Vd/Vt) ratio is approximately 0.3. In a patient on invasive mechanical ventilation, the Vd/Vt ratio can be up to 0.7 or 0.8 due to an increase in anatomical dead space from the addition of instrumental dead space (Fig. 6).

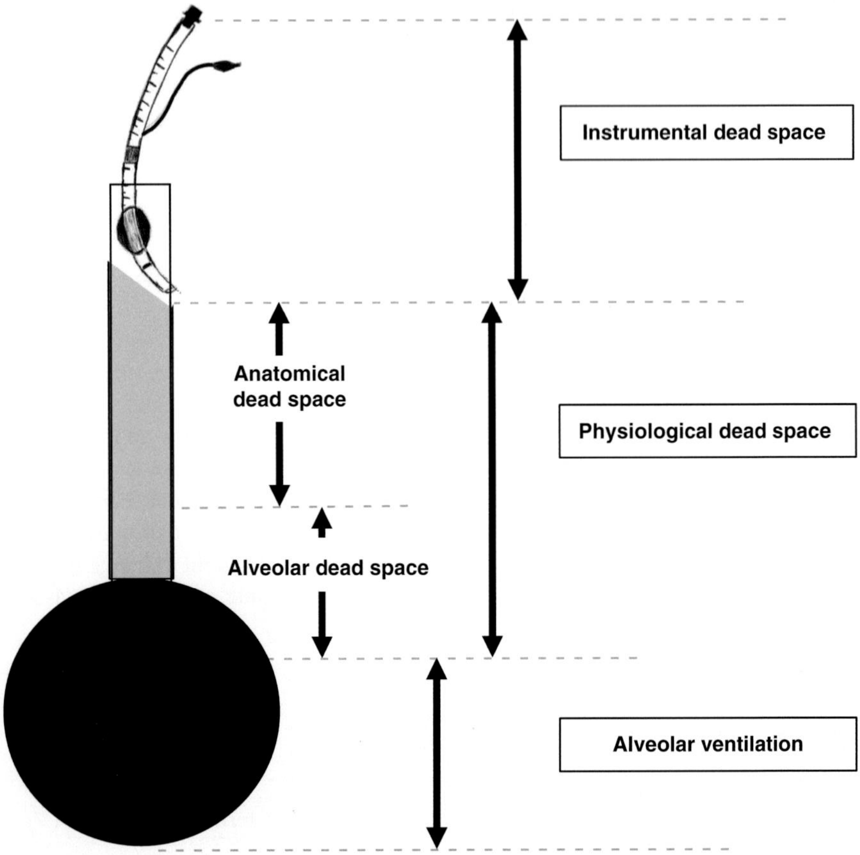

Fig. 6 Pictorial representation of total dead space

The partial pressure of arterial carbon dioxide ($PaCO_2$) is dependent on minute ventilation. Minute ventilation, defined by the total volume that enters lung in one minute, is the product of tidal volume and respiratory rate. However, the total volume of gas reaching the alveoli is not equivalent to tidal volume and must factor the gas in the anatomical dead space. Hence, the fraction of minute ventilation reaching the alveoli per unit time called alveolar ventilation is more important to consider in hypercarbia (Fig. 5):

$$\textbf{Alveolar ventilation} = (\textbf{Vt} - \textbf{Vd}) \times \textbf{respiratory rate}$$

The Bohr equation can be used to calculate the physiological dead space:

$$\textbf{Vd} = \textbf{Vt} \times (\textbf{PaCO}_2 - \textbf{PeCO}_2) / \textbf{PaCO}_2$$

$PeCO_2$: partial pressure of expired carbon dioxide.

The second half of this equation represents the dead space fraction. The diffusion of gases across the alveolar membrane is so rapid that $PaCO_2$ equals alveolar PCO_2 ($PACO_2$). $PeCO_2$ represents diluted $PACO_2$ with dead-space gases (which are usually inspired gases and devoid of CO_2).

In case of increased physiological dead space in patients on invasive mechanical ventilation, the instrumental dead space can be reduced by removing the number of connections like catheter mount, connectors, and closed suction. Using a heated humidifier instead of HME filter, cut the endotracheal tube without compromising safety, or change to tracheostomy (reduce the dead space by 10–12 mL).

Instrumental dead space may be very high (above 100 mL) with multiple connections like HME, catheter mount, connectors, and endotracheal tube. HME filter has a volume above 50 mL (up to 90 mL), catheter mount (20–60 mL), many connectors may be used in patients (CO_2 cuvette for end-tidal CO_2 monitoring, closed suction and other adaptors for inhalation therapies) and may represent an essential additional dead space [20].

16 Measuring Patient Effort and Work of Breathing

Spontaneous breathing in patients on invasive mechanical ventilation has been shown to induce both positive and negative effects. The patient's spontaneous breathing may help in the recruitment of basal lung fields, prevent disuse atrophy of the diaphragm and other respiratory muscles, reduce sedation requirements, and facilitate earlier weaning. However, the undue high respiratory drive can generate high tidal volume or pressure and may cause harm in the form of patient self-inflicted lung injury (P-SILI) similar to VILI [21]. The positive effect of early use of neuromuscular blocking agents (especially cisatracurium) in patients with ARDS is possibly related to abolishing spontaneous respiratory effort [22]. Thus, the monitoring of the breathing effort might be valuable in better understanding respiratory mechanics and precision-based mechanical ventilation.

Mechanical work is defined as the product of force and distance and is measured in Joules (J).

However, the assessment of breathing effort is difficult without complex diagnostic techniques. The "gold standard" parameters for the assessment of respiratory effort are the work of breathing (WOB) and pressure-time product (PTP), which are more research tools and require esophageal or gastric pressure. Recently, diaphragm electromyography and ultrasound have been tried to assess breathing effort with good results [23–25].

In respiratory physiology, work is the product of pressure (representing the force) and volume (representing the distance). It represents the energy required to move tidal volume at a given pressure (spontaneous, mechanical, or both). WOB is often reported in the work per liter (J/L) unit, obtained by dividing the work per breathing cycle by tidal volume.

The patients on neuromuscular blocking agents and invasive mechanical ventilation, and plots of airway pressure versus tidal volume, indicate the total amount of work needed to inflate the respiratory system. It represents the work done by the ventilator and not the work performed by the respiratory muscles.

The WOB calculation can be used to evaluate weaning failure, effects and titration of different modes, therapeutic interventions, and ventilator performance (like triggering and flow delivery).

Different components contribute to the total WOB: elastic, resistive, and intrinsic PEEP.

Elastic work: WOB to overcome the elastic recoil of the lung or chest wall.

Resistive work: Work done to overcome the airway, chest wall, or lung parenchyma resistance.

The total WOB in a healthy adult is from 0.3 to 0.6 J/L. In patients with either severe obstructive or restrictive lung disease, WOB is increased by two to three times at rest, and a marked increase is seen during exertion.

The pressure-time product (PTP) is the time integral of the pressure performed by the respiratory muscles (P_{MUS}) during inspiration.

The PTP is calculated as the time integral of the P_{MUS}:

$$\mathbf{PTP} = \mathbf{P}\left(\mathbf{cmH_2O}\right) \times \mathbf{t}\left(\mathbf{s}\right) = \int \mathbf{Pdt}\left(\mathbf{cmH_2O^*s}\right)$$

The PTP for global respiratory muscles can be calculated using this equation if esophageal pressure is available. The PTP will help to calculate effort for all three forces: elastic, resistive, and intrinsic PEEP (threshold). The PTP of the diaphragm needs gastric pressure measurement. The PTP is independent of volume and flow, helpful to calculate effort during isovolumic contractions. This is also a limitation of PTP as the effort for inefficient muscle contractions generated during higher flows and volume cannot be calculated [26].

17 Airway Occlusion Pressure (P0.1)

Airway occlusion pressure (P0.1) is the pressure generated in the occluded airway 100 milliseconds (ms) after the onset of inspiration to monitor the respiratory drive during mechanical ventilation.

P0.1 was first described by Whitelaw et al., who found decreased airway pressure during the first 100 ms after end-expiratory occlusion, and it correlates to end-tidal CO_2. There is also a good correlation between P0.1 and inspiratory effort compared to measured either by WOB or PTP. There is no effect of the patient's effort, lung or thoracic wall recoil, or airway resistance on inspiratory effort calculation as flow is interrupted, so resistance disappears.

The normal value of P0.1 in healthy subjects varies between 0.5 and 1.5 cmH_2O. However, a significant breath-to-breath variability is seen with P0.1 calculation, and an average of 3–4 values is taken.

The ventilators use different methods to measure P0.1, breath-to-breath estimation (using a trigger window), or a temporary end-expiratory occlusion only when a measurement is required.

P0.1 can be helpful in the precision-based adjustment of ventilatory support due to its close correlation with inspiratory effort. The higher values of P0.1 imply inadequate ventilatory support, while lower values correspond to excessive assistance (using a cutoff of $\leq$1.6 cmH_2O) both during control and spontaneous modes of ventilation. Recently, ventilator modes using a target P0.1 and closed-loop algorithm to automatically adjust the level of support have been developed.

P0.1 can also be used to adjust PEEP in patients with dynamic hyperinflation. Application of an external PEEP less than intrinsic PEEP is one of the recommended measures for dynamic hyperinflation. The decrease in P0.1 after the addition of external PEEP indicates a decreased intrinsic PEEP and WOB. P0.1 has extensively been tried during weaning. An increase in P0.1 along with other variables during spontaneous breathing trial can be taken as a surrogate of failure [27].

18 Mechanical Power

Mechanical power represents the energy transformed from a mechanical ventilator to the respiratory system over a given time. It includes all parameters (pressures, volume, flow, respiratory rate) associated with VILI. Different complex mathematical equations are available to calculate mechanical power. This includes the area under the quasi-static pressure-volume curves to more complex equations based on the static and dynamic components [28]. A simple equation to calculate the mechanical power on volume-controlled ventilation is given below:

$$\mathbf{Mechanical\ Power} = \mathbf{VE} \times \left(\mathbf{Peak\ Pressure} + \mathbf{PEEP} + \boldsymbol{F}/\mathbf{6}\right)\mathbf{20}$$

VE: Minute ventilation, F: inspiratory flow.

Mechanical power is expressed in Joules/minute.

Studies showed that mechanical power above 12 J/min was associated with reduced survival [29].

19 Conclusion

19.1 Stress Index

A simple and reliable approach to assess SI at the bedside is to examine the pressure-time curve on the ventilator screen. This simplification may aid in implementing SI in clinical practice in order to personalize mechanical ventilation. In constant flow-volume ventilation, the stress index is used to assess the pressure-time curve. A linear increase in pressure (constant compliance, stress index = 1) indicates adequate alveolar recruitment without overdistention. During inflation, compliance may worsen (progressive decrease in compliance, upward concavity, stress index > 1), suggesting overdistention, for which it is recommended to lower the PEEP or VT. A progressive increase in compliance (downward concavity, stress index < 1), along with the potential for additional recruitment, suggesttidal recruitment, and PEEP should be increased [30].

The knowledge of respiratory mechanics is crucial for the safe application of mechanical ventilation; it reduces VILI risk, helps in troubleshooting, and may improve outcome. The equation of motion and calculation of Pplat, driving pressure, resistance, compliance, and TCexp is helpful during LPV. The calculation of respiratory effort using airway occlusion pressure, ultrasound, or PTP is helpful to diagnose various conditions, weaning failure, and personalized mechanical ventilation settings. Mechanical power is a new tool in the armamentarium to monitor the risk of VILI and reduced survival.

References

1. Mauri T, Lazzeri M, Bellani G, Zanella A, Grasselli G. Respiratory mechanics to understand ARDS and guide mechanical ventilation. Physiol Meas. 2017;38(12):R280–303.
2. Barberis L, Manno E, Guérin C. Effect of end-inspiratory pause duration on plateau pressure in mechanically ventilated patients. Intensive Care Med. 2003;29:130–4.
3. Terragni PP, Filippini C, Slutsky AS, et al. Accuracy of plateau pressure and stress index to identify injurious ventilation in patients with acute respiratory distress syndrome. Anesthesiology. 2013;119(4):880–9.
4. Terragni PP, Rosboch G, Tealdi A, Corno E, Menaldo E, Davini O, Gandini G, Herrmann P, Mascia L, Quintel M, Slutsky AS, Gattinoni L, Ranieri VM. Tidal hyperinflation during low tidal volume ventilation in acute respiratory distress syndrome. Am J Respir Crit Care Med. 2007;175(2):160–6.
5. Amato MB, Meade MO, Slutsky AS, Brochard L, Costa EL, Schoenfeld DA, Stewart TE, Briel M, Talmor D, Mercat A, Richard JC, Carvalho CR, Brower RG. Driving pressure and survival in the acute respiratory distress syndrome. N Engl J Med. 2015;372(8):747–55.
6. Ladha K, Vidal Melo MF, McLean DJ, Wanderer JP, Grabitz SD, Kurth T, Eikermann M. Intraoperative protective mechanical ventilation and risk of postoperative respiratory complications: hospital based registry study. BMJ. 2015;(351):h3646.
7. Neto AS, Hemmes SN, Barbas CS, Beiderlinden M, Fernandez-Bustamante A, Futier E, et al. Association between driving pressure and development of postoperative pulmonary complications in patients undergoing mechanical ventilation for general anaesthesia: a meta-analysis of individual patient data. Lancet Respir Med. 2016;4(4):272–80.
8. Williams EC, Motta-Ribeiro GC, Vidal Melo MF. Driving pressure and transpulmonary pressure: how do we guide safe mechanical ventilation? Anesthesiology. 2019;131(1):155–63.
9. Aldenkortt M, Lysakowski C, Elia N, Brochard L, Tramer MR. Ventilation strategies in obese patients undergoing surgery: a quantitative systematic review and meta-analysis. Br J Anaesth. 2012;109:493–502.
10. Cortes-Puentes GA, Keenan JC, Adams AB, Parker ED, Dries DJ, Marini JJ. Impact of chest wall modifications and lung injury on the correspondence between airway and transpulmonary driving pressures. Crit Care Med. 2015;43:e287–95.

11. Keenan JC, Cortes-Puentes GA, Zhang L, Adams AB, Dries DJ, Marini JJ. PEEP titration: the effect of prone position and abdominal pressure in an ARDS model. Intensive Care Med Exp. 2018;6:3.
12. Pelosi P, Vargas M. Mechanical ventilation and intra-abdominal hypertension: "Beyond Good and Evil". Crit Care. 2012;16:187.
13. Cinnella G, Grasso S, Spadaro S, Rauseo M, Mirabella L, Salatto P, De Capraris A, Nappi L, Greco P, Dambrosio M. Effects of recruitment maneuver and positive end-expiratory pressure on respiratory mechanics and transpulmonary pressure during laparoscopic surgery. Anesthesiology. 2013;118:114–22.
14. Desai JP, Moustarah F. Pulmonary compliance. [Updated 2020 Sep 18]. In: StatPearls [internet]. Treasure Island: StatPearls Publishing; 2021. https://www.ncbi.nlm.nih.gov/books/NBK538324/
15. Stenqvist O, Odenstedt H, Lundin S. Dynamic respiratory mechanics in acute lung injury/acute respiratory distress syndrome: research or clinical tool? Curr Opin Crit Care. 2008;14(1):87–93.
16. Fry DL, Hyatt RE. Pulmonary mechanics. A unified analysis of the relationship between pressure, volume and gas flow in the lungs of normal and diseased human subjects. Am J Med. 1960;29:672–89.
17. Volta CA, Marangoni E, Alvisi V, Capuzzo M, Ragazzi R, Pavanelli L, et al. Respiratory mechanics by least squares fitting in mechanically ventilated patients: application on flow-limited COPD patients. Intensive Care Med. 2002;28(1):48–52.
18. Lucangelo U, Bernabé F, Blanch L. Respiratory mechanics derived from signals in the ventilator circuit. Respir Care. 2005;50(1):55–65.
19. Arnal JM, Garnero A, Saoli M, Chatburn RL. Parameters for simulation of adult subjects during mechanical ventilation. Respir Care. 2018;63(2):158–68.
20. Lellouche F, Delorme M, Brochard L. Impact of respiratory rate and dead space in the current era of lung protective mechanical ventilation. Chest. 2020;158(1):45–7.
21. Brochard L, Slutsky A, Pesenti A. Mechanical ventilation to minimize progression of lung injury in acute respiratory failure. Am J Respir Crit Care Med. 2017;195(4):438–42.
22. Papazian L, Forel JM, Gacouin A, Penot-Ragon C, Perrin G, Loundou A, Jaber S, Arnal JM, Perez D, Seghboyan JM, Constantin JM, Courant P, Lefrant JY, Guérin C, Prat G, Morange S, Roch A, ACURASYS Study Investigators. Neuromuscular blockers in early acute respiratory distress syndrome. N Engl J Med. 2010;363(12):1107–16.
23. Bellani G, Mauri T, Coppadoro A, et al. Estimation of patient's inspiratory effort from the electrical activity of the diaphragm. Crit Care Med. 2013;41:1483–91.
24. Zambon M, Greco M, Bocchino S, et al. Assessment of diaphragmatic dysfunction in the critically ill patient with ultrasound: a systematic review. Intensive Care Med. 2017;43:29–38.
25. de Vries H, Jonkman A, Shi ZH, Spoelstra-de Man A, Heunks L. Assessing breathing effort in mechanical ventilation: physiology and clinical implications. Ann Transl Med. 2018;6(19):387.
26. Akoumianaki E, Maggiore SM, Valenza F, Bellani G, Jubran A, Loring SH, et al. The application of esophageal pressure measurement in patients with respiratory failure. Am J Respir Crit Care Med. 2014;189(5):520–31.
27. Telias I, Damiani F, Brochard L. The airway occlusion pressure ($P_{0.1}$) to monitor respiratory drive during mechanical ventilation: increasing awareness of a not-so-new problem. Intensive Care Med. 2018;44(9):1532–5.
28. Giosa L, Busana M, Pasticci I, Bonifazi M, Macrì MM, Romitti F, Vassalli F, Chiumello D, Quintel M, Marini JJ, Gattinoni L. Mechanical power at a glance: a simple surrogate for volume-controlled ventilation. Intensive Care Med Exp. 2019;7(1):61.
29. Silva PL, Ball L, Rocco PRM, Pelosi P. Power to mechanical power to minimize ventilator-induced lung injury? Intensive Care Med Exp. 2019;7(Suppl 1):38.
30. Sun XM, Chen GQ, Chen K, Wang YM, He X, Huang HW, Luo XY, Wang CM, Shi ZH, Xu M, Chen L, Fan E, Zhou JX. Stress index can be accurately and reliably assessed by visually inspecting ventilator waveforms. Respir Care. 2018;63(9):1094–101. https://doi.org/10.4187/respcare.06151. Epub 2018 Jun 26. PMID: 29945907.

Principles of Mechanical Ventilation

Gabriela Alvarado, Jorge Hidalgo, Allyson Hidalgo, and Jorge E. Sinclair De Frías

1 Less Is More in Mechanical Ventilation

1.1 History of Ventilation

The management of patients with respiratory failure has undergone a constant transformation throughout the history of medicine; technological advances in recent decades have made it possible to better adapt ventilators to the needs of the patient and monitor the changes that occur in real time.

From the first records in ancient Egypt in the Papyrus of Ebers, one of the oldest medical treatises, it is mentioned how Isis, the goddess of mystery and wisdom, resurrected Osiris with a breath of life pushing air inside with her wings.

There are several mentions of ventilation in the Bible, where healing properties are attributed to air; in the Old Testament, it is narrated how the prophet Elisha performs a mouth-to-mouth resuscitation maneuver on a child. Hippocrates known as the father of medicine describes in his treatise about air tracheal intubation as a method to artificially ventilate the lungs of a human being.

In 175 BC, Galen, the prominent Greek physician and scientist, promoted the study of anatomy to understand the interaction of the lung and the heart, describing

G. Alvarado
Hospital Regional de Occidente, Quetzaltenango, Guatemala

J. Hidalgo (✉)
Critical Care Division, Belize Healthcare Partners, Belize, Belize

A. Hidalgo
Biochemistry, Arizona State University, Phoenix, AZ, USA

J. E. Sinclair De Frías
Faculty of Medicine, University of Panama, Panama City, Panama

J. Hidalgo et al. (eds.), *Personalized Mechanical Ventilation*,
https://doi.org/10.1007/978-3-031-14138-6_2

how the physical act of breathing causes the heart to beat. Andreas Vesalius, a medical researcher, published in 1543 a treatise on anatomy where he makes the first reference to positive-pressure ventilation: "But that life may be restored to the animal, an opening must be attempted in the trunk of the trachea, into which a tube of reed or cane should be put; you will then blow into this, so that the lung may rise again and take air."

Paracelsus in the years 1493 and 1541 carried out numerous experiments reviving a patient by placing a tube in the mouth and blowing air through a bellows. Robert Hooke in 1667 kept a dog alive by supplying a continuous flow of oxygen by applying positive pressure.

Mechanical ventilation began in the 1700s with the discovery of oxygen and subsequently the importance of respiration in the delivery of oxygen. William Tossach reported in 1774 the first case where mouth-to-mouth resuscitation was applied in a miner rescued from a coal mine.

The first mechanical apparatus used to provide noninvasive mechanical ventilation was introduced by Chassier in 1780, a bag-and-mask manual ventilator [1]. In 1827, Leroy demonstrated that positive-pressure ventilation had its hazards and that damage could be caused to the lungs by overinflation.

The first description of a negative-pressure ventilator was of a full-body-type ventilator. This "tank ventilator" was first described by the Scottish physician John Dalziel in 1838. It consisted of an airtight box, with the patient maintained in the sitting position, and negative pressure was established by manually pumping air into and out of the box [2].

Marshall Hall and Silverten, in 1857 and 1858, respectively, disclosed the method of chest pressure and arm lift used to fill the lungs of a suffocated person with fresh air. In the nineteenth century, ventilation was provided using subatmospheric pressure applied around the patient to replace or increase the work done by the respiratory muscles. The first viable iron lung was introduced in 1876 by the Frenchman Woillez and was called a manually operated spirophore.

In 1904, Sauerbruch even developed a negative-pressure operating chamber. The patient's body, except for the head, was maintained inside the chamber [3]. The chamber was large enough so that the surgeon was able to perform surgery while also in the chamber. The patient's lower body was encased in a flexible sack so that positive pressure could be applied to this part of the body, preventing blood from accumulating in the abdomen and lower extremities, causing what was referred to as "tank shock" [4].

Another approach to providing noninvasive mechanical ventilation was introduced by Green and Janeway in 1910 [1]. They referred to their device as a "rhythmic inflation apparatus." The patient's head was placed into the apparatus, and a seal was secured around the patient's neck with positive pressure applied to the patient's head.

In 1911, Dräger had already created a positive-pressure ventilation device, which became known as the Pulmotor, which used a cylinder of oxygen or compressed air as a source of energy for its operation and delivered a mixture of these gases and ambient air to the patient, through a nasobuccal mask.

In 1929, Drinker and McCann built an electric cabinet fan; later developed models of the iron lung were used extensively in the treatment of polio for nearly 30 years. Negative-pressure ventilation became a much greater clinical reality with the development of the iron lung; this approach to ventilatory support reached its pinnacle during the worldwide poliomyelitis epidemic from 1930 to 1960. The first ICUs were set up to manage in some cases dozens of patients, of all ages, requiring negative-pressure ventilation [5].

Although mechanical ventilators are generally classified as negative- and positive-pressure ventilators, negative-pressure ventilators are rarely used today. Available engineering advancements made it possible to switch from first-generation devices that initially were only volume controlled, had no alarms or monitors, and could not detect the breaths triggered by the patient.

In the second-generation devices, the trigger of the patients was possible, and some parameters such as respiratory rate could be monitored. Intermittent mandatory ventilation (IMV) began to be used, and pressure-controlled and pressure-assisted ventilation was used in clinical practice.

The third-generation devices have microprocessors. Flow triggering was introduced, and gas delivery and monitoring were possible. Synchronized intermittent mandatory ventilation (SIMV) was applied, and pressure support could be given. Today's complex and modern devices are known as fourth-generation devices, and the most important feature of these devices is the wide variety of modes and options they have [6].

The modern ventilator devices have made it possible to perfect the art of ventilation and provide patients with increasingly complete support, which has gone through several changes and has evolved until reaching the great technological advances that critical medicine currently has at its disposal.

1.2 Definition

Respiration is a fundamental biological function in the life of a human being; the gaseous exchange of oxygen and carbon dioxide takes place in the pulmonary alveoli and has as an indispensable requirement the correct functioning of each element of the respiratory system.

The ability to provide enough oxygen to the body and preserve gas exchange can be affected by multiple life-threatening medical conditions. With the development and evolution of mechanical ventilation, it is possible to provide artificial support to patients with loss of respiratory function, which can potentially save their lives.

Mechanical ventilation is a procedure that allows a mechanical device to help or replace the respiratory function, preserving lung mechanics and gas exchange. This respiratory assist machine integrates volume, pressure, time, and flow to deliver a tidal breath under positive pressure to replace the respiratory process during the time it takes to recover the patient's hemodynamics and respiratory autonomy.

Ventilatory support in critically ill patients is one of the most widely used life support strategies in intensive care units around the world. Its routine application has improved the quality of care for these patients and has had a significant impact on the survival. In recent years, the implementation of protective mechanical ventilation has improved the care of patients with acute respiratory failure, making ventilatory support safer and more effective.

One of the medical conditions where the benefits and applications of mechanical ventilation have been most demonstrated is in patients with acute respiratory distress syndrome (ARDS); 50 years after its initial description, this disease continues to be a common and lethal form of respiratory insufficiency.

Acute respiratory distress syndrome is defined as acute hypoxemia, non-cardiogenic pulmonary edema, reduced lung compliance, increased work of breathing, and need for ventilation; mortality remains high even in highly specialized centers.

ARDS most often develops in the context of pneumonia (bacterial, viral, and fungal), nonpulmonary sepsis, aspiration of gastric contents, and trauma. Several other causes are also associated with the development of ARDS, including acute pancreatitis, transfusions, hemorrhagic shock, or reperfusion injury and smoke inhalation.

In the global COVID-19 pandemic and ARDS secondary to a lung infection, ventilatory support became the cornerstone of currently available therapy. Given the rapid spread of COVID-19 and the lack of targeted medical therapy, the only globally accepted therapy is protective ventilation in any of its modalities.

1.3 Epidemiology

Mechanical ventilation is one of the most common interventions employed in critical patients. Annually, over 240,000 patients in the USA needs mechanical ventilation [7]. The number of patients requiring mechanical ventilation is expected to increase substantially. In the United States, approximately 310 persons per 100,000 adults undergo invasive ventilation for nonsurgical indications [8].

The mortality in intensive care unit from ARDS is 35.3%, and hospital mortality is 40% [9]. COVID-19 ARDS appears to have worse outcomes than ARDS from other causes. The mortality ranged between 26 and 61.5%, and in patients who received mechanical ventilation, the mortality can range between 65.7 and 94% [10].

In patients with COVID-19, it is estimated that 14% will develop a severe disease that requires oxygen and 5% require admission to intensive care and mechanical ventilation [11]. Although noninvasive ventilation has been used more frequently in intensive care units in recent years, it is not always available. It has been suggested that helmet NIMV may decrease intubation and improve mortality in ARDS patients; [12] however, its use in patients with COVID-19 has not yet been sufficiently studied.

1.4 Types of Ventilation

During the poliomyelitis epidemic, negative-pressure mechanical ventilation was widely used and saved many lives; this led to the creation of intensive care units specialized in the management of patients with respiratory failure.

The creation of the first intensive care rooms made it possible to evaluate the effects of ventilation on patients, leaving behind the use of negative pressure over time and improving mechanical ventilators over the last 70 years so that they are safe and effective.

The evolution of mechanical ventilation has made it possible to increasingly adapt ventilators to the patient and their pathophysiological characteristics. The incorporation of trigger allowed ventilated patients to improve synchrony with the ventilator.

Critically ill patients who require ventilatory support can use mainly two types of ventilation: invasive mechanical ventilation and noninvasive mechanical ventilation. The choice of the type of ventilation is made according to the specific requirements of each patient, their hemodynamic status, and their clinical condition. The type of respiratory failure and the possible benefits of each technique should also be considered.

Invasive mechanical ventilation	Noninvasive mechanical ventilation
• Support of patients in shock, hemodynamic instability, and cardiac arrest • Reduces work of breathing and oxygen consumption • Allows muscle rest • Correction of respiratory disorders • Ventilatory support and constant oxygen supply • Does not require patient collaboration • Decreases intracranial pressure in neurocritical patients	• Decreases the use of sedation and analgesia • Less days of hospitalization • Preserves swallowing and speech • Greater patient comfort • Avoids muscle atrophy • Lower risk of infections • Allows intermittent use • Helps in early extubation • Benefits in COPD, cardiogenic pulmonary edema, and immunosuppressed patients

To start invasive mechanical ventilation, it is necessary to establish an artificial airway; this is done through an orotracheal tube or a tracheostomy. In emergencies, supraglottic devices and emergency cricothyrotomy can be used.

Invasive mechanical ventilation is carried out by means of an artificial respirator that allows for a temporary replacement of respiration, providing the patient with a programmed volume of air with a certain frequency and with a certain pressure; it also has a constant oxygen supply, graphics, and alarms that allow monitoring. There are several modes of invasive ventilation, and they all have in common the ability to preserve gas exchange and assist the patient continuously for as long as required.

Noninvasive mechanical ventilation is carried out through an interface which can be nasal, nasobuccal, facial, and helmet type; it consists of providing a continuous positive pressure in the airway that allows the patient to reduce their respiratory effort and preserve their spontaneous breathing.

The choice of the type of mechanical ventilation is the first step in the care of the critical patient; the follow-up in the first hour can provide important information about the improvement or not of the patient and the need to change the ventilation mode. Invasive or noninvasive ventilation methods can be used in the same patient at different times. Adequate monitoring allows deciding the most appropriate interventions.

1.5 Objectives

Mechanical ventilation has several purposes in clinical practice; the initial objective is to provide ventilatory support to critically ill patients who have respiratory failure and who have a life-threatening clinical condition.

The primary objective is to maintain or correct gas exchange, providing continuous and controlled support that allows the reestablishment of the patient's hemodynamics, reduces work of breathing, and corrects the problem that triggered respiratory failure.

In patients with severe respiratory distress, mechanical ventilation can also substitute the action of respiratory muscles and decrease their oxygen demands. The main goal in most cases is to save the life of patients by temporarily replacing breathing.

Other goals of mechanical ventilation include optimizing oxygen delivery to the main organs, achieving synchrony, preserving muscle strength, avoiding iatrogenic complications, minimizing dynamic hyperinflation, and monitoring the biological reactions [13].

1.6 Indications

Critically ill patients who require mechanical ventilation can present a series of hemodynamic disorders that prevent them from preserving gas exchange. Most of these disorders have respiratory failure and the inability to spontaneously carry out the breathing process as a common presentation.

Although ventilatory support can temporarily replace pulmonary mechanics and provide enough time to perform interventions and reestablish the patient's hemodynamics, in many cases, it subjects the patient to potential complications, so the decision to initiate ventilation must be individualized by considering factors such as cause of ventilatory failure, patient's condition, life expectancy, and available resources into consideration.

The first aspect to take into account in the initial evaluation of all critical patients is the assessment of the airway, in patients with trauma, neoplasms, infections, obstruction, and airway edema; intubation is performed with the aim of ensuring the patency of the airway and preserving oxygenation. In some cases, patients can maintain spontaneous breathing after intubation, so this procedure is not always accompanied by ventilator-assisted ventilation.

The clinical assessment of the patient allows us to evaluate the type of mechanical ventilation that is required and the need or not for intubation; the neurological state allows to identify if the patient is able to collaborate and follow instructions, maintain spontaneous breaths, and preserve protective reflexes; in patients with cerebral edema and intracranial hypertension, the management should include assisted ventilation and use of sedatives and analgesics in order to reduce secondary brain injury.

The work of breathing and the contraction of the respiratory muscles should be constantly evaluated; an increase in the work of breathing and the respiratory rate together with alterations in the concentration of oxygen and carbon dioxide should be in most cases taken as an indicator of initiation of invasive or noninvasive ventilation. By decreasing respiratory work, mechanical ventilation allows oxygen to be rerouted from the respiratory muscles to other vulnerable tissues.

The classification of the type of respiratory failure must be carried out in a timely and early manner; the current availability of supplementation of oxygen at different concentrations and flows may be sufficient to treat patients who manifest hypoxemia without other clinical data of severity. Using the arterial alveolar gradient or the PaO_2/FiO_2 ratio can help classify the patient and determine their need for oxygen therapy.

The main indication to start both invasive and noninvasive mechanical ventilation is the impossibility of maintaining the metabolic demands of the body; in most cases, the decision is based on clinical judgment and physician experience, influenced by oxygen saturation, dyspnea, respiratory rate, chest radiograph, and other factors [14].

Many patients who require mechanical ventilation have relatively normal arterial blood gases but have clinical signs of increased work of breathing: nasal flaring; vigorous activity of the sternomastoid muscles; tracheal tug; recession of the suprasternal, supraclavicular, and intercostal spaces; paradoxical motion of the abdomen; and pulsus paradoxus [14].

The evaluation of oxygen saturation by means of pulse oximetry may differ from the actual saturation by about 4% [15]. Interpretation of readings of SpO_2 above 90% becomes difficult because of the oxygen dissociation curve.

Hypoxemia accompanied by a normal alveolar-to-arterial oxygen gradient and increase in $PaCO_2$ signifies hypoventilation. In patients with COVID-19, the main finding in arterial blood samples is hypoxemia with increased alveolar-to-arterial oxygen gradient; this translates into an imbalance of perfusion and ventilation or increases in pulmonary shunts; some of these patients improve their PO_2 concentrations only with oxygen supplementation, while others will require assisted ventilation [16].

The current trend to use less invasive techniques leaves noninvasive ventilation as one of the first options to be considered in patients who do not have any contraindication. It can be used from the beginning or as an aid in ventilator withdrawal in patients who have undergone invasive intubation. NIMV is usually a safe and well-tolerated technique, and its use reduces the rate of complications associated with ventilation.

An additional factor that must be assessed prior to intubation is the prognosis of the patient and the wishes they have regarding respiratory assistance; many patients with chronic medical problems share with their families their decision not to intubate, and this has often been supported legally. In patients who do not want invasive ventilation, NIMV can provide temporary support, respecting their wishes and allowing them to be more comfortable.

1.7 Duration of Mechanical Support

Ventilatory support can be provided to critically ill patients for as long as required; there is no limit to the duration of ventilation; however, complications associated with ventilation are directly related to the days of use of mechanical ventilator.

The vast majority of patients who undergo mechanical ventilation can discontinue ventilatory support within a few days. Sometimes, the disorders they present are acquired and rapidly reversible and are not associated with a serious underlying lung disease. In other cases, ventilation is used temporarily during surgical procedures and can be discontinued when the patient is able to maintain spontaneous breathing.

In critically ill patients who present with hemodynamic instability in whom it is not possible to maintain adequate perfusion, mechanical ventilation is used to reduce oxygen consumption and improve perfusion; in these patients, ventilation is continued until normal physiological parameters are recovered and the state of shock is reversed.

In patients neurocritical with intracranial hypertension, ventilation is an essential part in the management of cerebral edema; it is continued until the risk of secondary brain damage decreases and the neurological status of the patient allows him or her to regain his or her ability to breathe without assistance; sometimes, these patients suffer significant brain damage and are not able to protect their airway and must undergo a tracheostomy before being removed from the ventilator.

In the context of pneumonia and ARDS, ventilation with lung protection parameters is maintained until the infectious and inflammatory process improves; in these cases, the duration of ventilation is highly variable and the extent of lung damage will determine the moment of withdrawal of ventilation.

In recent years, the number of patients requiring prolonged mechanical ventilation or greater than 21 days has increased; [17] with improvements in the management of critically ill patients, it is increasingly common for patients with chronic diseases to survive and remain ventilated; this implies the need for performing tracheostomy and being transferred to care centers for chronic patients; in some cases, there is even a need to continue with ventilatory assistance at home.

The costs involved for health institutions to get a patient ventilated and risks of complications associated with ventilation make the priority in the management of patients with respiratory failure to be maintaining mechanical ventilation as short time as possible and using methods less invasive, although each case presents its own challenges and clinical characteristics.

1.8 Limitations

There are many limitations that can affect the correct implementation of mechanical ventilation in patients with respiratory failure; worldwide access to mechanical ventilators has been improving over the years; however, it is still possible, especially in developing countries, to find hospitals without enough mechanical ventilators and full intensive care services; these institutions need to use manual ventilation and transfer patients to other referral hospitals exposing patients to potential complications.

Many hospitals do not have the necessary equipment to administer noninvasive mechanical ventilation and high-flow oxygen, so all patients with ventilatory failure receive the same management, exposing them to the complications of invasive mechanical ventilation. On the other hand, intubation can sometimes be delayed in patients with noninvasive ventilation or high-flow oxygen if an adequate clinical assessment is not performed.

Modern ventilators allow the use of modalities adapted to the needs of the patient; systems such as neurally adjusted ventilatory assist (NAVA) allow the patient to interact with the ventilator and provide proportional ventilatory support; unconventional modes such as airway pressure-release ventilation or APRV make it possible to reduce the level of sedation used and preserve the patient's spontaneous ventilations; unfortunately, these ventilatory modes are not available in all ventilators and patients cannot always benefit from their use.

Patients with ventilatory support need to be monitored in intensive care services; these services have monitoring equipment and specialized personnel; in many cases, unstable patients with ventilatory support remain for long periods in emergency services or are in bed, increasing their mortality [7] and making its monitoring and management difficult.

Ventilated patients are not always managed by critical care specialists; in some places, there are not enough specialized personnel and ventilation is carried out by personnel with little experience; this affects the decisions made regarding ventilation and affects evolution of the patient; the current recommendation is to train all medical and paramedical personnel in the initial management of the critical patient and in concepts of protective mechanical ventilation.

In many institutions, mechanical ventilation protocols are implemented, despite the benefits that standardizing some procedures may have; in the case of mechanical ventilation, the decision to intubate and initiate support must be individualized; it is necessary to know the available options and use clinical judgment to decide the option that best suits and benefits the patient.

The mechanically ventilated patient also needs to be closely monitored; his or her hemodynamic and ventilatory parameters must be constantly evaluated to carry out timely interventions. The graphs present in the ventilator must be interpreted carefully as they provide additional information that allows detecting events associated with ventilation.

Each institution faces challenges and limitations in the management of patients with mechanical ventilation; a correct distribution and use of resources with a periodic and constant evaluation of its quality indicators can improve patient care. Quality medical education and training programs can positively influence the prognosis of patients and the incidence of complications.

1.9 Complications

In medicine, the aphorism "Primum non nocere" (The first thing is to do no harm) is well known. This reminds that any intervention or therapy implemented that can cause harm must be evaluated and avoided. When ventilatory support is started in a critically ill patient, the main challenge is to avoid any type of complication associated with ventilation.

Although mechanical ventilation can potentially save a patient's life and give them more time to recover, it can also expose them to other medical problems that can worsen their clinical condition; the continuous application of positive pressure in the airway is not physiological; its use even for short periods can cause lung damage and expose the patient to infectious and noninfectious complications.

Mechanical ventilation does not produce lung healing but has the potential to aggravate or even initiate lung injury. The progress made in the field of mechanical ventilation and in the management of the critical patient has made it possible to improve both patient monitoring and its safety and effectiveness, reducing risks and implementing lung protection strategies.

One of the initial strategies to prevent complications is to avoid intubation as much as possible; the availability of noninvasive ventilation modes and high-flow oxygen delivery devices can avoid this invasive procedure and improve the patient's condition at the same time. In the context of the COVID-19 pandemic, intubation has been associated with higher mortality, so it is important not to use it as the first option in all patients with respiratory failure.

The duration of assisted ventilation should be as short as possible; only the time necessary to reestablish the patient's hemodynamics and the ability to breathe spontaneously, daily suspension of sedatives, and spontaneous breathing tests can reduce the days of ventilation and avoid the appearance of delirium and agitation.

Mechanical ventilation is an essential procedure in patients treated in intensive care; however, there are many complications related to its use; complications are frequent and are associated in part with the excessive use of sedation, analgesics, muscle relaxants, and paralyzing agents.

Patients with invasive mechanical ventilation are at higher risk of acquiring infections; ventilator-associated pneumonia is common and is considered secondary to microaspiration of the contents of the oropharynx and to decreased protective reflexes and impaired mucociliary clearance. Its management includes broad-spectrum antibiotics and cultures that allow identifying the causative microorganisms.

The adverse effects of mechanical ventilation may be secondary to excessive and unphysiological transpulmonary positive pressure and relate to excessive and unphysiological variation of pleural pressure [13]. There are several types of ventilator-induced lung damage (VILI) as described in the following table:

Barotrauma	Lung damage induced by excessive airway pressure
Volutrauma	Overdistension-mediated lung injury
Atelectrauma	Mechanical injury caused by cyclical opening and collapse of atelectatic but recruitable lung units
Biotrauma	Broad pro-inflammatory biological response, predisposing to multi-organ failure

By identifying the role that mechanical forces play in the pathogenesis of lung injury and the different types of lung damage induced by the ventilator, the concept of lung-protective ventilation arises; this strategy seeks to optimize ventilator support and reduce the incidence of ventilator-induced lung injury with specific interventions. The main determinants of VILI include high pressures, high tidal volumes, and cyclical opening and closing of respiratory units; therefore, a fundamental part in the programming and monitoring of ventilation includes using a low tidal volume, maintaining plateau pressure under 30 cmH_2O, using positive pressure at the end of each breath, and minimizing the oxygen concentration used.

It is important to identify the events associated with the ventilator to treat them promptly and to actively implement prevention strategies. Establishing safety limits in patients on ventilatory support and closely monitoring them may allow the use of mechanical ventilation without causing further lung damage.

Early rehabilitation and psychological support of the critical patient are essential for their recovery; complications derived from emotional stress and the psychological effects that mechanical ventilation and their stay in intensive care have on the patient have been described; this complication is known as post-intensive care syndrome and is characterized by the appearance of physical difficulties, cognitive alterations, and emotional problems.

The main goal in the critical patient is to provide life support that is increasingly effective, comfortable, and safe, minimizing risks and complications to the maximum. Mechanical ventilation is an art that must be perfected through experience and physiological knowledge of lung function and gas exchange.

2 Personalized Mechanical Ventilation Tailored to Lung Morphology

2.1 Systemic Effects of the Mechanical Ventilation

The systemic effects of ventilation affect both the regional and systemic circulation, causing changes in the consumption and delivery of oxygen; these effects can manifest themselves at the cardiac, pulmonary, neurological, renal, and intestinal levels.

2.2 Cardiovascular System

The heart, the great vessels, and the pulmonary vascular tree are located within the thoracic cavity and can be affected by the changes in intrathoracic pressure that occur during ventilation; if we consider that the heart and the lungs work together within the thoracic cavity and that the thoracic cavity is a closed cavity, the heart is considered as a pressure chamber within another pressure chamber [18]. Increased intrathoracic pressure can affect cardiac function by decreasing afterload and right ventricular function.

The main objective of the heart is to maintain cardiac output to be able to meet oxygen demand; cardiac output undergoes variations in situations where oxygen demand is altered, such as in a severely ill patient. Cardiac output is determined by heart rate and by the volume of blood expelled by the left ventricle in each beat; stroke volume will depend on preload, afterload, and cardiac contractility.

The fall in cardiac output due to decreased venous return is frequent and is related to the ventilatory mode used and previous cardiac function. This depression of cardiac function may explain why the correction of oxygenation may not necessarily improve the supply of oxygen to the tissues.

Preload is a measure of the degree of maximum stretch or tension of the myocardial fibers before the onset of ventricular contraction and is determined by the mean length of the sarcomeres at the end of diastole [19]. As this length cannot be measured directly, other indices are used to evaluate it, such as ventricular end-diastolic volume or end-diastolic pressure. Preload is altered with variations in venous return and in cardiac diastolic dysfunction or with constrictive disorders that make ventricular filling difficult.

Changes in the diastolic volume of the right ventricle can increase the ejection force; according to the Frank-Starling law, there is a positive relationship between preload and stroke volume; this explains why the administration of intravenous solutions can increase preload temporarily. An important determinant of venous return is the magnitude of the circulating blood volume if it is decreased; positive-pressure ventilation causes systemic hypotension secondary to the pronounced decrease in cardiac output.

Mechanical ventilation can profoundly affect the cardiovascular system; both positive and negative pressures prevent the venous return of blood to the chest, which causes a reduction in cardiac output; in a patient ventilated with positive pressure, the return of blood to the chest depends on the difference between the peripheral venous pressure and the mean intrathoracic pressure. As airway pressure increases, intrathoracic pressure rises and venous return is prevented.

The return of blood to the thorax depends on the difference between the peripheral venous pressure and the intrathoracic pressure; even when the airway pressure remains equal to the atmospheric one, the venous return tends to decrease because the peripheral venous pressure is reduced by negative pressure.

The effects of positive-pressure ventilation on venous return depend on the magnitude and duration of the inspiratory pressure, and especially on the addition of pressure at the end of expiration (PEEP); capillary overdistension compresses the vascular bed, increasing resistances and reducing the afterload of the right ventricle.

When positive-pressure ventilation is started, there is a disparate effect on the preload of the right ventricle, which is reduced by a decrease in venous return, and on the preload of the left ventricle, which will increase due to an increase in venous return to the left atrium through the pulmonary veins [20].

Applying end-expiratory pressure (PEEP) during ventilation causes alveolar overdistension with compression of the pulmonary vascular bed and reduced afterload of the right ventricle, which redistributes blood flow. The systemic circulation can be profoundly altered by changes in intrathoracic pressure, while the pulmonary circulation is maintained unless the lung volumes also change [21].

Afterload is the pressure the heart must work against to expel blood during systole. The greater the afterload, the greater the pressure the ventricle must develop, which means more work and less efficiency of contraction. This pressure is directly related to systemic vascular resistance, and this in turn to changes in the diameter of the vessels.

Pleural pressure and airway pressure are negative in spontaneous respiration and act as the surrounding pressure of the lung and cardiac structures. During mechanical ventilation, these pressures increase along with the transpleural pressure. Ventilation primarily affects cardiac function by changing lung volume and intrathoracic pressure. This change will be made according to the resistance of the airways as well as the compliance of the lungs and the chest wall.

Intermittent positive pressure induces cyclical changes in left ventricular stroke volume. On inspiration, the increase in intrathoracic pressure decreases the preload of the right ventricle, causing a decrease in its ejection volume. At the same time, the blood volume contained in the pulmonary circuit is pushed towards the left ventricle, increasing its preload and its ejection volume during the inspiratory phase. Subsequently, the decrease in the stroke volume of the right ventricle causes a decrease in left ventricular filling and a reduction in its ejection volume during the expiratory phase.

Venous return can also decrease due to the presence of auto-PEEP in which the patient is unable to fully exhale the volume delivered in each breath, causing progressive hyperinflation, triggering an increase in intrathoracic pressure and decreased venous return.

The implementation of protective ventilation, with more controlled pressure values, new ventilatory modes, and new hemodynamic monitoring tools, has allowed better control of the cardiovascular changes induced by ventilation, improving its safety and benefits.

2.3 *Pulmonary System*

The open lung ventilation strategy has made it possible to significantly reduce the complications associated with mechanical ventilation, minimizing alveolar collapse and reducing overdistension; however, the beneficial effects of ventilation are associated with hemodynamic changes that can compromise lung function.

In all lungs, there is some degree of mismatch between ventilation and perfusion. In the normal lung in an upright position, this inequality takes the form of a regional pattern with a ventilation-perfusion relationship that decreases from the apex to the base. Disorganization of this pattern is observed in the diseased lung until finally, at the alveolar level, the normal relationships between ventilation and blood flow disappear.

Gas exchange occurs thanks to the coupling between ventilation and perfusion. Gaseous exchange occurs in the alveolar region through the alveolar-capillary unit, provided that ventilation is adequate. Ventilation-perfusion ratios (V/Q) vary considerably due to the hydrostatic effect and intraregional differences in blood flow distribution.

Areas with a high V/Q ratio cause ineffective ventilation, which is called the dead space effect. Areas with a low V/Q ratio, called shunt effect, cause hypoxemia due to perfusion of poorly ventilated areas.

Mechanical ventilation can increase dead-space ventilation and hypoventilated areas with greater blood perfusion due to differences in alveoli compliance, leading to ventilation and perfusion disturbances, overdistension of hyperventilated alveoli, and atelectasis in hypoventilated areas.

These alterations are of little clinical significance in patients with healthy lungs and are corrected with the use of adequate tidal volumes or the addition of PEEP. In patients with ARDS or with increased shunts, the improvement in gas exchange results from the reopening of collapsed alveoli; this beneficial effect of PEEP results from the redistribution of blood flow from severely injured areas to poorly or normally ventilated alveolar units.

2.4 *Renal System*

The kidney participates directly in the delivery of oxygen, since it regulates aspects such as fluid balance (preload), vascular tone (renin-angiotensin system, afterload, and ejection volume), hydroelectrolyte balance, acid-base balance, and production of erythropoietin.

The extensive pulmonary capillary network that receives all cardiac output allows the lung to interact with other organs. In the critically ill patient, lung-kidney communication exerts reciprocally and simultaneously, allowing a damaged lung to remotely affect the kidney (lung-kidney interaction) and vice versa.

Patients requiring mechanical ventilation often have kidney failure, which may be caused by the underlying disease or related to the treatment used; however, in recent years, the understanding mechanics of kidney damage directly induced by ventilation has improved [22].

The use of PEEP produces a decrease in urinary flow, sodium excretion, and creatinine clearance in response to the decrease in cardiac output and intrathoracic blood volume, observing a redistribution of intrarenal blood flow, with maintenance of total blood flow [23].

The distribution of intrarenal blood flow is reversed with ventilation, with the flow of the inner renal cortex being greater than that of the outer cortex, which releases vasoactive agents which contribute to the decrease in diuresis. Increased intrathoracic pressure causes arterial hypotension, decreased renal plasma flow, decreased glomerular filtration rate, and urinary excretion.

2.5 Neurological System

The patient under mechanical ventilation may present neurological alterations associated with decreased cerebral perfusion and increased intracranial pressure. The decrease in cardiac output and the presence of arterial hypotension directly affect tissue and cerebral perfusion.

As the brain is one of the most oxygen-dependent organs, this reduction in perfusion rapidly translates into cognitive deterioration and neurological manifestations, which can cause long-term sequelae.

In the ventilated patient, in addition to presenting cognitive alterations, symptoms of anxiety and depression are also frequent, which is frequently associated with asynchrony with the ventilator, which can extend the ventilation time and require a greater amount of sedatives.

2.6 Adaptation of the Patient to the Mechanical Ventilation

The initiation of ventilatory support requires continuous assessment of tolerance by the patient; with an adequate airway, the programming and sedation used are the factors that determine the patient's comfort during the time that ventilatory support is required.

The monitoring that is carried out includes the evaluation of the level of sedation and the adjustment of medications to allow adequate pain control and an optimal level of sedation that allows meeting the goals of lung protection but at the same time reducing the incidence of delirium and adverse effects associated with medication.

The development of new ventilation modalities has made it possible to provide ventilatory support proportional to the needs of the patient, allowing the ventilation to be adjusted to the characteristics of the patient and the desired objectives. Knowledge of the lung-heart interaction and the pathophysiology of pulmonary disorders has allowed the development of the concept of protective ventilation in critically ill patients.

When ventilation is not adequately adapted to the patient, asynchronies occur, which are characterized by a dissociation between the programmed volume delivery on the ventilator and the patient. Asynchronies have been related to an increase in complications in critically ill patients and greater morbidity. Inadequate programming can cause excess respiratory work and gasometric disturbances.

The identification of the type of asynchrony can guide the clinician about the modifications that must be made; an ineffective ventilatory effort can cause a poor adaptation of the patient to the ventilator; it can improve by modifying the sensitivity of the trigger, reducing air trapping, and modifying the level of assistance provided and the level of sedation.

On some occasions, a double cycling may occur causing ineffective additional breaths that must be compensated and causing an increase in the patient's respiratory rate and air trapping. Modifying the inspiratory time and trigger can correct this problem along with changes in the patient's sedation level.

Another problem that can occur during ventilation is the appearance of reverse trigger, which begins with diaphragmatic contraction in response to insufflation of the lungs; this problem can be corrected by improving air trapping and the level of sedation. Patients with pain and dyspnea may increase their inspiratory effort causing inadequate airflow.

Asynchronies can be detected with a clinical assessment of the patient in conjunction with visual evaluation of the volume, pressure, and flow curves present on the ventilator monitor. Modifications in the level of sedation and analgesia and some therapeutic interventions can improve patient synchrony and significantly improve prognosis.

References

1. Mushin WW, Rendell-Baker L, Thompson PW, Mapleson WW. Automatic ventilation of the lungs. Oxford: Blackwell Scientific; 1980.
2. Dalziel J. On sleep and apparatus for promoting artificial respiration. Br Assoc Adv Sci. 1838;1:127.
3. Sauerbruch F. Zur Pathologie des offenen pneumothorax und die Grundlagen meines Verfahrens zu seiner Ausschaltung. Mitteilungenaus den Grenzgebieten der Medizin und Chirugie. 1904;13:999–1004.
4. Pierson DJ. Noninvasive positive pressure ventilation: history and terminology. Respir Care. 1997;42(4):370–9.
5. Hodes HL. Treatment of respiratory difficulty in poliomyelitis. In: Poliomyelitis: papers and discussions presented at the third international poliomyelitis conference. Philadelphia: Lippincott; 1955. p. 91–113.
6. Kacmarek RM. The mechanical ventilator: past, present, and future. Respir Care. 2011;56(8):1170–80.
7. Bayram B, Şancı E. Invasive mechanical ventilation in the emergency department. Turk J Emerg Med. 2019;19(2):43–52. https://doi.org/10.1016/j.tjem.2019.03.001.
8. Mehta AB, Syeda SN, Wiener RS, Walkey AJ. Epidemiological trends in invasive mechanical ventilation in the United States: a population-based study. J Crit Care. 2015;30(6):1217–21.
9. Bellani G, Laffey JG, Pham T, et al. Epidemiology, patterns of care, and mortality for patients with acute respiratory distress syndrome in intensive care units in 50 countries. JAMA. 2016;315:788–800.
10. Wu C, Chen X, Cai Y, et al. Risk factors associated with acute respiratory distress syndrome and death in patients with coronavirus disease 2019 pneumonia in Wuhan, China. JAMA Intern Med. 2020;180(7):934–43. https://doi.org/10.1001/jamainternmed.2020.0994. [Epub ahead of print]

11. Wu Z, McGoogan JM. Characteristics of and important lessons from the coronavirus disease 2019 (COVID-19) outbreak in China: summary of a report of 72314 cases from the Chinese center for disease control and prevention. JAMA. 2020;323:1239. https://doi.org/10.1001/jama.2020.2648.
12. Patel BK, Wolfe KS, Pohlman AS, Hall JB, Kress JP. Effect of noninvasive ventilation delivered by helmet vs face mask on the rate of endotracheal intubation in patients with acute respiratory distress syndrome: a randomized clinical trial. JAMA. 2016;315:2435–41.
13. Gattinoni L, Marini JJ, Collino F, Maiolo G, Rapetti F, Tonetti T, Vasques F, Quintel M. The future of mechanical ventilation: lessons from the present and the past. Crit Care. 2017;21(1):183. https://doi.org/10.1186/s13054-017-1750-x.
14. Laghi F, Tobin MJ. Indications for mechanical ventilation. In: Tobin MJ, editor. Principles and practice of mechanical ventilation. 3rd ed. New York: McGraw-Hill; 2013. p. 129–62.
15. Tobin MJ. Respiratory monitoring. JAMA. 1990;264:244–51.
16. Tobin MJ. Basing respiratory management of COVID-19 on physiological principles. Am J Respir Crit Care Med. 2020;201(11):1319–20. https://doi.org/10.1164/rccm.202004-1076ED.
17. White AC. Long-term mechanical ventilation: management strategies. Respir Care. 2012;57(6):889–99. https://doi.org/10.4187/respcare.01850.
18. Tobin MJ. Chapter 36. Effect of mechanical ventilation on heart-lung interactions principles and practice of mechanical ventilation, 3rd ed. New York: McGraw Hill; 2012.
19. Guyton AC, Hall JE. Textbook of medical physiology. 12th ed. Philadelphia: Elsevier Saunders; 2011.
20. Parillo J, Dellinge P. Principles of diagnosis and management in the adult. 3rd ed. Maryland Heights: Mosby; 2008.
21. Mahmood SS, Pinsky MR. Heart-lung interactions during mechanical ventilation: the basics. Ann Transl Med. 2018;6(18):349. https://doi.org/10.21037/atm.2018.04.29.
22. Koyner JL, Murray PT. Mechanical ventilation and the kidney. Blood Purif. 2010;29:52–68.
23. Ranieri VM, et al. Effect of mechanical ventilation on inflammatory mediators in patients with acute respiratory distress syndrome: a randomized controlled trial. JAMA. 1999;282:54–61.

Humidification and Ventilator Circuit

Yasser Zahghloul and Anthony Navarrete

1 Humidity

Humidity is a general term used to describe the amount of water vapor in a gas. Some definitions should be known to understand the normal physiological humidity and humidification of the inspired gases.

Absolute humidity: is the mass of water vapor present in a volume of gas and expressed in milligrams of water per liter of gas.

Relative humidity: is the amount of water vapor at a particular temperature expressed as a percentage of the amount that would be held if the gas were saturated.

Dew point: the temperature at which gas is 100% saturated.

Water vapor pressure: humidity may also be expressed as the pressure exerted by water vapor in a gas mixture.

Isothermal saturation boundary (ISB): the point at which gases reach alveolar conditions (37 °C and 100% relative humidity).

Humidity varies with the temperature; the warmer the temperature, the more the water vapor that can be held in a gas [1].

Humidification and filter of the inspired air occur primarily in the nasopharynx, and gases that reach the alveolar level are 100% saturated at body temperature. In 24 h, the respiratory tract loses approximately 1470 J of heat and 250 mL of water.

A spontaneously breathing individual's inspired air is typically conditioned down to the fourth or fifth generation of subsegmental bronchi (i.e., the isothermic saturation boundary). Under normal circumstances, conditioning of inspired air occurs as

Y. Zahghloul (✉)
Sheikh Khalifa Medical City, Abu Dhabi, UAE

A. Navarrete
Facultad de Ciencias Medicas, Universidad Francisco Marroquin, Guatemala City, Guatemala
e-mail: anthonynavarrete@ufm.edu

J. Hidalgo et al. (eds.), *Personalized Mechanical Ventilation*,
https://doi.org/10.1007/978-3-031-14138-6_3

air passes through the nose and upper airway. Because these are bypassed during invasive ventilation, a humidity source must be added to the ventilator circuit [1].

The humidification system used during mechanical ventilation should provide at least 30 mg H_2O/L of absolute humidity at a temperature range of about 31–35 °C. Some clinicians prefer a delivered temperature range of 35–37 °C.

Water is intentionally removed from medical gases so that gases from pipelines to ventilators are dry and at room temperature, so gases should be warmed and humidified before going to the lungs.

The dry cold gases have many adverse effects on the respiratory system, e.g., dryness of the mucosa, thick secretion, sequestration of epithelium, mucus plugs, ciliary dysfunction, impaired surfactant activity atelectasis, and airway obstruction [2].

On the other hand, over-humidification of the inspired gases has many side effects, e.g., ciliary degeneration, impaired oxygenation, and decreased lung compliance, and may cause volume overload and pulmonary edema.

For noninvasive ventilation (NIV), inefficient gas conditioning may lead to increased nasal airway resistance, structural and functional damage to the nasal mucosa, increased work of breathing, difficulty in intubation, discomfort, and poor compliance to noninvasive ventilation [3].

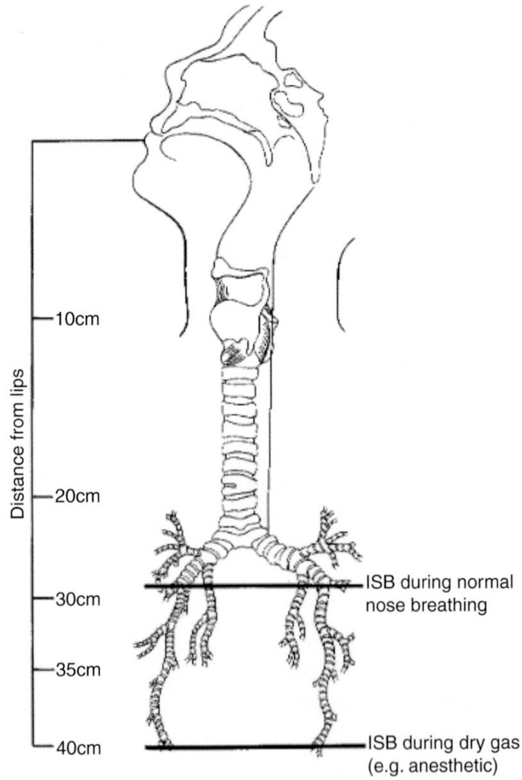

Position of the isothermic saturation boundary (ISB) during normal nose breathing and inhalation of dry gases (during intubation). (Redrawn from [4])

2 Methods of Humidification

The types of humidifiers include passover, vapor phase, wick, and active heat and moisture exchanger. With a closed-feed system, the water level in the reservoir is maintained either manually by adding water from a bag through a fill port or by a float-feed system that maintains a relatively constant water level. An advantage of the closed-feed system is that the water temperature can be better regulated and avoid the need to open the ventilator circuit to refill the device and thus reducing the risk of potential contamination.

3 Heat and Moisture Exchanger (HME)

It is also named condenser humidifier, artificial nose, passive humidifier, moisture exchanger, and vapor condenser. When combined with a filter for bacteria and viruses, it is named HMEF.

HME is a disposable device that includes an exchanging medium enclosed in a plastic housing and varies in size and shape. Each has a 15-mm female connection port at the patient end and a 15-mm male port at the other end; the patient port may also be 22-mm male fitting. It may have a port to attach the gas sampling line for a respiratory gas monitor or an oxygen line; one type utilizes a ceramic heating element with a water input port, a membrane, and an aluminum grid that vaporizes the water [5].

There are two types of HME, hydrophilic and hygroscopic. The hydrophilic HME has a membrane with small pores and is pleated to increase the surface area, providing moderately good, inspired humidity. The hygroscopic HME contains a wool/foam/paperlike material coated with moisture-retaining chemicals and may be impregnated with a bactericide [5].

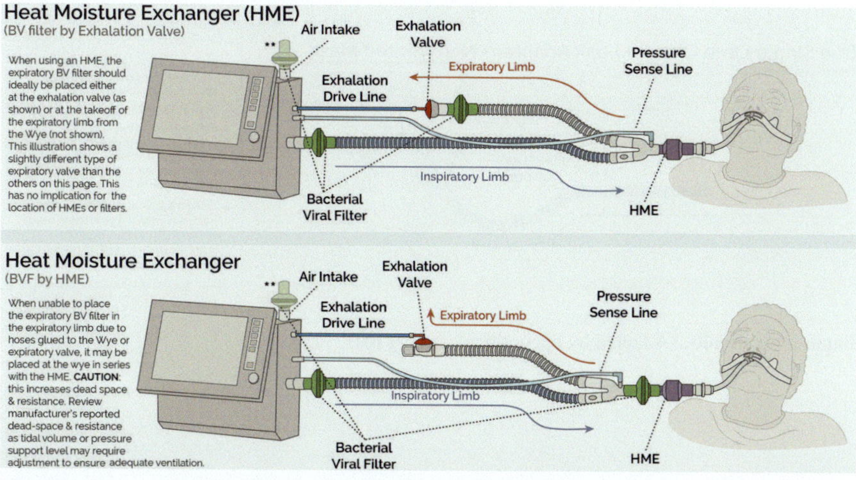

Heat moisture exchanger. (Adapted from OpenCriticalCare.org [6])

Heated humidifiers typically include a servo-controlled heater with a temperature probe that is placed close to the patient airway. These devices are typically equipped with a temperature display and a temperature alarm. The high-temperature alarm is set at 37–38 °C so that the inspired gas does not exceed 37 °C.

Whenever the temperature in the patient circuit is less than the temperature of the gas leaving the humidifier, condensate accumulates in the circuit. Notice that condensate accumulation (rain-out) will increase as the room temperature becomes cooler. Using heated wire circuits on the inspiratory and expiratory lines of the circuit can significantly reduce the amount of rain-out.

High-flow delivery systems, such as the high-flow nasal cannula, can deliver oxygen at a rate of 40 L/min. Patients tolerate such high flows because the inspired gas is humidified and warmed to 99.9% relative humidity and 37 °C.

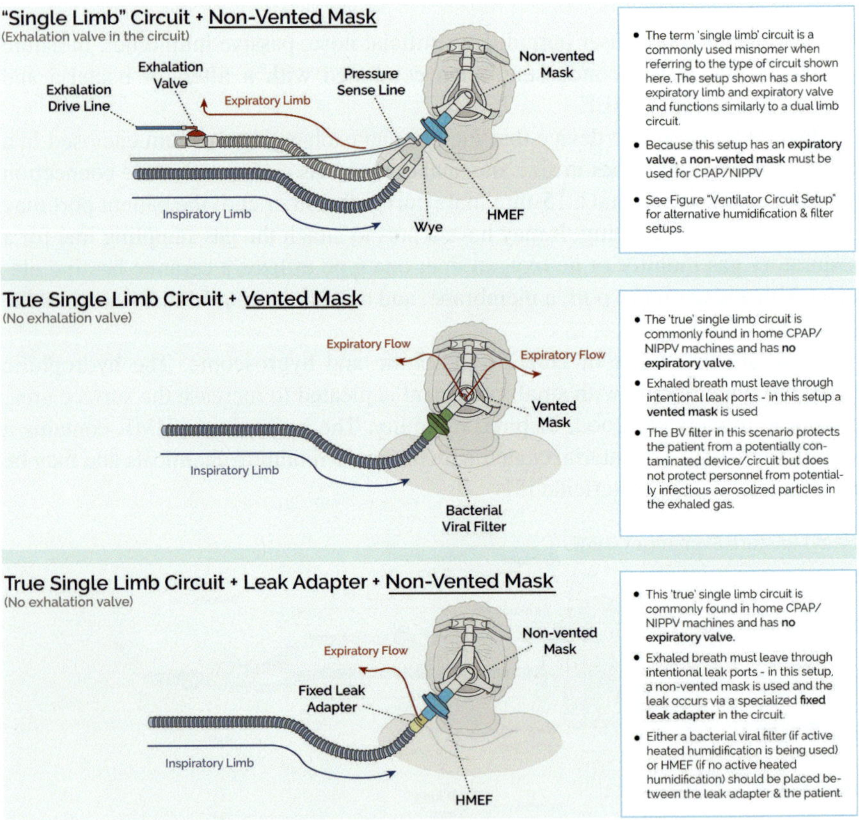

Single-limb circuits. (Adapted by opencriticalcare.org [6])

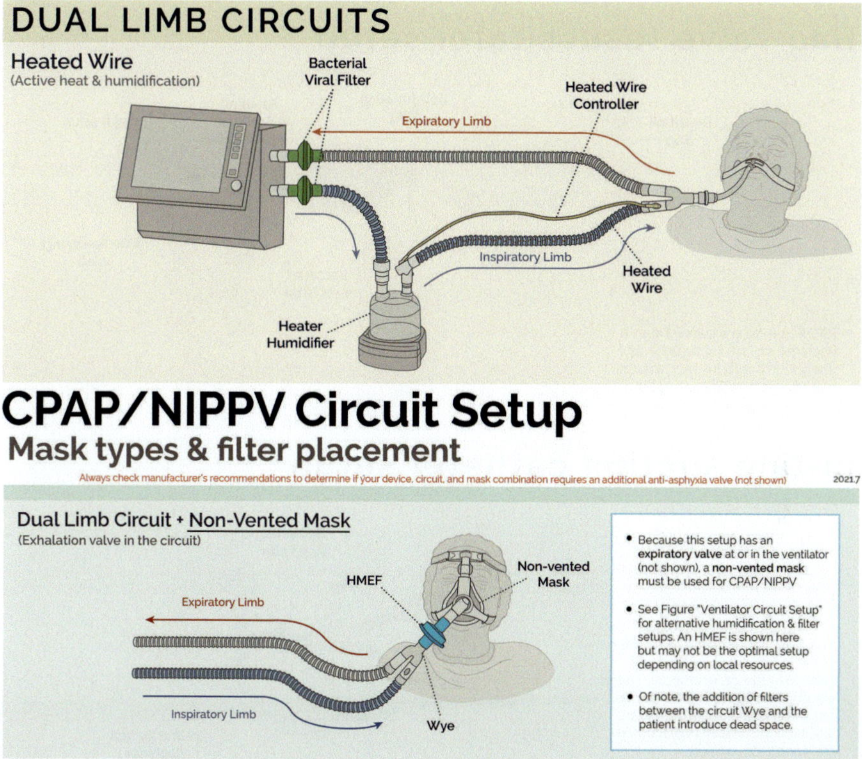

Dual-limb circuits. (Adapted by OpenCriticalCare.org [6])

4 Ventilator Circuit

The ideal ICU ventilator circuit should have some specifications; it should be simple, lightweight, biologically inert, single-use, disposable, gas-impermeable, and cheap to manufacture with low resistance and low compliance.

The inspiratory limb has a slightly larger volume because of the humidifier attachment. All connections are standardized, as should be the case for all such circuits. There is an ISO-mandated international understanding that all respiratory circuit components and airway equipment will have standardized sizes of connectors [7].

The circuit is made of inert plastic, which does not react with respiratory gas or water. The circuits are disposable to prevent cross-contamination between patients.

The tubing is 22 mm in diameter and has an internal volume of approximately 380 mL per meter. Each limb of the circuit is usually about 1.5–1.8 m long, so the total volume is around 1100–1400 mL.

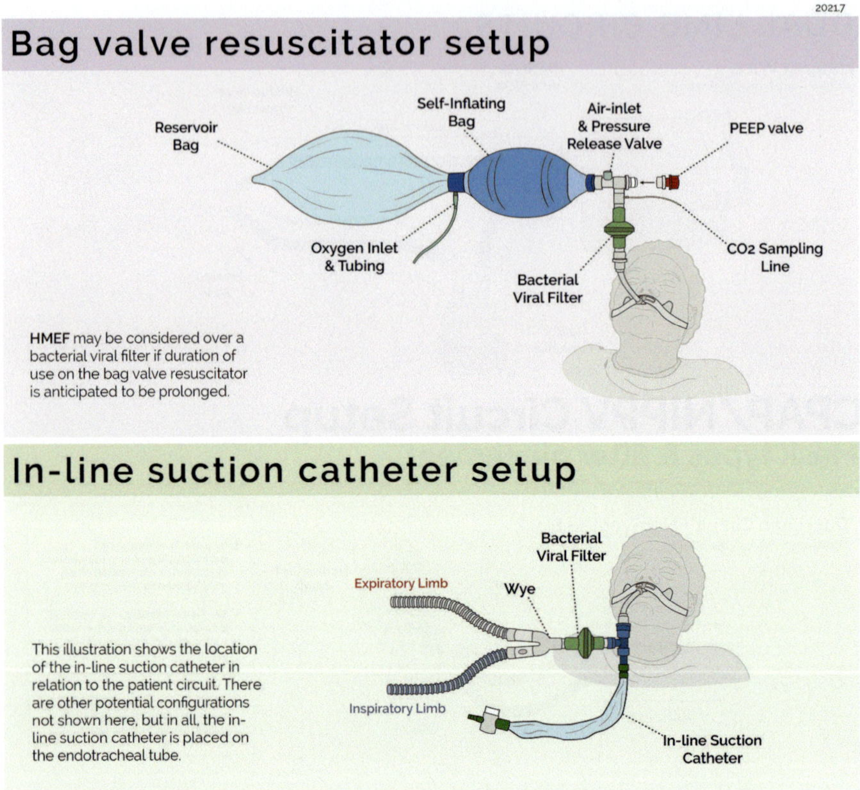

Position of the humidifier in a ventilator circuit. (Adapted by OpenCriticalCare.org [6])

With pressure applied to the circuit in inspiration, the tubing produces movement because of expansion. The more pressure is applied, the more tube movement there will be, and this is often seen in patients who need high peak airway pressure during ventilation, like in patients with poor lung compliance and patients with acute severe asthma.

The change in volume in response to distending pressure is described as circuit compliance. With high circuit compliance, the delivered tidal volume is reduced in mandatory ventilation because some of the flow and pressure are "wasted" on distending the tubing [7].

In spontaneous ventilation with high respiratory effort, the patient may also inhale gas from the expiratory tubing if it is insufficiently rigid. Circuits designed for specialized high-pressure applications (for example HFOV) have the least compliance and are usually not corrugated.

International standards recommend circuit compliance ideally no greater than 1 mL per every 1 cm H_2O distending pressure for every 1 m of tubing. Thus, when ventilated with a driving pressure of 10 cmH_2O, a typical 3.6 m ventilator circuit should change volume only by 30–40 mL.

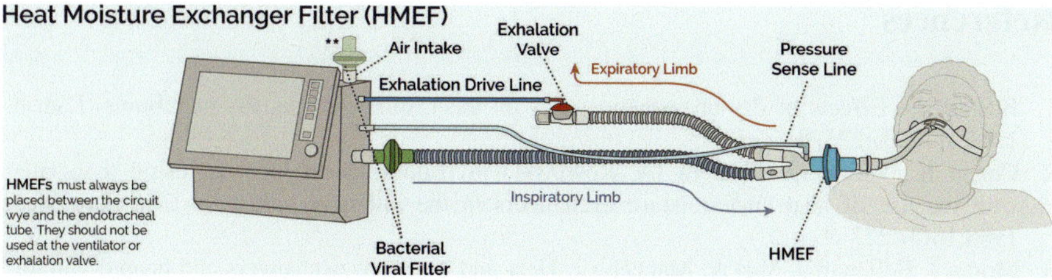

Heat moisture exchange filter. (Adapted by OpenCriticalCare.org [6])

The tubing has a wide diameter to minimize resistance; the resistance to flow through a typical ventilator circuit generates a pressure of less than 0.5 cmH_2O at 30 L/min flow rate.

The resistance to flow and compliance increase with increasing the length of tubing. Extra lengths of tubing are needed during some situations like in MRI and CT rooms.

Resistance may occur at the expiratory filter, which is a fine mesh filter designed to dehumidify the gas entering the expiratory cassette, decrease its bacterial colonization, and improve the longevity of its electronic components. In the presence of high circuit humidity, this filter can rapidly become waterlogged, resulting in high circuit resistance and high peak inspiratory pressure [8].

Regular maintenance of the ventilator circuit:

- Ventilator circuits should not be changed routinely for infection control purposes. The maximum duration of time that circuits can be used safely is unknown.
- Evidence is lacking related to ventilator-associated pneumonia (VAP) and issues of heated versus unheated circuits, type of heated humidifier, and technique for clearing condensate from the ventilator circuit [7].
- Although the available evidence suggests a lower VAP rate with passive humidification than with active humidification, other issues related to the use of passive humidifiers (resistance, dead-space volume, airway occlusion risk) preclude a recommendation for the widespread use of passive humidifiers [5].
- Passive humidifiers do not need to be changed daily for reasons of infection control or technical performance. They can be safely used for at least 48 h, and with some patient populations [5].
- The use of closed-suction catheters should be considered as part of a VAP prevention strategy, and they do not need to be changed daily for infection control purposes. The maximum duration of time that closed-suction catheters can be used safely is unknown.
- Clinicians caring for mechanically ventilated patients should be aware of the risk factors for VAP (e.g., nebulizer therapy, manual ventilation, and patient transport) [9].

References

1. Burton JD. Effects of dry anaesthetic gases on the respiratory mucous membrane. Lancet. 1962;1(7223):235–8.
2. Cohen IL, Weinberg PF, Fein IA, Rowinski GS. Endotracheal tube occlusion associated with the use of heat and moisture exchangers in the intensive care unit. Crit Care Med. 1988;16(3):277–9.
3. Moran I, Bellapart J, Vari A, Mancebo J. Heat and moisture exchangers and heated humidifiers in acute lung injury/acute respiratory distress syndrome patients. Effects on respiratory mechanics and gas exchange. Intensive Care Med. 2006;32(4):524–31.
4. Branson RD, Campbell RS, Johannigman JA, et al. Comparison of conventional heated humidification with a new active hygroscopic heat and moisture exchanger in mechanically ventilated patients. Respir Care. 1999;44:912–7.
5. Lellouche F, Qader S, Taille S, Lyazidi A, Brochard L. Influence of ambient temperature and minute ventilation on passive and active heat and moisture exchangers. Respir Care. 2014;59(5):637–43.
6. The OpenCriticalCare.org Project. https://opencriticalcare.org/about.
7. Pelosi P, Severgnini P, Selmo G, et al. In vitro evaluation of an active heat-and-moisture exchanger: the hygrovent gold. Respir Care. 2010;55(4):460–6.
8. Kelly M, Gillies D, Todd DA, Lockwood C. Heated humidification versus heat and moisture exchangers for ventilated adults and children. Cochrane Database Syst Rev. 2010;4:CD004711.
9. Ari A, Alwadeai KS, Fink JB. Effects of heat and moisture exchangers and exhaled humidity on aerosol deposition in a simulated ventilator dependent adult lung model. Respir Care. 2017;62(5):538–43.

Airway Management During Mechanical Ventilation: COVID-19

Carlos Sánchez, Jorge Hidalgo, Allyson Hidalgo, and Jorge E. Sinclair De Frías

1 Introduction

Viral diseases have become a real health problem and have had a very important increasing incidence in recent years, with outbreaks that have led health systems and governments from sporadic events to complex situations that are often difficult to sustain. However, this same situation has led to its detailed study, which in a certain way has allowed us to understand and predict its real impact in the short, medium, and long terms in a more or less reliable way [1].

In December 2019, the Wuhan Municipal Health Commission in the People's Republic of China published a report of 27 human cases of viral pneumonia with a somewhat different and more aggressive behavior than what we were used to when talking about viral pneumonia. Of these, seven patients were in critical condition. The disease had as its etiology a new human pathogen with high zoonotic capacity, perhaps due to transmission from the bat, and was provisionally designated as 2019 novel coronavirus (2019-nCoV) [2].

The disease caused by the new SARS-CoV-2 (severe acute respiratory syndrome coronavirus-2) spread rapidly through Asia and in a few days throughout the planet, being declared by the World Health Organization (WHO) as an international public health emergency in January 2020 [3] and as a pandemic in March [4].

C. Sánchez
IESS Quevedo General Hospital, Quevedo, Ecuador

J. Hidalgo (✉)
Critical Care Division, Belize Healthcare Partners, Belize, Belize

A. Hidalgo
Biochemistry, Arizona State University, Phoenix, AZ, USA

J. E. Sinclair De Frías
Faculty of Medicine, University of Panama, Panama City, Panama

J. Hidalgo et al. (eds.), *Personalized Mechanical Ventilation*,
https://doi.org/10.1007/978-3-031-14138-6_4

The virus can elicit a violent, dysregulated host immune response mediated by a "cytokine storm" released by immune effector cells that can lead to severe results in most of these older patients as ARDS, multiple-organ failure, and death [5].

Acute respiratory distress syndrome (ARDS) is defined as hypoxemia secondary to a rapid onset of non-cardiogenic pulmonary edema [6].

2 Epidemiology

The prevalence of hypoxic respiratory failure in COVID-19 patients globally stands at around 19% [7]. Recent reports from China showed that between 4 and 13% of COVID-19 patients in studies received ventilation with noninvasive positive pressure (NIPPV) and that between 2.3 and 12% required invasive mechanical ventilation [7–11]. The elderly and people with comorbidities have a higher risk of death, mainly those who have diseases associated with the lung and the cardiovascular system, perhaps due to the impact during the heart-lung interaction and diabetic patients. The death appeared to be primarily ARDS related [12].

3 Approach to the Intubated Patient

The invasion of the airway in the patient with COVID-19 should be carried out considering several aspects; firstly, the real possibility of improvement of the patient once he or she is intubated and later is connected to mechanical ventilation and availability of resources. We also refer to the personnel, the availability of ventilators, and the experience of the health team.

Arterial blood gas can help when deciding which patient should go to mechanical ventilatory assistance; however, it is not recommended that it be the only or most important criterion of evaluation to make decisions [6, 13].

We recommend classifying hypoxia, based on the index SpO_2/FiO_2 [10, 12] mainly in situations where resources are limited or decisions must be made very quickly [11].

Once it is decided to intubate the patient, intubation should be carried out using a rapid induction sequence, which will reduce the cough reflex and exposure time; mask ventilation should be avoided whenever possible, but if necessary, it must be carried out by two people, one serving as a mask seal and the other ventilating, [14, 15] reducing the risk of transmission from patient to staff [16].

When signs of respiratory distress are associated with severe hypoxemia, the following ventilatory strategies represent the opinion of experts; based on the current evidence, the rapid evolution of the patient with coronavirus acute respiratory distress syndrome (CARDS) should be managed as soon as possible; however, more data are required to confirm the efficacy of these maneuvers [17].

4 ARDS Phenotypes in COVID-19

It is important to note that the interaction between different factors and properties of pulmonary mechanics can lead to the development of a spectrum of affectations of the lung parenchyma related to time within two primary "phenotypes": type L, characterized by low elastance (that is, high compliance), low ventilation-to-perfusion ratio, low lung weight, and low recruitment capacity and type H, characterized by high elastance, high tolerance to the right shunt, high lung weight, and high recruitment capacity [18].

5 Respiratory Treatment

Although these severely hypoxemic patients share the same etiology (SARS-CoV-2) and meet most of the conditions by definition of Berlin ARDS, they can be quite different from each other; the same disease actually offers an impressive lack of uniformity [19].

Although the common denominator is severe hypoxemia, findings range from silent hypoxemia with normal breathing to pronounced dyspnea, from deep hypocapnia (less common) to hypercapnia, and from those who respond to high pressures or benefit from the prone position to those who do not; that is why the management of mechanical ventilation must be personalized without this meaning that we free ourselves from protocols and do what we want, but rather it must be a ventilation focused on the patient's lung condition, his or her phenotype, time of evolution, hemodynamic status, and desired goal, among many other things.

To improve results and develop treatment protocols for ARDS, the National Heart, Lung, and Blood Institute of the National Institutes of Health (Bethesda, Maryland) funded a series of multicenter clinical trials, which formed a research collaboration called the ARDS Network (http://ardsnet.org, accessed July 22, 2020) [20] and which are the basis for many of the behaviors currently taken to ventilate critically injured lung, as in ARDS for SARS-CoV-2.

6 Small Tidal Volumes

Among the best established guidelines for the management of ARDS patients is the use of small tidal volumes during mechanical ventilation (either in volume-controlled or pressure-controlled ventilation), which appears to be one of the most important goals. In 2000, researchers from the ARDSNet Lower Tidal Volume (ARMA) test reported significantly decreased mortality rates (31.0% vs. 39.8%) in patients with ARDS ventilated with 6 mL/kg of predicted tidal body weight volumes versus those with 12 mL/kg of predicted body weight [21]; this improvement seems to be related to the lower alveolar distention to which the respiratory functional unit is subjected, both in the most affected areas and those with less compromise.

At that point, it must be carefully analyzed and interpreted if hypoxemia is caused by direct lung damage in a patient with COVID-19 or if, on the contrary, it is a patient with non-severe COVID-19 who shows hypoxemia associated with another medical condition; if that is the case, as demonstrated in 2018, protective ventilation in patients without the ARDS test (PReVENT), ventilation with low tidal volumes, may not be more effective than intermediate volumes in intensive care without ARDS unit patients [22].

7 Positive End-Expiratory Pressure (PEEP)

Ashbaugh et al. reported that the improvement in hypoxemia and atelectasis observed in patients with ARDS was achieved through the implementation of positive end-expiratory pressure (PEEP) with different values depending on the level of lung involvement and the time of the disease [23].

Since then, PEEP continues to be used in the management of ARDS as one of the most important tools to use and continues to be the focus of many clinical research efforts.

Conceptually, PEEP is given to reduce atelectrauma (repetitive opening and closing of alveoli) by recruitment of collapsed alveoli [24]. Much attention has been paid to the levels at which PEEP is applied, with clinical evidence producing mixed results. Several trials reporting protective benefits of higher versus lower PEEP targets used higher tidal volumes in their control (lower PEEP), which perhaps introduced biases in their conclusions [25, 26]. This is why determining the optimal level of PEEP, the way this value is reached, and the return to an average value is still a challenge not fully elucidated in treating the patient with ARDS.

Trials that have controlled for low tidal volumes (6 mL/kg), including 2004 ARDS Network Higher vs. Lower PEEP (ALVEOLI) trial, have failed to establish a survival benefit for higher PEEP [27, 28]. Subgroup analysis, however, suggests that higher PEEP is associated with better survival among the subgroup of patients with ARDS who respond to objectively increased PEEP (patients showing better oxygenation in response to increased PEEP) [29].

However, it is still a long way to walk; it has yet to be shown whether survival in selected patients improves with increased PEEP in large randomized trials.

8 Plateau Pressure

There are no clinical trials examining the effect of plateau pressure (limitation in induced COVID-19 ARDS). However, there is a large amount of indirect evidence in patients with ARDS. In conjunction with low Vt ventilation, Pplat limitation is a lung protection strategy to limit VILI [30]. A systematic review and the RCT meta-analysis found that the use of a lung protection strategy that included a protocolized low Vt and Pplat 30 cmH_2O (9 RCTs and 1629 patients) reduced the risk of death (0.80 95% CI, 0.66–0.98) by 92%. A subsequent meta-analysis of RCTs comparing ventilation strategies with low and high Pplat in patients with ARDS (15 studies) found that short-term mortality was higher in patients with Pplat 32 cmH_2O during the first week in the ICU (day 1: RR 0.77 95% CI: 0.66–0.89; day 3: RR 0.76 95% CI 0.64 0.90; day 7: RR 0.78 95% CI 0.65 0.93) [31].

Based on the available body of evidence, several guidelines recommended keeping Pplat 30 cmH_2O in patients with ARDS 99; the panel considered the magnitude of the benefit to be moderate, the cost low, the patient values consistent, and the intervention acceptable and feasible to implement, and therefore issued a strong recommendation to keep Pplat at 30 cmH_2O when ventilating patients with ARDS [32].

9 Prone Position

It is considered that the beneficial effects of the prone position during mechanical ventilation of patients with ARDS establish a more uniform distribution of gravitational force on pleural pressure, which allows better ventilation of the dorsal pulmonary space [33] and limits overdistention of the lungs and alveoli [34].

The trial of patients with ARDS with severe proning (PROSEVA), conducted by Guerin et al., demonstrated a significant reduction in mortality at 28 and 90 days in patients with ARDS [35]. A recent systematic review and a meta-analysis of 9 RCTs (2129 patients) showed that ventilation in the prone position for at least 12 h in patients with moderate-to-severe ARDS reduced mortality (5 RCTs; RR 0.74, 95% CI 0.56–0.99), but had no effect on mortality in studies using ventilation in the prone position for <12 h (3 RCTs, RR 1.03, 95% CI 0.88–1.20). On the other hand, ventilation in the prone position increased the risk of pressure ulcers (RR 1.22, 95% CI 1.06–1.41) and endotracheal tube obstruction (RR 1.76, 95% CI 1.24–2.50) [36]. Other systematic reviews carried out reached similar conclusions [37, 38].

However, there are no available studies that describe the clinical evolution of COVID-19 patients ventilated in the prone position, including an aspect as relevant as how many times could a patient become prone during hospitalization or what are the parameters that must be taken into account to suspend pronation. In the light of current knowledge, there appear to be unanswered questions.

The main obstacle continues to be its implementation and generalization among each institution. The nursing and respiratory therapy staff is the most important factor for obtaining satisfactory results, since serious life events such as self-extubation, hemodynamic instability, lack of adequate sedation, and pressure ulcers can occur at any time. [39, 40] It is evident that this procedure, like most of those we carry out with our patients, is based on the practice and correct application of the technique; the management of this group of patients during the COVID-19 pandemic has shown us that the more patients we prone, the more the technique is improved; this leads us to think that simulation could lead to better results and a decrease in adverse events.

With regard to neuromuscular blockade, in an effort to avoid fan asynchrony, adjust tidal volumes, and decrease airway resistance to decrease parenchymal inflammation, neuromuscular blocking agents were introduced as part of alternative therapies for severe ARDS, thereby improving asynchrony, avoiding unwanted increases in the airway, and thereby improving patient survival [41].

The Surviving Sepsis Campaign recommends the use of intermittent doses of neuromuscular blocking agents to facilitate lung-protective ventilation in COVID-19 patients [39]. It is important to assess the need or not to use the neuromuscular blocking agent while the patient is in the supine position between pronation cycles or once the patient remains in the supine position, this with the aim of avoiding the unwanted effects of prolonged exposure to these drugs.

10 Tracheostomy

We first consider the role of tracheostomy in respiratory disease and failure. Approximately 8–13% of patients admitted to modern ICUs who require mechanical ventilation have a tracheostomy [42].

The indication for tracheostomy remains the facilitation of mechanical ventilation for a prolonged period while minimizing the complications of a translaryngeal endotracheal tube and weaning from ventilation. Tracheostomy may also be required for actual cases of airway obstruction, laryngeal edema (which may be an emerging feature of COVID-19) [43], or failed extubation due to weakness, poor cough, persistent secretions, or a combination of these factors.

Decision-making about access to intensive care and tracheostomy during the COVID-19 pandemic is based primarily on existing standards of practice, although the evidence base for timing of tracheostomy in those who are critically misguided is not substantial [44].

Decision makers may have to consider the opportunity to embark on a tracheostomy, with associated healthcare resources, in the context of shortages of personnel, equipment, medications, and installations. Although delaying tracheostomy for COVID-19 patients could reduce risks to staff, long-term translaryngeal intubation, sedation, mechanical ventilation, and ICU stay associated with such delays can lead to complications. However, premature extubation exposes patients and staff to the risks associated with emergency rescue oxygenation and reintubation strategies.

A conservative approach is recommended to test extubation, limited to those predicted to have a high probability of being extubated; it is suggested that the tracheostomy be delayed until at least day 10 of mechanical ventilation, and it is considered only when patients show signs of clinical improvement [45].

Regarding the technique to use, it is recommended to use the one with which the work team feels most familiar, either an open or a percutaneous technique.

References

1. Millan-Oñate J, Rodríguez-Morales AJ, Camacho-Moreno G, Mendoza Ramírez H, Rodríguez-Sabogal IA, Álvarez-Moreno C. A new emerging zoonotic virus of concern: the 2019 novel coronavirus (COVID-19). Infection [Internet]. 2020 [05/15/2020];24(3).
2. Palacios Cruz M, Santos E, Velázquez Cervantes MA, León JM. COVID-19, a global public health emergency. Rev Clin Esp [Internet]. 2020 [05/15/2020].
3. World Health Organization. 2019-nCoV outbreak is an emergency of international concern [Internet]. World Health Organization, Regional Office for Europe; 2020 [cited 31 Jan 2020].
4. World Health Organization. WHO Director-General's opening remarks at the media briefing on COVID-19—11 March 2020 [Internet]. World Health Organization; 2020 [cited 11 Mar 2020].
5. Down B, Kulkarni S, Ahmed Khan AH, Barker B, Tang I. Novel coronavirus (COVID-19) infection: what a doctor on the frontline needs to know. Ann Med Surg (Lond). 2020;55:24.
6. Sánchez DJ, Peniche MK, Martínez RE, Cortés RJ, Rivera SG, Diaz PG, et al. False beliefs of acid-base disorders. Coulomb Minute Intensive Care. 2018; https://doi.org/10.1016/j.acci.2018.06.006.
7. Wu Z, McGoogan JM. Characteristics of and important lessons from the coronavirus disease 2019 (COVID-19) outbreak in China: summary of a report of 72 314 cases from the Chinese Center for Disease Control and Prevention. JAMA. 2020;323(13):1239–42. https://doi.org/10.1001/jama.2020.2648.
8. Guan WJ, Ni ZY, Hu Y, Liang WH, Ou CQ, He JX, Liu L, Shan H, Lei CL, Hui DSC, Du B, Li LJ, Zeng G, Yuen KY, Chen RC, Tang CL, Wang T, Chen PY, Xiang J, Li SY, Wang JL, Liang ZJ, Peng YX, Wei L, Liu Y, Hu YH, Peng P, Wang JM, Liu JY, Chen Z, Li G, Zheng ZJ, Qiu SQ, Luo J, Ye CJ, Zhu SY, Zhong NS, China Medical Treatment Expert Group for Covid-19. Clinical characteristics of coronavirus disease 2019 in China. N Engl J Med. 2020;382:1708–20. https://doi.org/10.1056/NEJMoa2002032.
9. Yang X, Yu Y, Xu J, Shu H, Xia J, Liu H, Wu Y, Zhang L, Yu Z, Fang M, Yu T, Wang Y, Pan S, Zou X, Yuan S, Shang Y. Clinical course and outcomes of critically ill patients with SARS-CoV-2 pneumonia in Wuhan, China: a single-centered, retrospective, observational study. Lancet Respir Med. 2020;8(5):475–81. https://doi.org/10.1016/S2213-2600(20)30079-5.
10. Phan LT, Nguyen TV, Luong QC, et al. Importation and human-to-human transmission of a novel coronavirus in Vietnam. N Engl J Med. 2020;382(9):872–4.
11. Riviello ED, Kiviri W, Twagirumugabe T, Mueller A, Banner-Goodspeed VM, Officer L, et al. Hospital incidence and outcomes of ARdS using the Kigali modification of the Berlin definition. Am J Respir Crit Care Med. 2016;193(1):52–9.
12. Wang D, Hu B, Hu C, Zhu F, Liu X, Zhang J, Wang B, Xiang H, Cheng Z, Xiong Y, Zhao Y, Li Y, Wang X, Peng Z. Clinical characteristics of 138 hospitalized patients with 2019 novel coronavirus-infected pneumonia in Wuhan, China. JAMA. 2020;323(11):1061–9. https://doi.org/10.1001/jama.2020.1585.
13. Rice TW, Wheeler AP, Bernard GR, Hayden DL, Schenfeld DA, Warre LB, et al. Comparison of the SpO2/FiO2 ratio and the PaO2/FiO2 ratio in patients with acute lung injury or ARDS. Chest. 2007;132:410–7.
14. Wax RS, Christian MD. Practical recommendations for critical care and anesthesiology teams caring for novel coronavirus (2019-nCoV) patients. Can J Anaesth [Internet]. 2020 [cited 05/15/2020];67.
15. Jin Y-H, Cai L, Cheng Z-S, Cheng H, Deng T, Fan YP, et al. A rapid advice guideline for the diagnosis and treatment of 2019 novel coronavirus (2019-nCoV) infected pneumonia (standard version). Mil Med Res [Internet]. 2020 [cited 05/15/2020];7.
16. Cheung JC, Ho LT, Cheng JV, Cham EYK, Lam KN. Staff safety during emergency airway management for COVID-19 in Hong Kong. Lancet Respir Med [Internet]. 2020 [cited 05/15/2020];8.

17. Ranieri VM, Rubenfeld GD, Thompson BT, Ferguson ND, Caldwell E, Fan E, Camporota L, Slutsky AS, Force ADT. Acute respiratory distress syndrome: the Berlin definition. JAMA. 2012;307:2526–33.
18. Gattinoni L, et al. COVID-19 pneumonia: different respiratory treatments for different phenotypes? Intensive Care Med. 2020;46(6):1099–102. https://doi.org/10.1007/s00134-020-06033-2.
19. Chen N, Zhou M, Dong X, Qu J, Gong F, Han Y, Qiu Y, Wang J, Liu Y, Wei Y, Xia J, Yu T, Zhang X, Zhang L. Epidemiological and clinical characteristics of 99 cases of 2019 novel coronavirus pneumonia in Wuhan, China: a descriptive study. Lancet. 2020;395:507–13.
20. Thompson BT, Bernard GR. ARDS Network (NHLBI) studies: successes and challenges in ARDS clinical research. Crit Care Clin. 2011;27:459–68.
21. Brower RG, Matthay MA, Morris A, Schoenfeld D, Thompson BT, Wheeler A, Acute Respiratory Distress Syndrome Network. Ventilation with lower tidal volumes as compared with traditional tidal volumes for acute lung injury and the acute respiratory distress syndrome. N Engl J Med. 2000;342:1301–8.
22. Writing Group for the PReVENT Investigators. Effect of a low vs intermediate tidal volume strategy on ventilator- free days in intensive care unit patients without ARDS: a randomized clinical trial. JAMA. 2018;320:1872–80.
23. Ashbaugh D, Boyd Bigelow D, Petty T, Levine B. Acute respiratory distress in adults. Lancet. 1967;290:319–23.
24. Tremblay LN, Slutsky AS. Ventilator-induced lung injury: from the bench to the bedside. Intensive Care Med. 2006;32:24–33.
25. Amato MB, Barbas CS, Medeiros DM, Magaldi RB, Schettino GP, Lorenzi-Filho G, Kairalla RA, Deheinzelin D, Munoz C, Oliveira R, Takagaki TY, Carvalho CR. Effect of a protective-ventilation strategy on mortality in the acute respiratory distress syndrome. N Engl J Med. 1998;338:347–54.
26. Villar J, Kacmarek RM, Pérez-Méndez L, Aguirre-Jaime A. A high positive end-expiratory pressure, low tidal volume ventilatory strategy improves outcome in persistent acute respiratory distress syndrome: a randomized, controlled trial. Crit Care Med. 2006;34:1311–8.
27. Brower RG, Lanken PN, MacIntyre N, Matthay MA, Morris A, Ancukiewicz M, Schoenfeld D, Taylor Thompson B, National Heart, Lung, and Blood Institute ARDS Clinical Trials Network. Higher versus lower positive end-expiratory pressures in patients with the acute respiratory distress syndrome. N Engl J Med. 2004;351:327–36.
28. Meade MO, Cook DJ, Guyatt GH, Slutsky AS, Arabi YM, Cooper DJ, Davies AR, Hand LE, Zhou Q, Thabane L, Austin P, Lapinsky S, Baxter A, Russell J, Skrobik Y, Ronco JJ, Stewart TE, Lung Open Ventilation Study Investigators. Ventilation strategy using low tidal volumes, recruitment maneuvers, and high positive end-expiratory pressure for acute lung injury and acute respiratory distress syndrome: a randomized controlled trial. JAMA. 2008;299:637–45.
29. Guo L, Xie J, Huang Y, Pan C, Yang Y, Qiu H, Liu L. Higher PEEP improves outcomes in ARDS patients with clinically objective positive oxygenation response to PEEP: a systematic review and meta-analysis. BMC Anesthesiol. 2018;18:172.
30. Yasuda H, Nishimura T, Kamo T, Sanui M, Nango E, Abe T, Takebayashi T, Lefor AK, Hashimoto S. Optimal plateau pressure for patients with acute respiratory distress syndrome: a protocol for a systematic review and meta- analysis with meta-regression. BMJ Open. 2017;7:e015091.
31. Fan E, Del Sorbo L, Goligher EC, Hodgson CL, Munshi L, Walkey AJ, Adhikari NKJ, Amato MBP, Branson R, Brower RG, Ferguson ND, Gajic O, Gattinoni L, Hess D, Mancebo J, Meade MO, McAuley DF, Pesenti A, Ranieri VM, Rubenfeld GD, Rubin E, Seckel M, Slutsky AS, Talmor D, Thompson BT, Wunsch H, Uleryk E, Brozek J, Brochard LJ, American Thoracic Society, European Society of Intensive Care Medicine, and Society of Critical Care Medicine. An official American Thoracic Society/European Society of Intensive Care Medicine/Society of Critical Care Medicine clinical practice guideline: mechanical ventilation in adult patients with acute respiratory distress syndrome. Am J Respir Crit Care Med. 2017;195:1253–63.

32. Rhodes A, Evans LE, Alhazzani W, Levy MM, Antonelli M, Ferrer R, Kumar A, Sevransky JE, Sprung CL, Nunnally ME, Rochwerg B, Rubenfeld GD, Angus DC, Annane D, Beale RJ, Bellinghan GJ, Bernard GR, Chiche JD, Coopersmith C, De Backer DP, French CJ, Fujishima S, Gerlach H, Hidalgo JL, Hollenberg SM, Jones AE, Karnad DR, Kleinpell RM, Koh Y, Lisboa TC, Machado FR, Marini JJ, Marshall JC, Mazuski JE, McIntyre LA, McLean AS, Mehta S, Moreno RP, Myburgh J, Navalesi P, Nishida O, Osborn TM, Perner A, Plunkett CM, Ranieri M, Schorr CA, Seckel MA, Seymour CW, Shieh L, Shukri KA, Simpson SQ, Singer M, Thompson BT, Townsend SR, Van der Poll T, Vincent JL, Wiersinga WJ, Zimmerman JL, Dellinger RP. Surviving sepsis campaign: international guidelines for management of sepsis and septic shock: 2016. Intensive Care Med. 2017;43:304–77.
33. Lamm WJ, Graham MM, Albert RK. Mechanism by which the prone position improves oxygenation in acute lung injury. Am J Respir Crit Care Med. 1994;150:184–93.
34. Broccard A, Shapiro RS, Schmitz LL, Adams AB, Nahum A, Marini JJ. Prone positioning attenuates and redistributes ventilator-induced lung injury in dogs. Crit Care Med. 2000;28:295–303.
35. Guerin C, Reignier J, Richard JC, Beuret P, Gacouin A, Boulain T, et al. Prone positioning in severe acute respiratory distress syndrome. N Engl J Med. 2013;368(23):2159–68.
36. Bloomfield R, Noble DW, Sudlow A. Prone position for acute respiratory failure in adults. Cochrane Database Syst Rev. 2015;2015:CD008095.
37. Mora-Arteaga JA, Bernal-Ramirez OJ, Rodriguez SJ. The effects of prone position ventilation in patients with acute respiratory distress syndrome. A systematic review and metaanalysis. Med Int. 2015;39:359–72.
38. Lee JM, Bae W, Lee YJ, Cho YJ. The efficacy and safety of prone positional ventilation in acute respiratory distress syndrome: updated study-level meta-analysis of 11 randomized controlled trials. Crit Care Med. 2014;42:1252–62.
39. Alhazzani W, Moller MH, Arabi YM, Loeb M, Gong MN, Fan E, et al. Surviving sepsis campaign: guidelines on the management of critically ill adults with coronavirus disease 2019 (COVID-19). Crit Care Med. 2020;48(6):e440–69. https://doi.org/10.1097/CCM.0000000000004363.
40. The Australian and New Zealand Intensive Care Society COVID-19 Guidelines. https://www.anzicscom.au/wp-content/uploads/2020/03/ANZICS-COVID-19-Guidelines-Version-1pdf. Accessed 17 June 2020.
41. Papazian L, Forel JM, Gacouin A, Penot-Ragon C, Perrin G, Loundou A, et al. Neuromuscular blockers in early acute respiratory distress syndrome. N Engl J Med. 2010;363(12):1107–16.
42. Mehta AB, Syeda SN, Bajpayee L, Cooke CR, Walkey AJ, Wiener RS. Trends in tracheostomy for mechanically ventilated patients in the United States. Am J Respir Crit Care Med. 2015;192:446–54.
43. McGrath BA, Wallace S, Goswamy J. Laryngeal oedema associated with COVID-19 complicating airway management. Anesthesia. 2020;75(7):972. https://doi.org/10.1111/anae.15092.
44. Hosokawa K, Nishimura M, Egi M, Vincent J-L. Timing of tracheotomy in ICU patients: a systematic review of randomized controlled trials. Crit Care. 2015;19:424–12.
45. McGrath BA, Brenner MJ, Warrillow SJ, Pandian V, Arora A, Cameron TS, Añon JM, Martínez GH, Truog RD, Block SD, Lui GCY, McDonald C, Rassekh CH, Atkins J, Qiang L, Vergez S, Dulguerov P, Zenk J, Antonelli M, Pelosi P, Walsh BK, Ward E, Shang Y, Gasparini S, Donati A, Singer M, Openshaw PJM, Tolley N, Markel H, Feller-Kopman DJ. Tracheostomy in the COVID-19 era: global and multidisciplinary guidance. Lancet Respir Med. 2020;8:717–25. https://doi.org/10.1016/S2213-2600(20)30230-7.

High-Flow Nasal Cannula

Prashant Nasa and Deven Juneja

1 Introduction

Supplemental oxygen is the first line of therapeutics for the management of hypoxaemia. Heated and humidified oxygen delivery through a high-flow nasal cannula (HFNC) is increasingly becoming popular for the management of acute respiratory failure. Since the last decade, evidence has accumulated on HFNC as an effective non-invasive respiratory support. The HFNC is referred to by various names in the literature like humidified high-flow therapy, nasal high-flow and high-flow nasal oxygen (HFNO). This chapter reviews HFNC for its physics and mechanism of action, indications, evidence and any adverse effects.

2 Set-Up and Mechanism of Action

Conventional oxygen therapy (COT) involves low-flow systems, like nasal cannula, face masks or high-flow systems, like a non-breathing face mask or venturi mask. However, all traditional oxygen delivery methods have a particular limitation of supply-demand mismatch in conditions with a high demand of inspiratory flows. Other limitations include inconsistent fraction of inspired oxygen (FiO_2) with air dilution. Besides, insufficient humidification and cold gases reduce tolerance due to the dry nose or throat discomfort. HFNC is an innovative tool for delivery of warmed

P. Nasa (✉)
Department of Critical Care Medicine, NMC Specialty Hospital, Dubai, UAE

D. Juneja
Institute of Critical Care Medicine, Max Super Specialty Hospital, Saket, New Delhi, India

J. Hidalgo et al. (eds.), *Personalized Mechanical Ventilation*,
https://doi.org/10.1007/978-3-031-14138-6_5

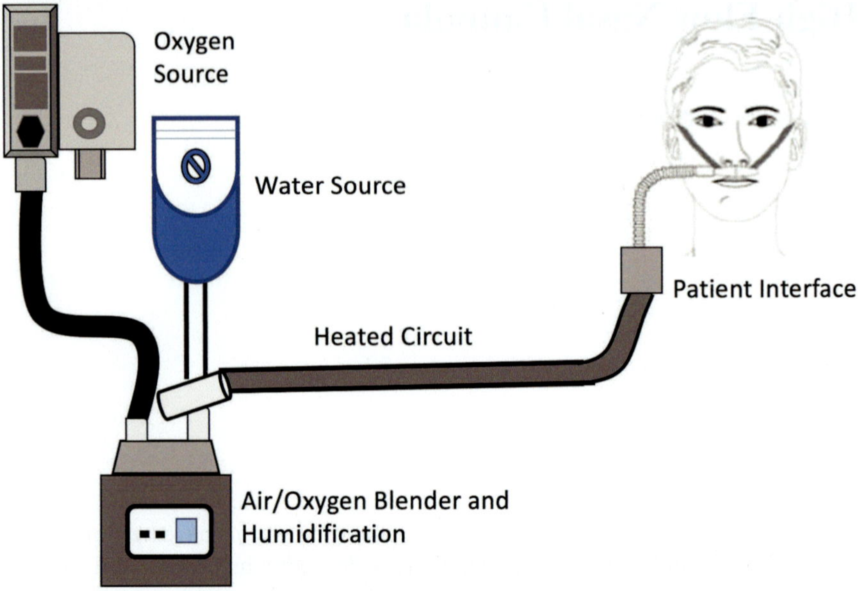

Fig. 1 Set-up of high-flow nasal cannula

and humidified oxygen through an open system using a special nasal cannula [1]. It can deliver consistent FiO_2 ranging between 0.21 and 1.0 and with a flow rate of up to 60 L/min (Fig. 1).

2.1 *Set-Up*

HFNC console comprises an active humidifier and air-oxygen blender, which connects to the patient's interface through a heated single-limb circuit.

Temperature and Humidification: The temperature of inspired gases is typically set between 31 and 39 °C to match an ideal body temperature. Active humidification up to 100% relative to the atmosphere is possible, and its delivery is ensured with a heated circuit to avoid condensation.

Flow and FiO_2: The flow rate is set up depending on the patient's inspiratory demands. Reliable delivery of FiO_2 is possible with careful selection of the flow rates. However, flow rates may reach higher than 60 L/min in patients with respiratory distress, causing entrapment of ambient air and impacting delivered FiO_2. Oxygen source in a hospital setting is usually a piped oxygen. There are inbuilt oxygen sensors to analyse the oxygen delivery of inspiratory gases, which can detect any discrepancy [2].

Interface: The nasal prongs used for HFNC are pliable and softer than the conventional nasal cannula. The nasal interface of HFNC is comfortable and better tolerated by patients [3]. Different sizes are available for paediatric and adult patients. Small, medium and large sizes are available for adults. An appropriate size selection of nasal cannula is crucial to optimise the nasal prongs-to-nares ratio and avoid the direct impact of positive-pressure ventilation on nasopharynx and upper airway [4]. Special interfaces are available for high-flow oxygen delivery through a tracheostomy in hospitals or domiciliary settings [5].

2.2 Mechanism of Action

The mechanism of action has been an area of research. There are various proposed physiological effects of HFNC.

Anatomical dead-space washout: High flow rates of HFNC reduce anatomical dead space by continuous flushing of exhaled gases in upper airways with fresh gases [6].

It enables a more significant proportion of delivered minute ventilation to participate in alveolar gas exchange and reduces rebreathing. This also facilitates the delivery of stable FiO_2, especially with mouth breathing (reservoir effect). HFNC can improve exercise endurance and oxygen saturation and reduces dyspnoea and leg fatigue during high-intensity exercise in patients with severe COPD [7].

Positive end-expiratory pressure (PEEP): Despite an open system, high flow rates of HFNC resist expiratory flow and produce PEEP. The amount of PEEP depends on the flow rate and mouth positions (close vs. open) and varies between 1 and 6 cmH_2O [8].

Mucociliary clearance: Conventional oxygen delivery with inadequate temperature and humidification alters the physiochemical properties of respiratory mucus, reducing ciliary clearance and precipitating bronchoconstriction [9]. Impaired mucociliary clearance also reduces lung compliance and increases work of breathing (WOB). Heated and humidified gases of HFNC improve mucociliary clearance. Effective clearance of secretions is helpful in patients with COPD and bronchiectasis.

Improved pulmonary mechanics: In patients with acute hypoxemic respiratory failure, the use of HFNO reduces WOB or inspiratory effort and increases lung volume or compliance [10]. On the other hand, in patients with acute exacerbation of COPD and hypercapnic respiratory failure, HFNC counterpoises a load of dynamic hyperinflation and reduces inspiratory effort compared to oxygen therapy [11]. In a randomised controlled trial (RCT) comparing HFNO with NIV in hospitalised patients with acute exacerbation of COPD, HFNC was found non-inferior to NIV in improving blood gas abnormalities [12].

Patient's comfort: The comfort and tolerability of the patient to HFNO are reported to be higher because of a soft and pliable nasal prong compared to low-flow nasal cannula or face masks [13].

3 Indications

Recently, the European Respiratory Society (ERS) guidelines on HFNC gave conditional recommendations on HFNC for the management of acute respiratory failure (AHRF) [14]. The American College of Physicians (ACP) also published guidelines for the management of acute respiratory failure in hospitalised patients [15]. The Cochrane meta-analysis reported no difference in treatment failure between HFNC and non-invasive ventilation (NIV) for the management of acute respiratory failure. On the other hand, HFNC had less treatment failure over conventional oxygen therapy (COT) [16]. There are few differences between these guidelines on recommendations for various non-invasive respiratory support (Tables 1 and 2). However, the evidence reported was of low certainty for most of the recommendations.

Table 1 European Respiratory Society recommendations on non-invasive respiratory support

Conditions	Recommendations	Certainty of evidence
Acute hypoxemic respiratory failure	HFNC over COT HFNC over NIV	Moderate certainty Very low certainty
Post-operative patients after extubation with		
Low risk of respiratory complications	HFNC or COT	Low certainty
High risk of respiratory complications	HFNC over COT	Low certainty
Non-surgical patients		
No high risk of extubation failure	HFNC over COT	Low certainty
High risk of extubation failure	NIV over HFNC	Moderate certainty
Acute hypercapnic respiratory failure	NIV over HFNC	Low certainty

Table 2 American College of Physicians recommendations on HFNO in the management of acute respiratory failure

Conditions	Recommendations	Certainty of evidence
Acute respiratory failure		
Acute hypoxemic respiratory failure	HFNO over NIV	Low certainty
Acute hypercapnic respiratory failure	HFNO over NIV	Insufficient evidence
Post-extubation		
Acute hypoxemic respiratory failure	HFNO over COT	Low certainty

4 Evidence

There is emerging literature on the clinical applications of HFNC in various settings. HFNC is increasingly being recommended for the management of different patient populations [14].

4.1 Acute Respiratory Failure

The current evidence favours the use of HFNC over COT in the management of patients with AHRF [14]. COT can cause unreliable FiO_2 delivery, may be ineffective in reducing WOB and may contribute to patient self-inflicted lung injury (P-SILI). Additionally, non-humidified COT may lead to oral or nasal dryness and patient discomfort [17, 18].

A meta-analysis of nine RCTs involving 2093 patients found no difference between HFNC and COT on mortality reduction, intensive care unit (ICU) and hospital length of stay (LOS). However, HFNC effectively reduced the need for endotracheal intubation and escalation of respiratory support (NIV or invasive mechanical ventilation) with low certainty of evidence [19].

HFNC has also been shown to reduce the WOB, patient discomfort and dyspnoea. The maximum benefit of HFNC may be observed in patients with severe disease requiring a high FiO_2, or at high risk of intubation [20].

Patients already on NIV for acute hypoxemic respiratory failure may require frequent breaks for relieving mask pressure, talking, eating or drinking. HFNC may also be preferred over COT during these NIV breaks as it provides better patient comfort, relieves tachypnoea or prevents desaturation oxygenation [21]. Additionally, the use of HFNC may be associated with lesser side effects like eye irritation [22].

Only a few studies have evaluated the cost-benefit of HFNC as compared to COT [23]. A recent study from the United Kingdom demonstrated an overall cost saving of 156£ with HFNC compared to COT. The authors even suggested that these savings may be higher in high-risk patients with severe disease [23].

Compared to NIV, the use of HFNC in managing patients with acute hypoxemic respiratory failure may lead to a reduced need for escalation to invasive mechanical ventilation (IMV). Although its impact on mortality remains ambiguous, a large multicentre RCT has reported improved mortality with HFNC [24]. In addition, the use of HFNC may be associated with shorter ICU LOS and better patient comfort in comparison to NIV [25, 26]. Recently, the ACP clinical guidelines on HFNC performed a meta-analysis of 29 RCTs comparing HFNC vs. NIV and found slight superiority of HFNC on patient-centred outcomes, reduction of all-cause mortality, intubation and hospital-acquired pneumonia. They also reported better patient comfort and improvement in dyspnoea with the initial use of HFNC [15]. The "clinically meaningful outcomes" have more robust evidence only for acute hypoxemic respiratory failure and not for COT or hypercapnic respiratory failure.

In managing COPD patients with mild-to-moderate hypercapnic respiratory failure, HFNC has been shown to be equally efficacious to NIV in reducing respiratory rate and for CO_2 removal [12]. However, HFNC has not been shown to reduce the intubation rate or mortality. Even though HFNC may be associated with better patient comfort, it offers no statistically significant difference in terms of length of stay in ICU or hospital [14].

In patients with COVID-19 infection, there are concerns about high aerosol generation with the use of HFNC, and the use of NIV with helmet mask is generally preferred. However, the use of HFNC may be associated with low risk of aerosol dispersion, which is comparable to that of COT [27]. An RCT comparing HFNC to helmet NIV in COVID-19 patients with AHRF showed a lesser need for intubation at 28 days in the NIV group but showed no difference in overall mortality [28].

4.2 Post-operative Patients

The trials comparing HFNC to COT in post-operative patients have failed to show any difference in ICU or hospital LOS, and overall mortality. No statistically significant effect on oxygenation, patient discomfort or improvement in respiratory rate has also been reported. However, the use of HFNC may be associated with a reduced need for escalation to IMV or NIV [14].

In post-operative patients with high risk of respiratory complications, either NIV or HFNC may be used. In a large multicentre RCT (BiPOP trial), HFNC was non-inferior to NIV in post-operative cardiothoracic patients at high risk for respiratory complications. There was no statistically significant difference in treatment failure rates or ICU mortality, but skin breakdown after 24 h was significantly more in the NIV group [29]. Recent guidelines also suggested for prophylactic HFNC compared to COT in post-operative patients (only after cardiac or thoracic surgery) with high risk of respiratory complications and/or who are obese. No difference was found in mortality reduction, ICU LOS or need for escalation of respiratory support in comparison to NIV. Guidelines were against the use of HFNC in other post-operative patients [30].

4.3 Post-extubation Respiratory Support in Non-surgical Patients

HFNC may be preferable to COT for providing respiratory support after extubation in non-surgical patients, as it may be associated with reduced incidence of re-intubation and need for escalation to NIV. However, no significant differences have been reported in mortality and ICU or hospital LOS [14]. Guidelines also recommend HFNC over COT in high-risk patients who were intubated for more than 24 h to reduce the risk of extubation failure. The high-risk patients have one or more of

the risk factors: age >65 years, congestive heart failure, moderate-severe COPD, APACHE II score >12, obesity (BMI >30), issue related to airway patency (e.g. clearance of airway secretion), difficulty in weaning, two or more comorbidities or duration of IMV >7 days [29].
HFNC has only been associated with better patient comfort but no difference in re-intubation rates compared to NIV. As there is no statistically significant difference in mortality rates, NIV may be a better therapeutic modality in this group of patients. However, HFNC may be applied in a select group of patients who do not tolerate NIV or have any contraindications for applying NIV [14, 29].

5 Contraindications

As with other types of non-invasive oxygen support, it is contraindicated to apply HFNC in patients with altered mental status unable to maintain their airways, patients with copious secretions at risk of aspiration and patients with severe hemodynamic instability (unstable arrhythmias and those with cardiorespiratory arrest). Most of these contraindications are relative. Physician discretion is required while exercising HFNC with contraindications. Patients with facial injuries or defects may also find it difficult to tolerate the nasal cannulas, and hence cautious use is advocated in these patients.

6 Adverse Effects

HFNC provides heated humidified oxygen at high flows, and patients generally tolerate it better than NIV support. However, some patients may not tolerate high-flow oxygen, and air leak may lead to loss of positive airway pressure effect. There is slight risk of nasal bleeding with nasopharynx structural abnormalities or coagulopathy [14]. Despite a recent increase in its use, HFNC is still not widely available, especially in resource-limited settings. In addition, it is more expensive than COT and requires training of healthcare staff for its proper application and monitoring. Close monitoring is required to watch for any deterioration and need for intubation and IMV.

7 Conclusions

HFNC is increasingly being applied in the management of acute hypoxemic respiratory failure and may be preferable to COT and NIV in managing these patients. It offers advantages like better patient comfort and less adverse effects while providing adequate oxygenation and reducing WOB. It can be instrumental in reducing the need for IMV and escalation of respiratory support. Its applications are now being expanded to managing post-operative risk of respiratory failure, post-extubation respiratory support and even acute exacerbation of COPD. Even though a few studies have shown HFNC to be equally efficacious in the initial management of COPD patients with mild-moderate hypercapnia, NIV remains the modality of choice. However, with increasing experience in managing patients on HFNC, it has become a viable alternative to NIV in most clinical situations where NIV is contraindicated or not tolerated.

References

1. Park S. High-flow nasal cannula for respiratory failure in adult patients. Acute Crit Care. 2021;36(4):275–85. https://doi.org/10.4266/acc.2021.01571.
2. Vargas F, Saint-Leger M, Boyer A, Bui NH, Hilbert G. Physiologic effects of high-flow nasal cannula oxygen in critical care subjects. Respir Care. 2015;60(10):1369–76. https://doi.org/10.4187/respcare.03814.
3. Roca O, Riera J, Torres F, Masclans JR. High-flow oxygen therapy in acute respiratory failure. Respir Care. 2010;55(4):408–13.
4. Sivieri EM, Gerdes JS, Abbasi S. Effect of HFNC flow rate, cannula size, and nares diameter on generated airway pressures: an in vitro study. Pediatr Pulmonol. 2013;48(5):506–14. https://doi.org/10.1002/ppul.22636.
5. Stripoli T, Spadaro S, Di Mussi R, Volta CA, Trerotoli P, De Carlo F, et al. High-flow oxygen therapy in tracheostomized patients at high risk of weaning failure. Ann Intensive Care. 2019;9(1):4. https://doi.org/10.1186/s13613-019-0482-2.
6. Möller W, Celik G, Feng S, Bartenstein P, Meyer G, Oliver E, et al. Nasal high flow clears anatomical dead space in upper airway models. J Appl Physiol (1985). 2015;118(12):1525–32. https://doi.org/10.1152/japplphysiol.00934.2014.
7. Cirio S, Piran M, Vitacca M, et al. Effects of heated and humidified high flow gases during high-intensity constant-load exercise on severe COPD patients with ventilatory limitation. Respir Med. 2016;118:128–32. https://doi.org/10.1016/j.rmed.2016.08.004.
8. Okuda M, Tanaka N, Naito K, Kumada T, Fukuda K, Kato Y, et al. Evaluation by various methods of the physiological mechanism of a high-flow nasal cannula (HFNC) in healthy volunteers. BMJ Open Respir Res. 2017;4(1):e000200. https://doi.org/10.1136/bmjresp-2017-000200.
9. Heaton RW, Henderson AF, Gray BJ, et al. The bronchial response to cold air challenge: evidence for different mechanisms in normal and asthmatic subjects. Thorax. 1983;38:506–11. https://doi.org/10.1136/thx.38.7.506.
10. Mauri T, Turrini C, Eronia N, et al. Physiologic effects of high-flow nasal cannula in acute hypoxemic respiratory failure. Am J Respir Crit Care Med. 2017;195:1207–15. https://doi.org/10.1164/rccm.201605-0916OC.
11. Elshof J, Duiverman ML. Clinical evidence of nasal high-flow therapy in chronic obstructive pulmonary disease patients. Respiration. 2020;99(2):140–53. https://doi.org/10.1159/000505583.
12. Cortegiani A, Longhini F, Madotto F, Groff P, Scala R, Crimi C, et al. High flow nasal therapy versus noninvasive ventilation as initial ventilatory strategy in COPD exacerbation: a multicenter non-inferiority randomized trial. Crit Care. 2020;24(1):692. https://doi.org/10.1186/s13054-020-03409-0.
13. Rittayamai N, Tscheikuna J, Rujiwit P. High-flow nasal cannula versus conventional oxygen therapy after endotracheal extubation: a randomized crossover physiologic study. Respir Care. 2014;59:485–90.

14. Oczkowski S, Ergan B, Bos L, Chatwin M, Ferrer M, Gregoretti C, et al. ERS clinical practice guidelines: high-flow nasal cannula in acute respiratory failure. Eur Respir J. 2022;59:2101574. https://doi.org/10.1183/13993003.01574-2021.
15. Baldomero AK, Melzer AC, Greer N, Majeski BN, MacDonald R, Linskens EJ, et al. Effectiveness and harms of high-flow nasal oxygen for acute respiratory failure: an evidence report for a clinical guideline from the American College of Physicians. Ann Intern Med. 2021;174(7):952–66. https://doi.org/10.7326/M20-4675.
16. Lewis SR, Baker PE, Parker R, Smith AF. High-flow nasal cannulae for respiratory support in adult intensive care patients. Cochrane Database Syst Rev. 2021;3(3):CD010172. https://doi.org/10.1002/14651858.CD010172.pub3. PMID: 33661521; PMCID: PMC8094160.
17. Brochard L, Slutsky A, Pesenti A. Mechanical ventilation to minimize progression of lung injury in acute respiratory failure. Am J Respir Crit Care Med. 2017;195(4):438–42.
18. Yoshida T, Grieco DL, Brochard L, Fujino Y. Patient self-inflicted lung injury and positive end-expiratory pressure for safe spontaneous breathing. Curr Opin Crit Care. 2020;26(1):59–65.
19. Rochwerg B, Granton D, Wang DX, Helviz Y, Einav S, Frat JP, et al. High flow nasal cannula compared with conventional oxygen therapy for acute hypoxemic respiratory failure: a systematic review and meta-analysis. Intensive Care Med. 2019;45(5):563–72. https://doi.org/10.1007/s00134-019-05590-5.
20. Bos LD, Artigas A, Constantin J-M, Hagens LA, Heijnen N, Laffey JG, et al. Precision medicine in acute respiratory distress syndrome: workshop report and recommendations for future research. Eur Respir Rev. 2021;30(159):200317.
21. Frat JP, Brugiere B, Ragot S, Chatellier D, Veinstein A, Goudet V, et al. Sequential application of oxygen therapy via high-flow nasal cannula and noninvasive ventilation in acute respiratory failure: an observational pilot study. Respir Care. 2015;60(2):170–8.
22. Spoletini G, Mega C, Pisani L, Alotaibi M, Khoja A, Price LL, et al. High-flow nasal therapy vs standard oxygen during breaks off noninvasive ventilation for acute respiratory failure: a pilot randomized controlled trial. J Crit Care. 2018;48:418–25.
23. Jahagirdar D, Picheca L. Heated humidified high flow oxygen for respiratory support: a review of clinical effectiveness, cost-effectiveness, and guidelines. 2019. https://www.ncbi.nlm.nih.gov/books/NBK544686/pdf/Bookshelf_NBK544686.pdf. Assessed 30 Mar 2022.
24. Frat JP, Thille AW, Mercat A, Girault C, Ragot S, Perbet S, et al. High-flow oxygen through nasal cannula in acute hypoxemic respiratory failure. N Engl J Med. 2015;372(23):2185–96.
25. Doshi P, Whittle JS, Bublewicz M, Kearney J, Ashe T, Graham R, et al. High-velocity nasal insufflation in the treatment of respiratory failure: a randomized clinical trial. Ann Emerg Med. 2018;72(1):73–83.e5.
26. Grieco DL, Menga LS, Raggi V, Bongiovanni F, Anzellotti GM, Tanzarella ES, et al. Physiological comparison of high-flow nasal cannula and helmet noninvasive ventilation in acute hypoxemic respiratory failure. Am J Respir Crit Care Med. 2020;201(3):303–12.
27. Li J, Fink JB, Ehrmann S. High-flow nasal cannula for COVID-19 patients: low risk of bio-aerosol dispersion. Eur Respir J. 2020;55:2000892.
28. Grieco DL, Menga LS, Cesarano M, Rosà T, Spadaro S, Bitondo MM, et al. Effect of helmet noninvasive ventilation vs high-flow nasal oxygen on days free of respiratory support in patients with COVID-19 and moderate to severe hypoxemic respiratory failure: the HENIVOT randomized clinical trial. JAMA. 2021;325(17):1731–43.
29. Stéphan F, Barrucand B, Petit P, Rézaiguia-Delclaux S, Médard A, Delannoy B, et al. High-flow nasal oxygen vs noninvasive positive airway pressure in hypoxemic patients after cardiothoracic surgery: a randomized clinical trial. JAMA. 2015;313(23):2331–9.
30. Rochwerg B, Einav S, Chaudhuri D, Mancebo J, Mauri T, Helviz Y, et al. The role for high flow nasal cannula as a respiratory support strategy in adults: a clinical practice guideline. Intensive Care Med. 2020;46(12):2226–37. https://doi.org/10.1007/s00134-020-06312-y.

Modes of Mechanical Ventilation

Ayman M. Eltoukhy Salem

1 Introduction

Mechanical ventilation has been introduced with the goal of reducing undue workload of respiration, unloading respiratory muscles, supporting gas exchange, and alleviation of dyspnea, while other treatment measures would control the cause leading to respiratory failure. The algorithm that describes the breathing pattern and the interaction between the patient and the ventilator is referred to as the mode [1].

Common modes of ventilation can be divided into three basic categories: conventional modes in which none of the settings is automatically regulated, adaptive modes in which one or more settings are automatically regulated, and biphasic ventilation modes which alternate intermittently between two positive pressure levels [2].

Proportional ventilation modes work by amplifying the spontaneous efforts of the patient's respiratory muscle activity to improve the imbalance between capacity and demand of the patient [3].

A mode should define five basic phase variables of a mechanical breath [2, 4]: triggering (cycle-on), control, target/limit, cycling (cycle-off), and baseline (Fig. 1).

1. Triggering: It refers to the initiation of the breath (inspiration) whether it is pressure, flow, or time set.
2. Target: It refers to the independent limits of the inspiratory excursion whether it is volume, pressure, flow, or a combination of these. Reaching the target variable during inspiration does not abort the inspiratory phase unlike the alarm limit.

A. M. E. Salem (✉)
Critical Care Department, Sheikh Khalifa Medical City, Abu Dhabi, UAE
e-mail: aymansalem@seha.ae

J. Hidalgo et al. (eds.), *Personalized Mechanical Ventilation*,
https://doi.org/10.1007/978-3-031-14138-6_6

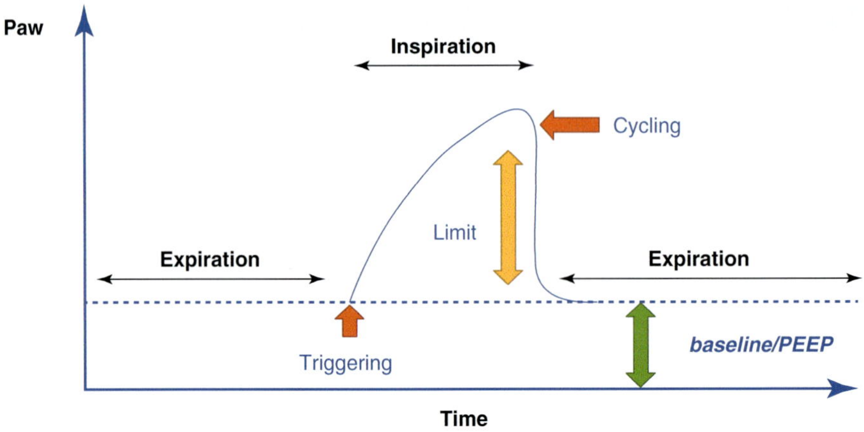

Fig. 1 The mechanical respiratory cycle

3. Cycling: It refers to the ending of inspiration giving way to passive exhalation. It could be time (for mandatory and assisted breath) or flow (for spontaneous breath) set.
4. Baseline (end-expiratory pressure/PEEP): It refers to the state of equilibrium of the respiratory system with the only thing happening is a slow bias gas flow out of the circuit via the expiratory valve.
5. The control variable is the variable which the ventilator uses as a feedback signal for controlling inspiration [5]. It is also defined in terms of the equation of motion [6]:

$$P_{vent} + P_{muscle} = Elastance \times tidal\ volume + Flow \times Resistance$$

Clearly, if one variable is predetermined, it becomes the control variable, and all other variables are simply dependent upon it. Since flow is volume over time, only volume and pressure are considered control variables.

2 Types of Mechanical Breath

1. Control breath: a breath initiated by the ventilator (i.e., time triggered) and terminated by the machine (i.e., time cycled) (Figs. 2 and 3).
2. Assist breath: a breath initiated by the patient (i.e., pressure or flow triggered) and terminated by the machine (i.e., time cycled) (Figs. 2 and 3).
3. Spontaneous (support) breath: a breath initiated by the patient (i.e., pressure or flow triggered) and terminated by the patient (i.e., flow cycled) (Fig. 4).

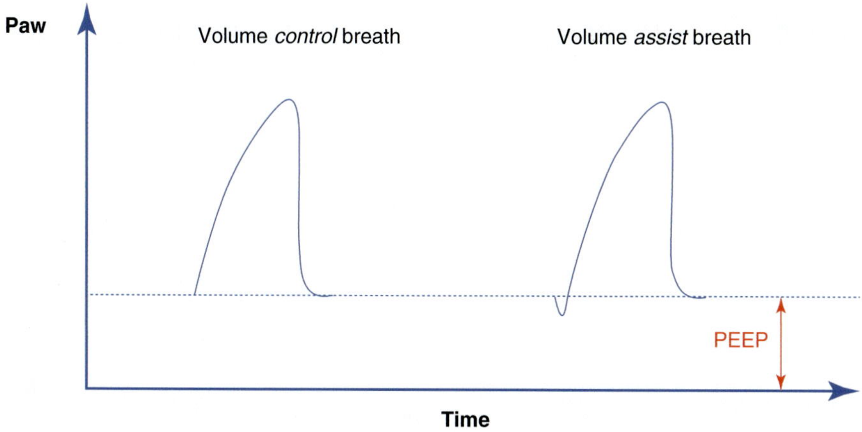

Fig. 2 Difference between control and assist breath in volume control mode on the pressure-time curve

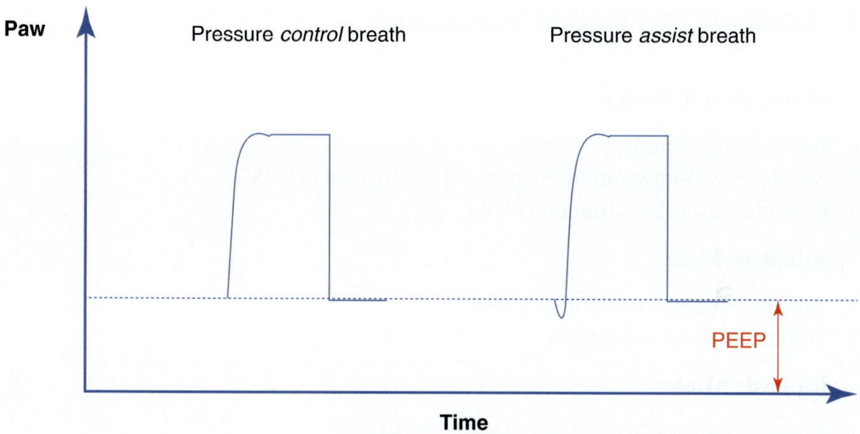

Fig. 3 Difference between control and assist breath in pressure control mode on the pressure-time curve

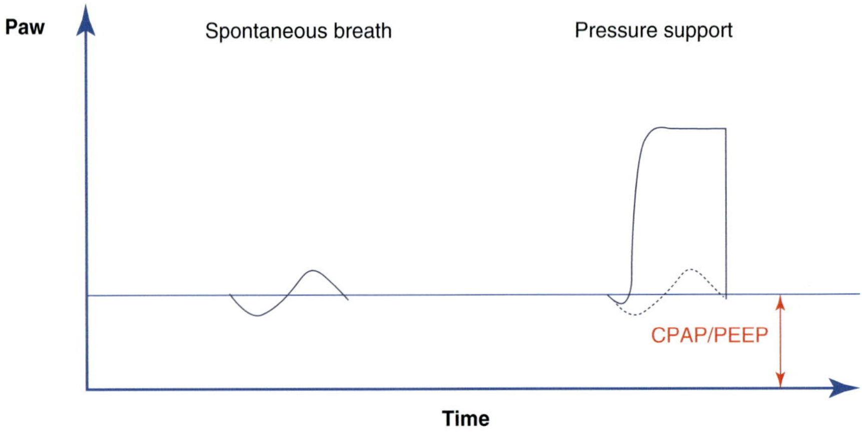

Fig. 4 Schematic representation of spontaneous breath while on CPAP (unsupported) and on pressure support ventilation

3 Modes of Mechanical Ventilation

Conventional Modes

1. Assist control modes
2. Synchronized intermittent mandatory ventilation (SIMV)
3. Pressure support ventilation (PSV)

Adaptive Modes

1. Adaptive support ventilation (ASV)
2. Volume support ventilation

Biphasic Modes

1. Airway Pressure Release Ventilation (APRV)

Proportional Modes

1. Neurally adjusted ventilatory assist (NAVA)
2. Proportional assist ventilation (PAV)

4 Conventional Modes of Ventilation

4.1 Assist Control Mode (A/C)

In A/C modes, mechanical breaths are delivered to the patient at a minimum set rate. It can be initiated by the ventilator at fixed intervals according to the set frequency (i.e., controlled breath) or can be triggered by the patient's inspiratory efforts (i.e.,

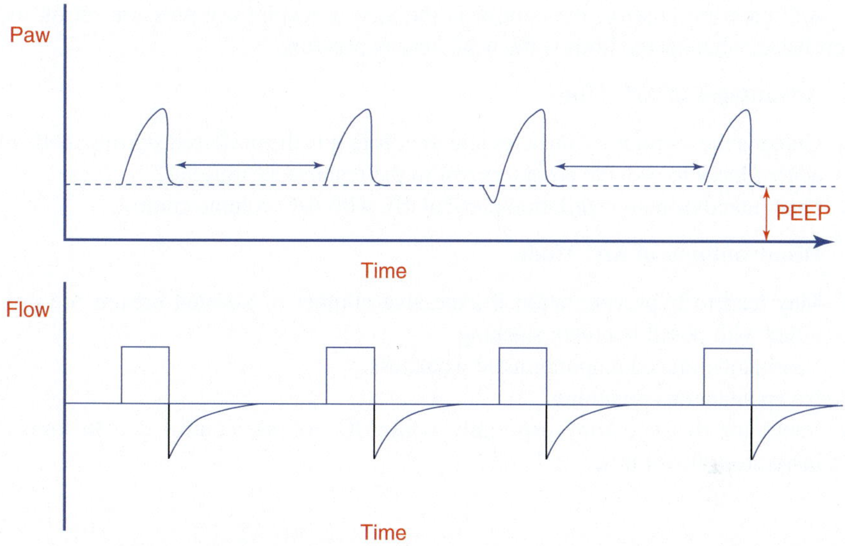

Fig. 5 A/C volume control pressure-time waveform and the corresponding flow-time waveform

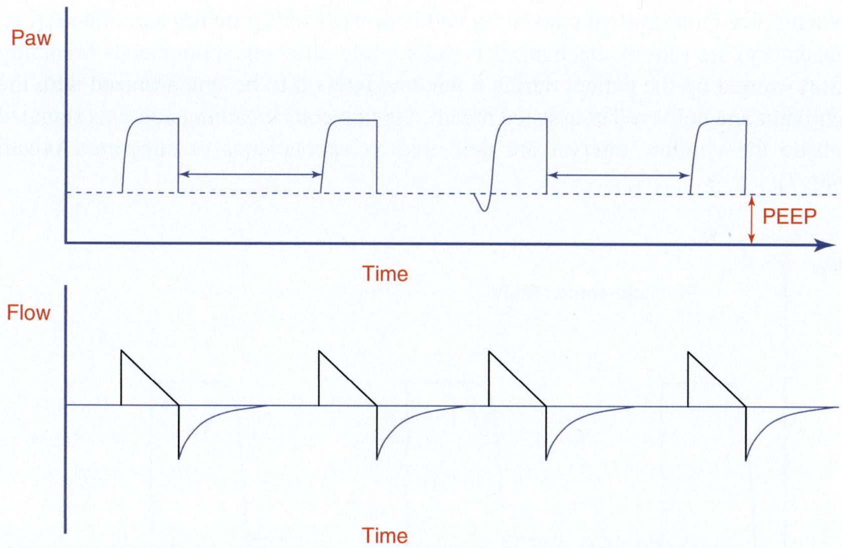

Fig. 6 A/C pressure control pressure-time waveform and the corresponding flow-time waveform

assisted breath) with subsequent increase in respiratory rate above the set frequency. Controlled and assisted breaths are identical with regard to the inspiratory time, flow waveform, control, and limit variables (Figs. 5 and 6).

A/C volume control: the control is the tidal volume set on the ventilator, whereas the limit is the peak inspiratory flow rate.

A/C pressure control: the control is the airway inspiratory pressure set on the ventilator, whereas the limit is the peak airway pressure.

Advantages of A/C Mode

1. Unloads the respiratory muscles and therefore it is the preferred starting mode in acute illness to provide complete rest to the respiratory muscles.
2. Guaranteed minute ventilation particularly with A/C volume control.

Disadvantages of A/C Mode

1. May lead to hyperventilation if excessive number of assisted breaths are provided with possible breath stacking.
2. Ventilator-induced diaphragmatic weakness.
3. No spontaneous breathing.
4. Ventilator dyssynchrony especially with A/C volume control due to limited inspiratory flow rates.

4.2 Synchronized Intermittent Mandatory Ventilation (SIMV)

Synchronized intermittent mandatory ventilation (SIMV) provides a minimum (i.e., mandatory) set rate of mechanical breaths while allowing spontaneous breathing effort exerted by the patient during a window interval to be synchronized with the ventilator and delivered as assisted breath. Spontaneous breathing attempts signaled outside the window interval are delivered as spontaneous or supported breath (Fig. 7).

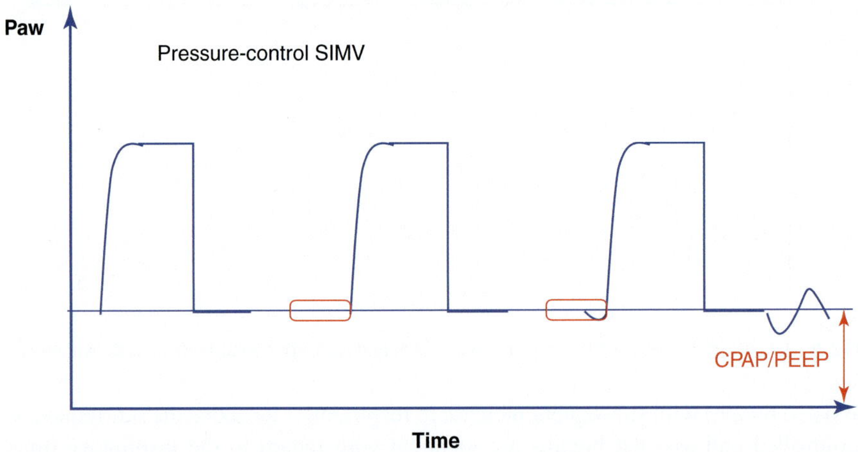

Fig. 7 Pressure SIMV pressure-time waveform demonstrating the imaginative triggering window (red box) for synchronization of assist breath

SIMV volume control: the control is the tidal volume set on the ventilator, and the limit is the peak inspiratory flow rate.

SIMV pressure control: the control is the airway inspiratory pressure set on the ventilator, and the limit is the peak airway pressure.

Advantages of SIMV Mode

1. It provides backup minute ventilation while allowing spontaneous breathing in synchrony with the mandatory breaths.
2. It is sometimes used as a weaning mode.

Disadvantages of SIMV Mode

1. Increased work of breathing even though the addition of pressure support may help reduce some of the work of breathing.
2. Reduces cardiac output particularly in patients with left ventricular dysfunction [7].

4.3 Pressure Support Ventilation (PSV)

PSV is a spontaneous mode of ventilation whereby the ventilator is triggered by a change in flow or pressure in the circuit caused by the patient's inspiratory efforts and provides a pressure-augmented breath to the target inspiratory level set on the ventilator. Cycling takes place when the inspiratory flow rate markedly declines to a certain percentage of the peak inspiratory flow rate, classically 25%.

The peak inspiratory flow rate, tidal volume, and respiratory rate are all dependent on the patient's effort, respiratory system compliance, and target pressure support (Fig. 8).

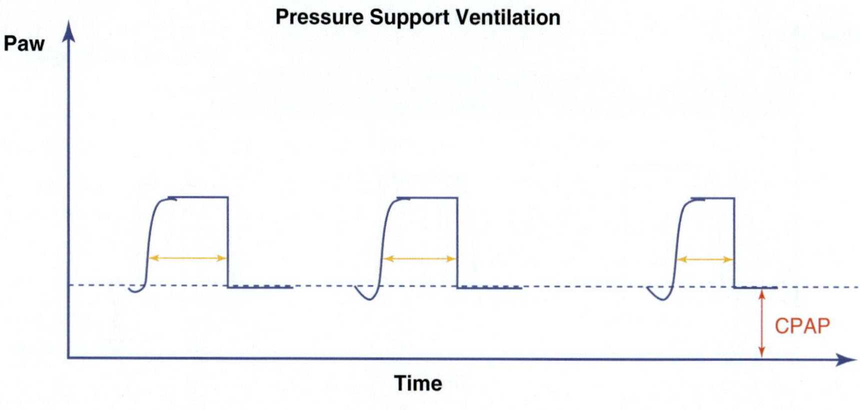

Fig. 8 Pressure-time waveform of spontaneous breaths in PSV showing variable inspiratory time and frequency but same pressure limit

Advantages of PSV

1. Better synchrony
2. Weaning mode
3. Less need for sedation

Disadvantages of PSV

1. Variable tidal volume and minute ventilation
2. Decreased cardiac output
3. Failed (ineffective) triggering
4. Over-assistance leading to diaphragmatic disuse atrophy
5. Sleep apnea
6. Auto-PEEP

5 Adaptive Modes of Ventilation

These are all pressure-controlled modes with attempts at adjustment of the tidal volume to meet specific minute ventilation requirements. Airway pressures may vary in between breaths but remain below a set limit usually 10 cmH_2O below the pressure alarm limit (known as *pressure regulation ceiling*) (Fig. 9).

The principle can be applied to the three main types of mechanical inspiratory breath, whether controlled, assisted, or spontaneous. The ventilator aims at checking the respiratory system compliance with each breath to make the adjustments in pressure to meet the target tidal volume. In case the target could not be achieved due to low compliance, high resistance, excessive tidal volumes, or relatively low pressure limits, or a combination of these factors, the ventilator provides an alert that the set tidal volume cannot be achieved.

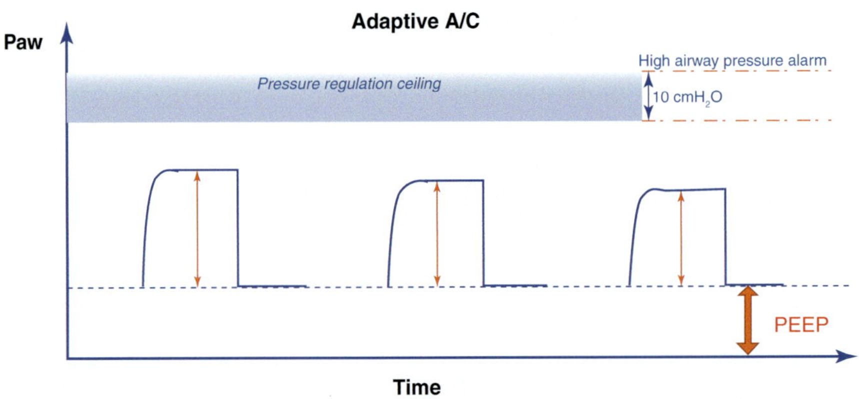

Fig. 9 A schematic representation of pressure-time waveform of adaptive A/C mode demonstrating variable airway pressure as well as the pressure regulation ceiling within 10 cmH_2O of the high-pressure alarm limit

5.1 *Adaptive A/C Mode*

Trigger: time, flow, or pressure
Limit: peak airway pressure, tidal volume
Cycle: time

5.2 *Adaptive SIMV*

Trigger: flow or pressure
Limit: peak airway pressure, tidal volume
Cycle: time or flow

5.3 *Adaptive Pressure Support (Volume Support)*

Volume support is a spontaneous mode where a target tidal volume is set on the ventilator. The ventilator adjusts the amount of pressure support to deliver with each breath to achieve the set tidal volume (Fig. 10). The respiratory rate is determined by the patient.

Trigger: flow or pressure
Limit: peak airway pressure, tidal volume
Cycle: flow

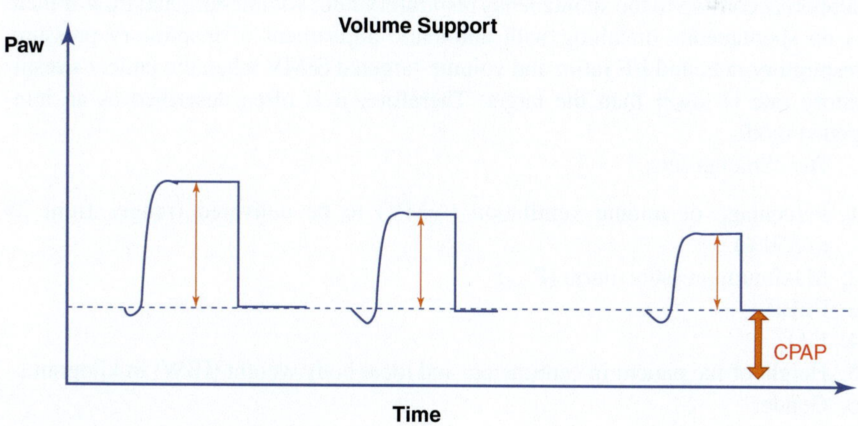

Fig. 10 Pressure-time waveform of volume support showing variable pressure support in relation to the patient's effort (inversely proportional)

Advantages

1. Almost guaranteed tidal volume
2. May provide better synchronization

Disadvantages

1. More sophisticated
2. Different names with different manufacturers may lead to some confusion
3. No significant advantage over conventional modes
4. No backup rate
5. The ventilatory support decreases as the patient demands and/or work of breathing increases

5.4 Adaptive Support Ventilation (ASV)

ASV is a positive-pressure mode of mechanical ventilation with a closed-loop control system that adjusts respiratory rate, tidal volume, and inspiratory time continuously depending on the patient's lung mechanics and effort.

ASV automatically determines an optimal tidal volume/respiratory rate combination based on the minimal work of breathing principle described by Otis [8, 9]. Lung mechanics are measured breath by breath, and expiratory time is determined according to the expiratory time constant in order to prevent dynamic hyperinflation.

ASV combines various ventilator modes: volume-targeted PSV if the patient's respiratory rate is more than the target with automatic adjustment of the pressure support according to the spontaneous respiratory rate; volume-targeted PCV if there is no spontaneous breathing with automatic adjustment of inspiratory pressure, respiratory rate, and I/E ratio; and volume-targeted SIMV when the patient's respiratory rate is lower than the target. Therefore, it is often described as an integrated mode.

The clinician sets:

1. Percentage of minute ventilation (%MV) to be delivered (ranges from 25 to 350%)
2. Maximum pressure alarm (P_{max})
3. PEEP
4. FiO_2
5. Height of the patient in centimeters and ideal body weight (IBW) in kilograms
6. Gender
7. Trigger
8. Tube resistance compensation

ASV automatically calculates minute ventilation and dead space based on the ideal body weight. It selects the respiratory pattern in terms of tidal volume, respiratory rate, and I/E ratio that provides the least work of breathing as configured by the Otis equation.

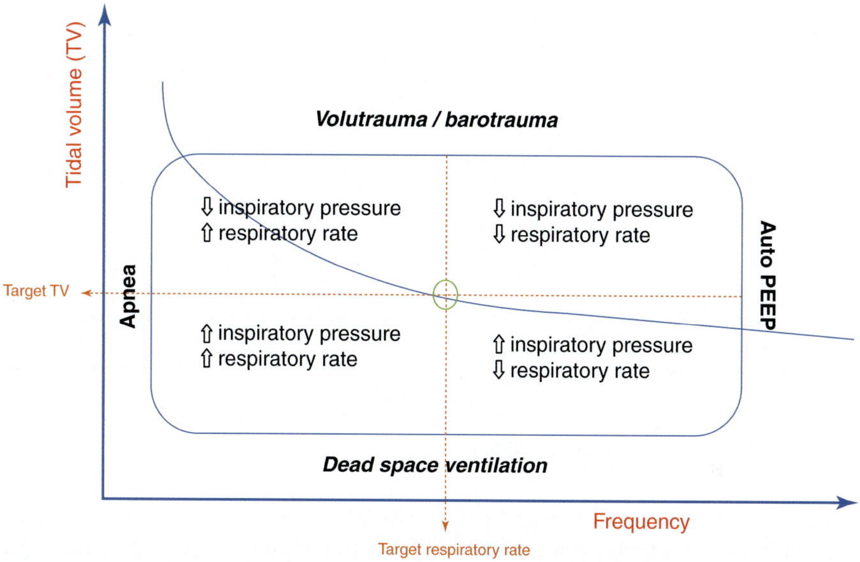

Fig. 11 Security boundaries determined by the operating principle of ASV

ASV is based on lung-protective strategies (i.e., volume and pressure limited), which aim to reach the target tidal volume and respiratory rate within a security boundary (Fig. 11) where the highest energy efficiency could be obtained and complications as volutrauma and barotrauma are avoided [10].

Advantages of ASV

1. Versatile, can be used to ventilate all intubated patients actively or passively
2. Adjusts to the patient's respiratory effort
3. Prevents auto-PEEP, barotrauma, and volutrauma
4. Decreased time on mechanical ventilation
5. Less labor intensive

Disadvantages of ASV

1. Tends to ventilate with low tidal volume and high respiratory rate
2. Tidal volume, respiratory rate, and I/E ratio cannot be set directly
3. Exclusive to Hamilton ventilators

6 Biphasic Ventilation

6.1 Airway Pressure Release Ventilation (APRV)

APRV is an inverse-ratio pressure-controlled mode of ventilation that delivers an almost continuous positive pressure with intermittent, time-cycled brief releases at a lower pressure allowing for spontaneous breathing throughout the cycle (Fig. 12).

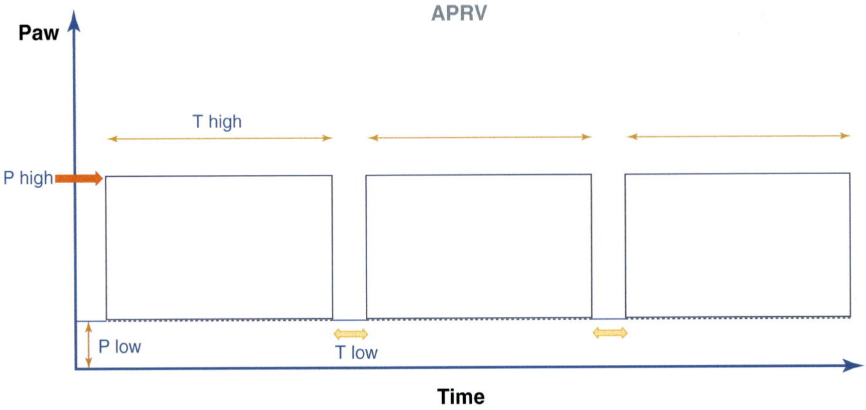

Fig. 12 Pressure-time waveform in APRV

The sustained positive pressure results in higher mean airway pressure with subsequent lung recruitment, whereas the brief releases keep the airway pressure high above the atmospheric pressure to prevent derecruitment resulting in an open-lung ventilation. Consequently, APRV has been particularly useful in the management of patients with acute hypoxemic respiratory failure and ARDS.

Settings

1. P_{high}: is the highest pressure applied to the respiratory system. It is usually based on the latest plateau pressure or mean airway pressure + 3 cmH_2O measured on conventional mode (usually in the range of 25–35 cmH_2O).
2. T_{high}: is the time spent at the highest pressure P_{high} (range 3–8 s).
3. P_{low}: is the lowest pressure applied to the respiratory system (usually set at zero).
4. T_{low}: is the time spent at the lowest pressure P_{low} (range 0.3–0.8 s) usually set at one time constant.
5. ATC: automatic tube compensation, usually set at 100%.
6. FiO_2.
7. Pressure support: is the amount of pressure supporting spontaneous breaths, usually set at zero.

Determinants of Oxygenation

1. P_{high}: to be increased by 2 cmH_2O to increase the mean airway pressure
2. T_{high}: to be increased by 0.5–1 s in order to increase the mean airway pressure
3. T_{low}: to be reduced by 0.2 s if T_{high} is more than 10 s
4. Increased FiO_2

Determinants of Ventilation

1. Frequency: reduce T_{high} by 0.2 s up to 3 s to increase the frequency.
2. The driving pressure (i.e., $P_{high} - Pl_{ow}$): increasing the driving pressure would increase the delivered tidal volume.

3. T_{low}: it is ideally set at 75% of the peak expiratory flow [11] to prevent derecruitment but no less than 40% of the peak expiratory flow (i.e., no more than 1 time constant).
4. Spontaneous breathing: titrate sedation to allow for 10–30% of the minute ventilation.

Weaning of APRV

1. Decrease FiO_2 until 40–50% while meeting target oxygenation.
2. Stretch and drop to achieve a CPAP of 15 cmH_2O, i.e., decrease P_{high} by 2 cmH_2O every 6 h while keeping FiO_2 at 40% and then increase T_{high} by 1–2 s once P_{high} is at 20 cmH_2O.
3. Once P_{high} is around 15–16 cmH_2O and T_{high} is 12–15 s, shift to CPAP of 15 cmH_2O with or without pressure support of 5 cmH_2O.

Advantages of APRV

1. Alveolar recruitment and improved oxygenation [12]
2. Potential lung-protective effect by reducing dynamic strain
3. Preservation of spontaneous breathing which maximizes recruitment of lung tissue specially the dependent lung units, promotes venous return to the heart, and prevents wasting of the respiratory muscles.
4. Less need for sedation.
5. Reduction in left ventricular transmural pressure with subsequent increase in cardiac output and reduction in myocardial work of contraction.

Disadvantages of APRV

1. Risk of volutrauma from increased transpulmonary pressure
2. Increased work of breathing due to spontaneous breathing
3. Decreased venous return and increased right ventricular afterload as well as worsening pulmonary hypertension
4. May worsen intracranial hypertension
5. Risk of dynamic hyperinflation and air leaks

7 Proportional Modes of Ventilation

Proportional modes of ventilation are novel spontaneous modes of closed-loop control of mechanical ventilation that deliver inspiratory assist in proportion to the patient's effort and, in contrast to all other modes (Fig. 13), would respond directly to changes in ventilatory needs in order to reduce the patient's effort, improve patient ventilator synchrony, and provide lung- and diaphragm-protective ventilation.

It comprises two proportional spontaneous breathing modes:

1. Proportional assist ventilation with load-adjustable gain factor (PAV+): it unloads a percentage of the work of breathing. The clinician sets the percentage

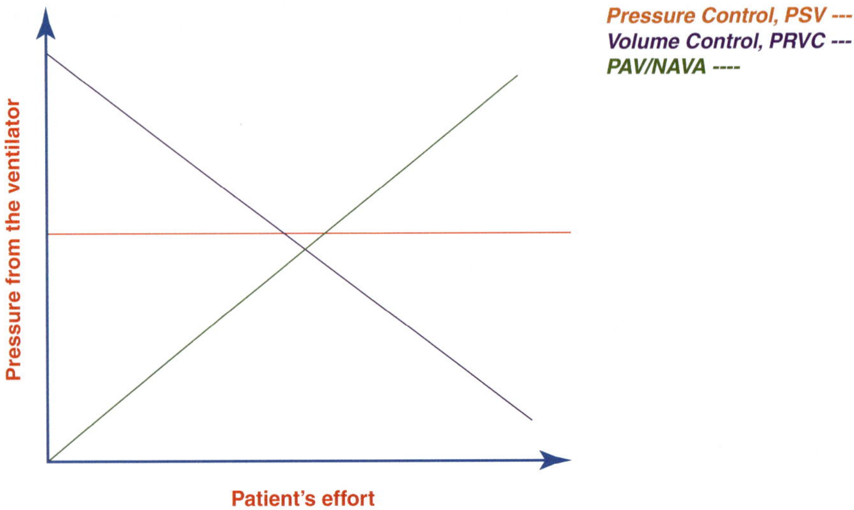

Fig. 13 The relationship between the patient's effort and the ventilator support during various modes of ventilation

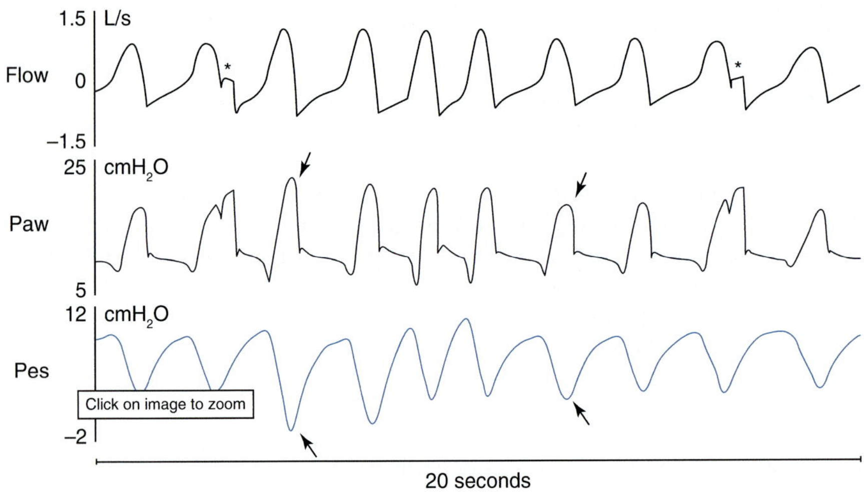

Fig. 14 In PAV+, short inspiratory occlusions are automatically performed (indicated by *) for the calculation of respiratory resistance and compliance. Arrows indicate that airway pressure (Paw) is delivered in proportion to the patient's effort (Pes) (Courtesy of Springer Nature from "Proportional modes of ventilation: technology to assist physiology" by Jonkman AH, Rauseo M, Carteaux G, et al. Intensive Care Med. 2020;46(12):2301–2313. https://doi.org/10.1007/s00134-020-06206-z)

of work of breathing to be provided by the ventilator. The ventilator uses intermittent end-inspiratory and end-expiratory pauses to calculate the compliance and resistance periodically (Fig. 14).

2. Neurally adjusted ventilatory assist (NAVA): it provides a level of inspiratory assist based on the magnitude of the diaphragmatic EMG activity.

Both have different settings from classical modes since they have different targets than flow, pressure, or volume which are brought to full control by the patient. Since tidal volume is mainly controlled by the respiratory center in the brain stem, it may not be affected by changing the level of assist.

7.1 Proportional Assist Ventilation (PAV+)

PAV+ delivers inspiratory assist in proportion to the instantaneous flow and volume generated by the patient's inspiratory effort (i.e., Pmus muscular pressure), which is estimated from semicontinuous automatic measurements of respiratory mechanics applying the equation of motion of the respiratory system [3]:

$$\mathit{Paw} + \mathit{Pmus} = \underset{(V)}{\mathit{Tidal\ volume}} \times \underset{(E)}{\mathit{Elastance}} + \underset{(R)}{\mathit{airway\ resistance}} \times \underset{(\dot{V})}{\mathit{flow}}$$

$$\mathit{Paw} = \%\mathit{assist} \times \mathit{Ptotal}$$

$$\mathit{Therefore}, \mathit{Paw} = \mathit{Pmus} \times \%\mathit{assist}\left(100 - \%\mathit{assist}\right)$$

PAV+ matches very well the patient's inspiratory demand at the onset of inspiration with no limit to flow delivery regardless of the PAV+ settings (i.e., as the patient demand increases, pressure will increase as well as the flow). Furthermore, cycling is also improved as the ventilator adjusts the flow at the end of inspiration in a similar manner. Therefore, patient ventilator synchrony is significantly improved [13].

PAV+ Variables

- Percentage work of breathing (%WOB) [range 5–95%]
- Trigger
- Cycle

Advantages of PAV+

1. Improved patient-ventilator synchrony and possibly a shorter duration of mechanical ventilation
2. Continuous measurement of respiratory system mechanics
3. Lung diaphragm-protective ventilation with decreased risk of lung overdistension as well as reduced risk of diaphragm disuse atrophy secondary to ventilator over-assistance
4. Less incidence of ineffective triggering and autotriggering than PSV
5. Potential improvement in sleep quality

Limitations of PAV+

1. Conditions that depress the respiratory system (e.g., sedatives, CNS disease, alkalosis) reduce the respiratory muscle output (e.g., muscle relaxants, fatigue, myasthenia gravis, Guillain-Barre syndrome) or decrease the force generated by the diaphragm (e.g., dynamic hyperinflation), all of which cause significant limitation of the patient's effort imposing a high risk of hypoventilation.
2. Excessive air leaks (e.g., bronchopleural fistula) lead to delayed cycling as the ventilator misinterprets the flow and volume escaping the circuit as a continuous patient effort.
3. Dynamic hyperinflation leads to underestimation of the calculated values of respiratory system compliance (Crs) and total airway resistance (RTOT). Moreover, auto-PEEP results in triggering delay with subsequent reduction of the assisted patient's effort.
4. Severe obstructive lung disease, when there is a large difference between the inspiratory and expiratory resistance as PAV+ tends to measure the respiratory system resistance (Rrs) during expiration.
5. Excessive assist (runaway), i.e., the ventilator continues to deliver inspiratory assist despite the fact that the patient has terminated his/her inspiratory effort. It occurs rarely and only when the percentage of assist is greater than the sum of elastic and resistive loads of the respiratory system at a particular point during inspiration (i.e., % assist ≥90%).

7.2 *Neurally Adjusted Ventilatory Assist (NAVA)*

NAVA delivers inspiratory assist in proportion to the diaphragm electrical activity (EAdi) measured via a dedicated nasogastric tube with embedded electrodes (Fig. 15).

Inspiratory assist in NAVA is proportional to EAdi *over the inspiratory cycle.* It is triggered for every EAdi increase more than 0.5 μV above the baseline and is terminated when EAdi falls at 70% of its peak value. Therefore, triggering is not affected by the presence of air leak or intrinsic PEEP. Unlike PAV+, NAVA greatly improves triggering and can be easily applied to noninvasive ventilation (NIV). Moreover, assisted breaths can be triggered by EAdi, pressure, or flow.

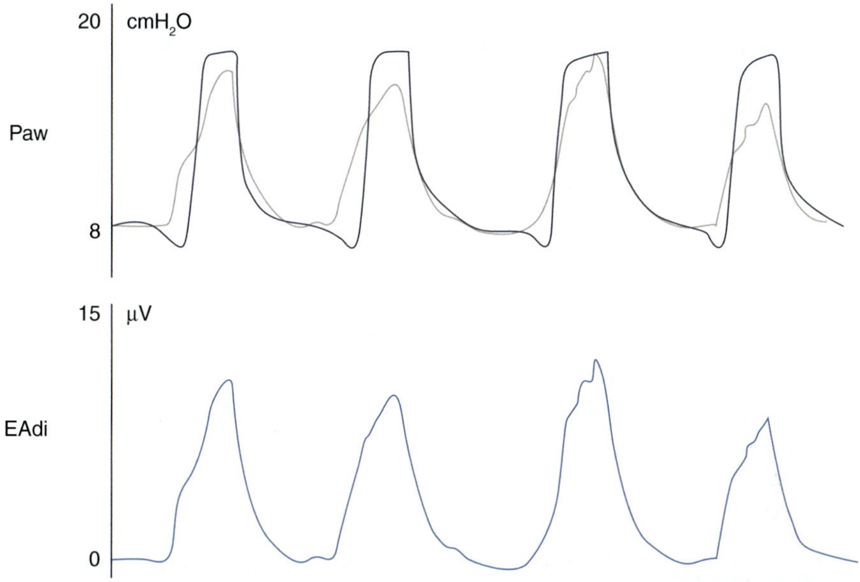

Fig. 15 Example of NAVA preview during pressure-support ventilation. The gray curve shows a preview of the estimated airway pressure (Paw) that would exist if the patient was ventilated in NAVA mode. The shape of this Paw curve resembles the diaphragm electrical activity (EAdi) curve (i.e., proportionality). The amount of assist depends on the EAdi amplitude and the selected NAVA level. (Courtesy of Springer Nature from "Proportional modes of ventilation: technology to assist physiology" by Jonkman AH, Rauseo M, Carteaux G, et al. Intensive Care Med. 2020;46(12):2301–2313. https://doi.org/10.1007/s00134-020-06206-z)

7.3 *NAVA Variable*

The pressure applied for each millivolt of EMG activity (i.e., the proportionality gain):

$$\text{Paw} = (\text{NAVA level} \times \text{EAdi}) + \text{PEEP}$$

Increased EAdi may be caused by:

- Increased mechanical load, e.g., increased airway resistance
- Increased ventilatory demand, e.g., increased dead space or increased CO_2 production
- Increased respiratory drive, e.g., sepsis

Advantages of NAVA

1. Improved patient-ventilator synchrony with better neuromuscular coupling and preserved breathing variability

2. Lung and diaphragm-protective ventilation
3. Effective triggering even in the presence of air leaks or with NIV

Limitations of NAVA

1. Suppressed respiratory drive, e.g., sedatives or CNS disease
2. Neuromuscular disease, phrenic nerve injury, or muscle relaxants
3. Improper placement of EAdi catheter, e.g., diaphragmatic hernia and esophageal atresia.

References

1. Chatburn RL. Classification of ventilator modes: update and proposal for implementation. Respir Care. 2007;52(3):301–23.
2. Lei Y. Medical ventilator system basics: a clinical guide. Oxford: Oxford University Press; 2017.
3. Jonkman AH, Rauseo M, Carteaux G, et al. Proportional modes of ventilation: technology to assist physiology. Intensive Care Med. 2020;46(12):2301–13. https://doi.org/10.1007/s00134-020-06206-z.
4. Chatburn RL, et al. Understanding mechanical ventilators. Expert Rev Respir Med. 2010;4(6):809–19.
5. Garnero AJ, et al. Pressure versus volume controlled modes in invasive mechanical ventilation. Med Intensiva (English Edition). 2013;37(4):292–8.
6. Chatburn RL. Classification of mechanical ventilators and modes of ventilation. In: Principles and practice of mechanical ventilation. 3rd ed. New York: McGraw-Hill; 2012.
7. Mathru M, Rao TL, El-Etr AA, Pifarre R. Hemodynamic response to changes in ventilatory patterns in patients with normal and poor left ventricular reserve. Crit Care Med. 1982;10(7):423–6. https://doi.org/10.1097/00003246-198207000-00001. PMID: 7044680.
8. Otis AB, Fenn WO, Rahn H. Mechanics of breathing in man. J Appl Physiol. 1950;2:592–607.
9. Tehrani FT. The origin of adaptive support ventilation. Int J Artif Organs. 2005;28:1051–2.
10. Fernández J, Miguelena D, Mulett H, Godoy J, Martinón-Torres F. Adaptive support ventilation: state of the art review. Indian J Crit Care Med. 2013;17(1):16–22. https://doi.org/10.4103/0972-5229.112149.
11. Jain SV, Kollisch-Singule M, Sadowitz B, et al. The 30-year evolution of airway pressure release ventilation (APRV). Intensive Care Med Exp. 2016;4(1):11. https://doi.org/10.1186/s40635-016-0085-2.
12. Zhou Y, Jin X, Lv Y, Wang P, Yang Y, Liang G, Wang B, Kang Y. Early application of airway pressure release ventilation may reduce the duration of mechanical ventilation in acute respiratory distress syndrome. Intensive Care Med. 2017;43(11):1648–59. https://doi.org/10.1007/s00134-017-4912-z. Epub 2017 Sep 22. PMID: 28936695; PMCID: PMC5633625.
13. Kacmarek RM. Proportional assist ventilation and neurally adjusted ventilatory assist. Respir Care. 2011;56(2):140–52.

Conventional Mechanical Ventilation in Acute Respiratory Failure

Bonnie R. Wang and Robert C Hyzy

1 What Is Mechanical Ventilation?

Conventional mechanical ventilation is the invasive delivery of positive pressure to the lungs through an endotracheal or tracheostomy tube. During inspiration, air is forced into the lungs and overcomes airway resistance and elastance of the lungs and chest wall to reach the alveoli. Positive intra-alveolar pressure increases until the end of inspiration. During expiration, air flows down the pressure gradient between the alveoli and the mouth to exit the lungs [1].

2 Objectives of Mechanical Ventilation

Positive-pressure ventilation is a life-sustaining supportive measure when used to maintain alveolar ventilation and gas exchange for homeostasis, which may have been otherwise refractory to alternative therapies such as heated high-flow nasal cannula or noninvasive ventilation. It is used to support the patient while practitioners attempt to diagnose and treat the underlying pathophysiology of respiratory and/or metabolic derangements but is not a curative therapy on its own.

B. R. Wang (✉)
University of Michigan, Ann Arbor, MI, USA
e-mail: wbonnie@med.umich.edu

R. C Hyzy
Division of Pulmonary and Critical Care Medicine, University of Michigan, Ann Arbor, MI, USA
e-mail: rhyzy@med.umich.edu

J. Hidalgo et al. (eds.), *Personalized Mechanical Ventilation*,
https://doi.org/10.1007/978-3-031-14138-6_7

Mechanical ventilation is often applied to optimize respiratory gas exchange by providing adequate alveolar ventilation and improving tissue oxygenation [2]. It relieves respiratory distress by increasing proximal airway pressure to drive inspiration, allowing for respiratory muscle rest with subsequent decrease in oxygen consumption by inspiratory muscles [3, 4]. The application of positive end-expiratory pressure (PEEP) can decrease intrapulmonary shunting through collapsed alveoli and physiologically increase lung compliance by transitioning lung mechanics to a more favorable portion of the pressure-volume curve [5, 6]. In addition, intubation and mechanical ventilation are commonly used for airway protection and procedural support when sedation and neuromuscular blockade may be required [2].

Timing to initiation of mechanical ventilation depends more on clinical judgement than precise science. Factors to consider include clinical assessment of increased work of breathing, trajectory of impending hypoxic and/or hypercapnic respiratory failure, underlying pathophysiology of disease if known, and/or need for anticipated procedures [1, 7]. In patients receiving heated high-flow oxygen therapy, a low ROX index (i.e., <5), measured as the ratio of oxygen saturation/FiO_2 to respiratory rate, is a strong predictor of intubation [8]. While there is no consensus on the exact timing to initiate mechanical ventilation, a key concept is that delaying intubation is associated with increased complications and mortality [9–12] (Fig. 1).

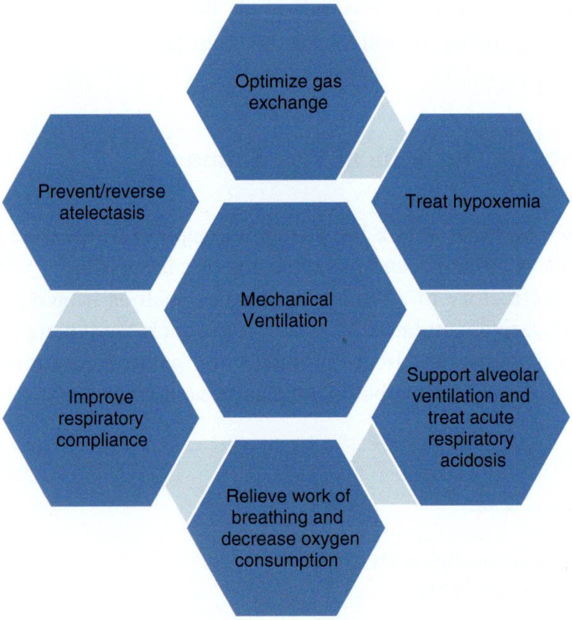

Fig. 1 Indications for mechanical ventilation when conditions are refractory to other measures. (Adapted from Slutsky, Chest 1993;104:1833 [2])

3 Basic Components of Ventilation

The following phase variables are important to consider when determining the initial mode [6, 13]:

- Trigger: what initiates inspiration
- Target: how gas is delivered during the inspiratory phase
- Cycle: what terminates inspiration
- Baseline: proximal airway pressure during the expiratory phase

There are different available selections for each phase variable (Table 1).

Table 1 Phase variables

Trigger	Target	Cycle	Baseline
Patient triggered • Ventilator delivers breath when patient triggers a breath via changes in pressure or flow	Flow	Inspiratory time	Positive end-expiratory pressure (PEEP)
Ventilator triggered • Ventilator delivers breath independent of the patient via set time	Inspiratory pressure	Volume	
		Flow • Reduction in inspiratory flow to set level (i.e., 25% of peak flow)	
		Pressure • Usually set as a safety mechanism to avoid injurious high airway pressures	

4 Basic Modes of Ventilation [1, 5, 7, 13]

Different modes of ventilation manipulate combinations of the above phase variables for breath delivery. The most common modes include:

- Volume-controlled assist control ventilation (VC-AC)
- Pressure-controlled assist control ventilation (PC-AC)
- Volume-synchronized intermittent mandatory ventilation (V-SIMV)
- Pressure-synchronized intermittent mandatory ventilation (P-SIMV)
- Pressure support ventilation (PSV)
- Autoflow
- Airway pressure release ventilation (APRV)

Volume assist control ventilation: The ventilator delivers a breath when the patient triggers a breath or independently if no breath is triggered within a predefined period of time. An inspiratory flow rate is set as the target variable, and inspiration ends when a fixed tidal volume (cycle variable) has been delivered (see Fig. 2).

Pressure-controlled assist control ventilation: The ventilator delivers a breath when the patient triggers a breath or independently if no breath is triggered within a predefined period of time. An inspiratory pressure is set as the target variable, and inspiration ends after a set inspiratory time (see Fig. 3).

Volume-synchronized intermittent mandatory ventilation (V-SIMV): Ventilator will deliver volume-controlled or volume-assisted breaths intermixed with spontaneous breaths that receive either no additional support or a set pressure support (see Fig. 4).

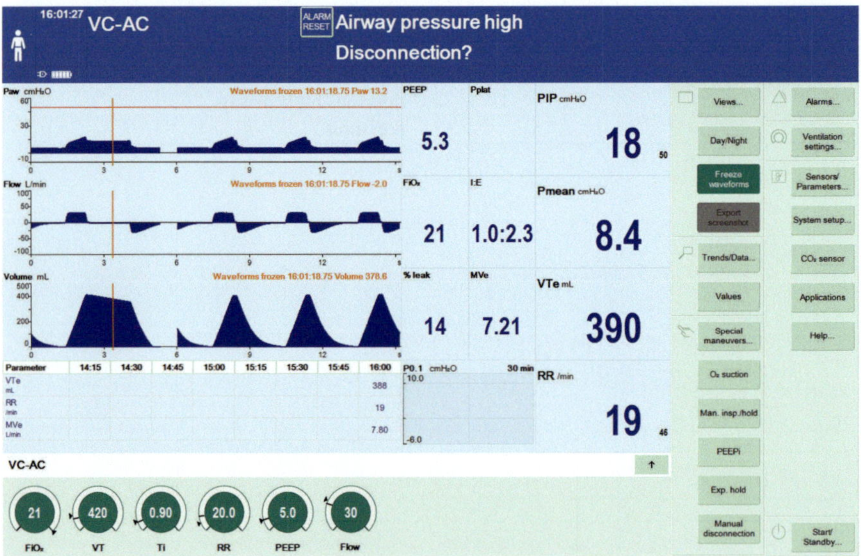

Fig. 2 Volume-controlled assist control ventilation mode. (Source: Dräger)

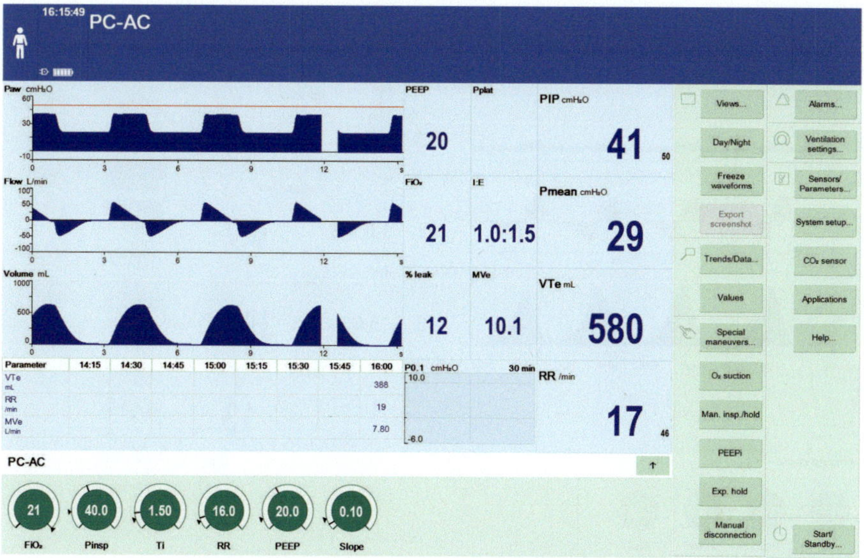

Fig. 3 Pressure-controlled assist control ventilation mode. (Source: Dräger)

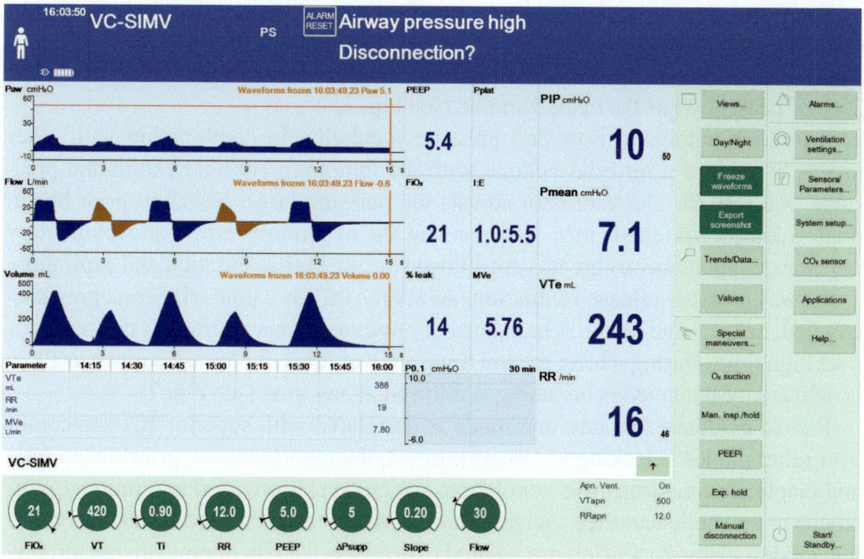

Fig. 4 Volume-synchronized intermittent mandatory ventilation mode. Spontaneous breaths are supported by set pressure support and shown in brown. (Source: Dräger)

Pressure-synchronized intermittent mandatory ventilation (P-SIMV): Ventilator will deliver pressure-controlled or pressure-assisted breaths intermixed with spontaneous breaths that receive either no additional support or a set pressure support.

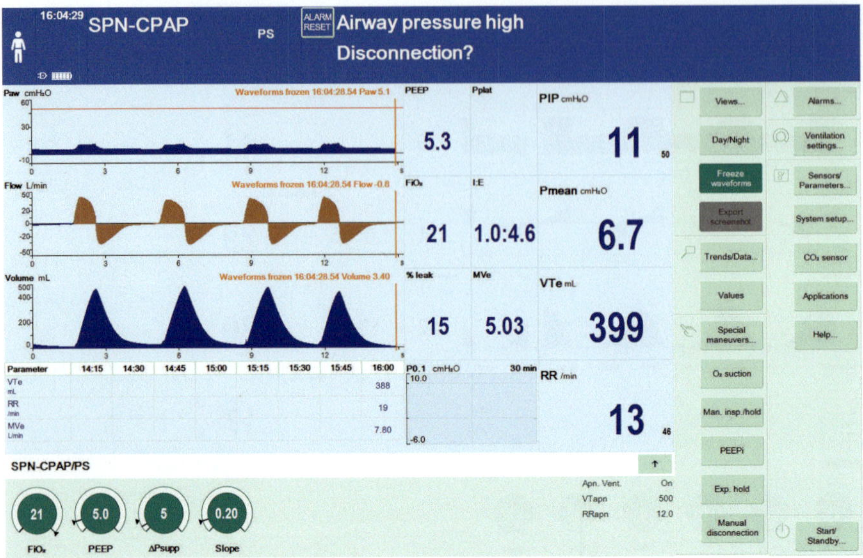

Fig. 5 Pressure support ventilation mode. (Source: Dräger)

Pressure support ventilation: Every breath is patient triggered. A level of airway pressure support is set as the target variable to augment every breath. Pressure is maintained at the set level until inspiratory flow diminishes below a set level (i.e., 25% of peak flow) as the cycle variable (see Fig. 5).

Autoflow: automatic flow and pressure regulation in combination with other modes to achieve a set tidal volume with the minimum possible ventilation pressures (see Fig. 6). The ventilator adjusts the pressure target based on prior breath tidal volumes, which in turn is dependent on inspiratory effort and pulmonary impedance. Spontaneous breaths are allowed during both inspiration and expiration.

Airway pressure release ventilation (APRV): APRV is a time-triggered, pressure-targeted, time-cycled mode. A high level of pressure known as Phigh is delivered for a set high time. During a brief release time, a lower level of pressure known as Plow is delivered. Spontaneous breathing is allowed at any time (see Fig. 7).

Robust evidence that any one mode is correlated with superior ICU outcomes over other modes is lacking [2, 14, 15]. Level of support needed, priorities of lung and diaphragmatic protective ventilation, patient synchrony, and institutional preference and experience often dictate initial ventilator modes. Modes that can maintain modest inspiratory effort are favored to decrease the risk of rapid disuse atrophy of diaphragm fibers in patients purely ventilated on control modes [16, 17].

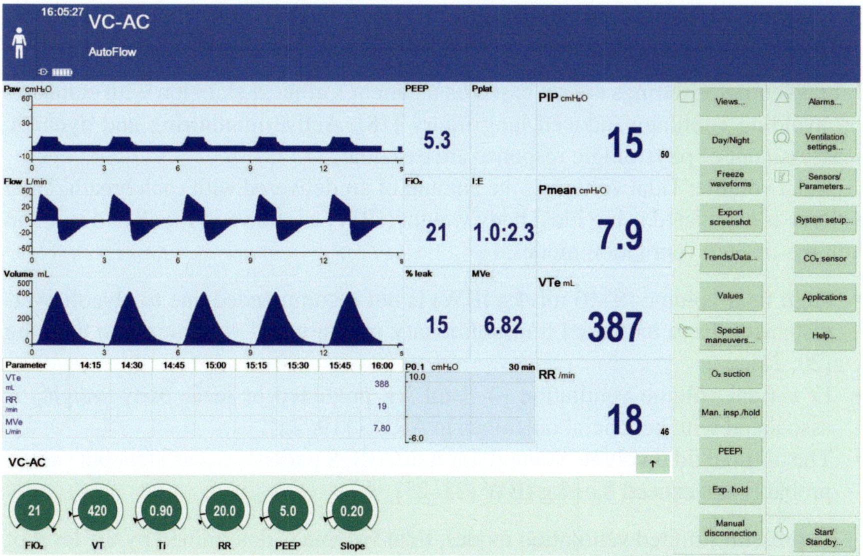

Fig. 6 Autoflow with volume-controlled assist control ventilation mode. Ventilator adjusts the pressure and flow based on changing compliance and resistance to reach the set tidal volume. (Source: Dräger©)

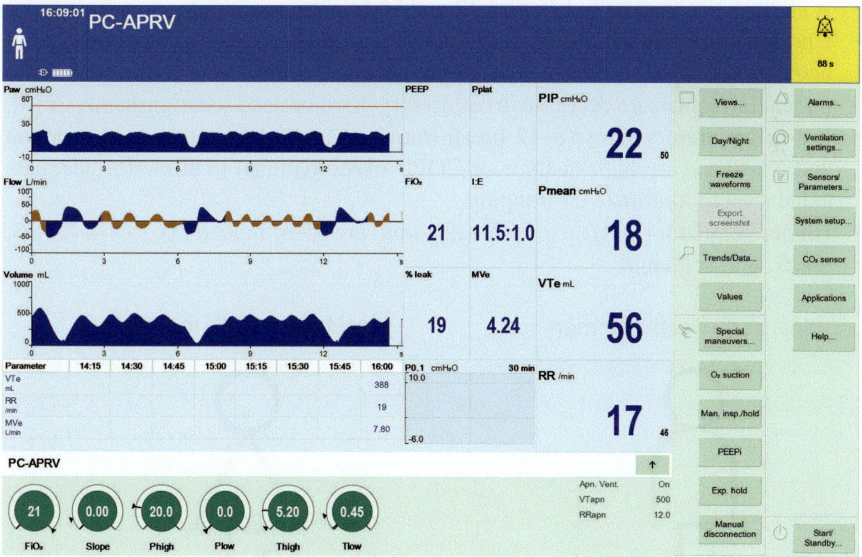

Fig. 7 Airway pressure release ventilation mode. Spontaneous breaths are shown in brown. (Source: Dräger)

5 General Ventilator Settings [1, 18]

Initial ventilator settings are set based on a patient's clinical situation with emphasis on avoiding ventilator-induced lung injury [18]. Active monitoring and dynamic reassessment of physiologic response are essential.

Tidal volume: Tidal volume is the amount of air delivered with each breath. Tidal volume is calculated using ideal body weight (IBW) as shown in Fig. 8 and is set on volume-limited ventilation modes.

- High tidal volume (9–10 mL/kg IBW) is not recommended due to alveoli overdistension from increased transpulmonary pressure and volutrauma to the lung [20, 21].
- Low tidal volume ventilation (4–8 mL/kg predicted or ideal body weight) is associated with beneficial outcomes in ARDS [19, 22].
- The optimal tidal volume strategy for non-ARDS patients is less clear but should probably not exceed 8 cc/kg IBW [23–25].

In pressure-limited ventilation modes, tidal volume is determined by the level of pressure set, patient's effort, and lung/chest wall compliance [5].

Ventilator rate: Ventilator rate is the number of breaths per minute delivered by the ventilator. Rate is set to achieve a minute ventilation necessary to match respiratory and metabolic needs.

- A starting rate is usually between 12 and 16 breaths per minute.
- One approach is to set the ventilator rate at 2–4 breaths/min less than the spontaneous rate so that ventilator will supply adequate minute ventilation should the patient have an acute decrease in respiratory drive or need sedation/paralysis [5].
- Lower respiratory rates (8–12 breaths/min) are used when airway obstruction and resistance are high (asthma or COPD exacerbations) to allow for adequate exhalation to minimize air trapping.
- Higher ventilator rates (up to 36 breaths/min) are often applied in cases of ARDS, shock, and acidemia.

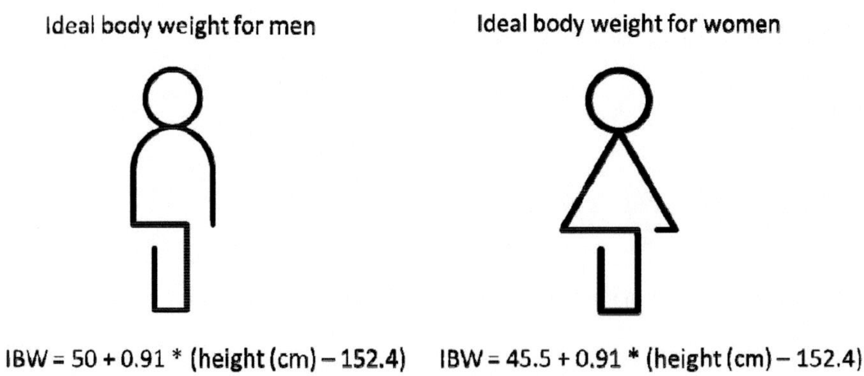

Fig. 8 Ideal body weight is dependent on gender and height [19]

Fractional concentration of inspired oxygen (FiO_2): set to maintain goals of arterial oxygen tension (PaO_2) of 60 mmHg or O_2 saturation of 90–96% [26, 27]. Hyperoxia (SpO_2 >96%) has potentially been associated with potential harm from toxic reactive oxygen species that can cause cell injury in the lungs, central nervous system, absorption atelectasis, coronary vasoconstriction, and reduced cardiac output [28–30]. However, studies in ARDS patients and in a more general population of hypoxemic patients, more than half of whom were receiving invasive mechanical ventilation, have failed to demonstrate a benefit to a conservative oxygen strategy based on PaO_2 or saturation, respectively [31, 32].

- Lower oxygen targets such as SpO_2 88–92% are considered for patients at risk of hypercapnic respiratory failure, including chronic obstructive pulmonary disease, obesity hypoventilation, neuromuscular respiratory diseases, and obstructive sleep apnea [33].
- Higher oxygen targets such as SpO_2 approaching 100% are considered for select groups such as carbon monoxide poisoning, cluster headaches, sickle cell crisis, and pneumothorax [26].

Positive end-expiratory pressure (PEEP): pressure in the alveoli at the end of expiration. PEEP improves arterial oxygenation by increasing alveolar recruitment and decreasing intrapulmonary shunting while reducing atelectrauma from cyclic opening and closing of alveoli [34, 35]. However, excessive PEEP can lead to overdistension, increased dead space and pulmonary vascular resistance, and impaired venous return [22]. PEEP titration strategies have included use of high/low FiO_2/PEEP tables, optimizing plateau pressure, compliance, driving pressure, pressure-volume curves, or stress index [19, 36–42]. Optimal method of PEEP titration is unknown, and ideal level of PEEP will vary based on the individual and clinical context [43].

- Extrinsic PEEP is set on the ventilator.
- Intrinsic PEEP or auto-PEEP is air that is trapped in the lungs resultant from an insufficient expiratory time (see Fig. 9).

Inspiratory flow: rate that inspired gas is delivered.

- With volume-limited modes of ventilation, flow is usually set at 40–60 L per minute with a ramp pattern to target an inspiratory:expiratory ratio of 1:2 or 1:3 to meet patient ventilatory demands and limit dyssynchrony.
- Higher rates up to 75 L per minute are considered for patients with obstructive lung disease and airflow obstruction to shorten inspiratory time and extend expiratory time to eliminate carbon dioxide and reduce dynamic hyperinflation from auto-PEEP. Note that higher flows may result in higher peak pressures [1].
- With pressure-limited modes, inspiratory flow is variable and dependent on the set inspiratory pressure limit, inspiratory time, compliance and resistance of the respiratory system, and patient effort.

Trigger sensitivity: Breaths can be initiated by the patient or the ventilator. Patient-triggered breaths are detected by changes in pressure or flow, usually −1

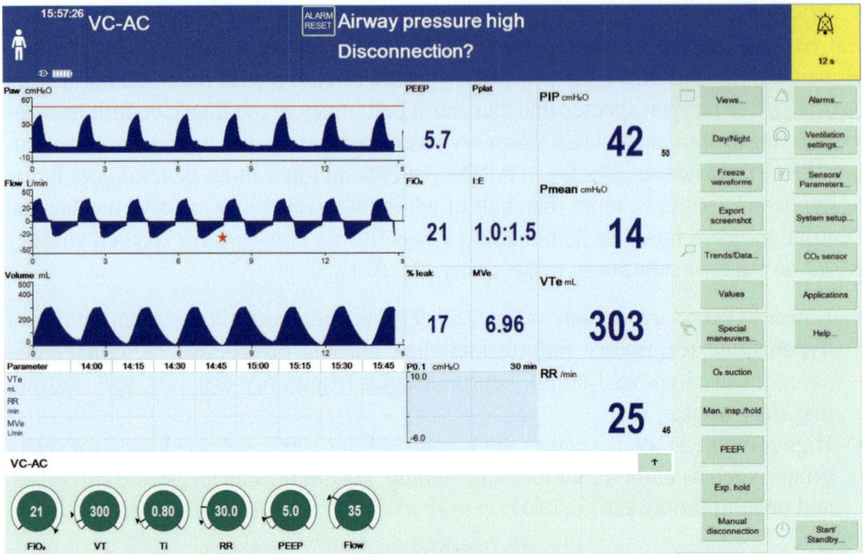

Fig. 9 Auto-PEEP is suggested by the persistence of airflow at the end of expiration. It reflects the pressure gradient between alveoli and the ventilator at the end of expiration. (Source: Dräger)

to −3 cm H_2O below end-expiratory pressure if a pressure trigger is used or 2 L/min if a flow trigger is used [7]. Trigger sensitivity does not need to be set for ventilator-triggered breaths, which are dependent on the set respiratory rate.

6 Potential Effects of Mechanical Ventilation

While positive-pressure ventilation can be a life-sustaining tool, adverse physiologic effects are not uncommon. As positive pressure is applied during inspiration, intrapleural and intrathoracic pressures increase and intrathoracic blood vessels and pericardium can become compressed. Venous return decreases which can subsequently decrease right ventricular preload and stroke volume. This in turn can reduce left ventricular preload and cardiac output [44].

High tidal volumes or levels of PEEP can narrow and compress nearby alveolar vessels under West zone 1 conditions. This increases pulmonary vascular resistance and right ventricular afterload, which can decrease RV output particularly in the setting of preexisting RV dysfunction. If RV dilation occurs, ventricular interdependence can lead to the decreased filling of the left ventricle, which can lower LV stroke volume and cardiac output [44, 45].

Conversely, cardiac transmural pressure, equivalent to intraventricular pressure minus intrathoracic pressure, is decreased with positive-pressure ventilation

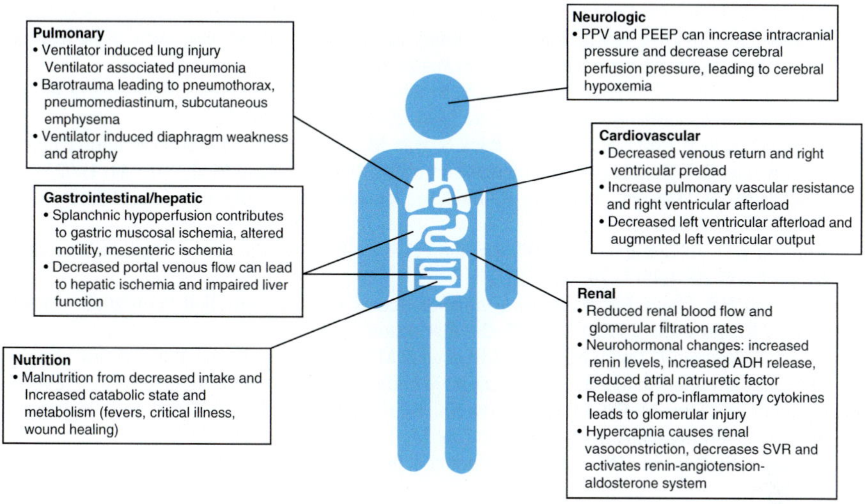

Fig. 10 Potential ventilator-associated effects on pulmonary, neurologic, renal, and gastrointestinal systems and nutritional status [1, 7, 20, 46]

compared to spontaneous breathing. Decreased cardiac transmural pressure translates to decreased left ventricular afterload and augmented LV output [1, 7].

Other potential effects of mechanical ventilation on several organ systems are detailed in Fig. 10.

References

1. Cairo JM. Pilbeam's mechanical ventilation physiological and clinical applications. 6th ed. Elsevier; 2016.
2. Slutsky AS. Mechanical ventilation. American College of Chest Physicians' consensus conference. Chest. 1993;104(6):1833–59.
3. Field S, Kelly SM, Macklem PT. The oxygen cost of breathing in patients with cardiorespiratory disease. Am Rev Respir Dis. 1982;126(1):9–13.
4. John B, West AML. West's respiratory physiology. 10th ed. Alphen aan den Rijn: Wolters Kluwer; 2016.
5. Tobin MJ. Mechanical ventilation. N Engl J Med. 1994;330(15):1056–61.
6. Poor H. Basics of mechanical ventilation. Springer; 2018.
7. Tobin MJ. Principles and practice of mechanical ventilation. 3rd ed. New York: McGraw-Hill Medical; 2013.
8. Roca O, Caralt B, Messika J, Samper M, Sztrymf B, Hernández G, et al. An index combining respiratory rate and oxygenation to predict outcome of nasal high-flow therapy. Am J Respir Crit Care Med. 2019;199(11):1368–76.
9. Mosier JM, Sakles JC, Whitmore SP, Hypes CD, Hallett DK, Hawbaker KE, et al. Failed noninvasive positive-pressure ventilation is associated with an increased risk of intubation-related complications. Ann Intensive Care. 2015;5:4.

10. Carrillo A, Gonzalez-Diaz G, Ferrer M, Martinez-Quintana ME, Lopez-Martinez A, Llamas N, et al. Non-invasive ventilation in community-acquired pneumonia and severe acute respiratory failure. Intensive Care Med. 2012;38(3):458–66.
11. Demoule A, Girou E, Richard JC, Taille S, Brochard L. Benefits and risks of success or failure of noninvasive ventilation. Intensive Care Med. 2006;32(11):1756–65.
12. Kang BJ, Koh Y, Lim CM, Huh JW, Baek S, Han M, et al. Failure of high-flow nasal cannula therapy may delay intubation and increase mortality. Intensive Care Med. 2015;41(4):623–32.
13. MacIntyre N. Design features of modern mechanical ventilators. Clin Chest Med. 2016;37(4):607–13.
14. Branson RD, Johannigman JA. What is the evidence base for the newer ventilation modes? Respir Care. 2004;49(7):742–60.
15. Campbell RS, Davis BR. Pressure-controlled versus volume-controlled ventilation: does it matter? Respir Care. 2002;47(4):416–24; discussion 24–6.
16. Levine S, Nguyen T, Taylor N, Friscia ME, Budak MT, Rothenberg P, et al. Rapid disuse atrophy of diaphragm fibers in mechanically ventilated humans. N Engl J Med. 2008;358(13):1327–35.
17. Goligher EC, Dres M, Patel BK, Sahetya SK, Beitler JR, Telias I, et al. Lung- and diaphragm-protective ventilation. Am J Respir Crit Care Med. 2020;202(7):950–61.
18. Slutsky AS, Ranieri VM. Ventilator-induced lung injury. N Engl J Med. 2013;369(22):2126–36.
19. Brower RG, Matthay MA, Morris A, Schoenfeld D, Thompson BT, Wheeler A. Ventilation with lower tidal volumes as compared with traditional tidal volumes for acute lung injury and the acute respiratory distress syndrome. N Engl J Med. 2000;342(18):1301–8.
20. Dreyfuss D, Soler P, Basset G, Saumon G. High inflation pressure pulmonary edema. Respective effects of high airway pressure, high tidal volume, and positive end-expiratory pressure. Am Rev Respir Dis. 1988;137(5):1159–64.
21. International consensus conferences in intensive care medicine: ventilator-associated lung injury in ARDS. This official conference report was cosponsored by the American Thoracic Society, the European Society of Intensive Care Medicine, and the Societé de Réanimation de Langue Française, and was approved by the ATS Board of Directors, July 1999. Am J Respir Crit Care Med. 1999;160(6):2118–24.
22. Fan E, Del Sorbo L, Goligher EC, Hodgson CL, Munshi L, Walkey AJ, et al. An official American Thoracic Society/European Society of Intensive Care Medicine/Society of Critical Care Medicine clinical practice guideline: mechanical ventilation in adult patients with acute respiratory distress syndrome. Am J Respir Crit Care Med. 2017;195(9):1253–63.
23. Simonis FD, Serpa Neto A, Binnekade JM, Braber A, Bruin KCM, Determann RM, et al. Effect of a low vs intermediate tidal volume strategy on ventilator-free days in intensive care unit patients without ARDS: a randomized clinical trial. JAMA. 2018;320(18):1872–80.
24. Serpa Neto A, Cardoso SO, Manetta JA, Pereira VG, Espósito DC, Pasqualucci Mde O, et al. Association between use of lung-protective ventilation with lower tidal volumes and clinical outcomes among patients without acute respiratory distress syndrome: a meta-analysis. JAMA. 2012;308(16):1651–9.
25. Neto AS, Simonis FD, Barbas CS, Biehl M, Determann RM, Elmer J, et al. Lung-protective ventilation with low tidal volumes and the occurrence of pulmonary complications in patients without acute respiratory distress syndrome: a systematic review and individual patient data analysis. Crit Care Med. 2015;43(10):2155–63.
26. Siemieniuk RAC, Chu DK, Kim LH, Güell-Rous MR, Alhazzani W, Soccal PM, et al. Oxygen therapy for acutely ill medical patients: a clinical practice guideline. BMJ. 2018;363:k4169.
27. Mackle D, Bellomo R, Bailey M, Beasley R, Deane A, Eastwood G, et al. Conservative oxygen therapy during mechanical ventilation in the ICU. N Engl J Med. 2020;382(11):989–98.
28. Chu DK, Kim LH, Young PJ, Zamiri N, Almenawer SA, Jaeschke R, et al. Mortality and morbidity in acutely ill adults treated with liberal versus conservative oxygen therapy (IOTA): a systematic review and meta-analysis. Lancet. 2018;391(10131):1693–705.

29. Helmerhorst HJ, Roos-Blom MJ, van Westerloo DJ, de Jonge E. Association between arterial Hyperoxia and outcome in subsets of critical illness: a systematic review, meta-analysis, and meta-regression of cohort studies. Crit Care Med. 2015;43(7):1508–19.
30. Girardis M, Busani S, Damiani E, Donati A, Rinaldi L, Marudi A, et al. Effect of conservative vs conventional oxygen therapy on mortality among patients in an intensive care unit: the oxygen-ICU randomized clinical trial. JAMA. 2016;316(15):1583–9.
31. Schjørring OL, Klitgaard TL, Perner A, Wetterslev J, Lange T, Siegemund M, et al. Lower or higher oxygenation targets for acute hypoxemic respiratory failure. N Engl J Med. 2021;384:1301–11.
32. Barrot L, Asfar P, Mauny F, Winiszewski H, Montini F, Badie J, et al. Liberal or conservative oxygen therapy for acute respiratory distress syndrome. N Engl J Med. 2020;382(11):999–1008.
33. Austin MA, Wills KE, Blizzard L, Walters EH, Wood-Baker R. Effect of high flow oxygen on mortality in chronic obstructive pulmonary disease patients in prehospital setting: randomised controlled trial. BMJ. 2010;341:c5462.
34. Mélot C. Contribution of multiple inert gas elimination technique to pulmonary medicine. 5. Ventilation-perfusion relationships in acute respiratory failure. Thorax. 1994;49(12):1251–8.
35. Caironi P, Cressoni M, Chiumello D, Ranieri M, Quintel M, Russo SG, et al. Lung opening and closing during ventilation of acute respiratory distress syndrome. Am J Respir Crit Care Med. 2010;181(6):578–86.
36. Talmor D, Sarge T, Malhotra A, O'Donnell CR, Ritz R, Lisbon A, et al. Mechanical ventilation guided by esophageal pressure in acute lung injury. N Engl J Med. 2008;359(20):2095–104.
37. Beitler JR, Sarge T, Banner-Goodspeed VM, Gong MN, Cook D, Novack V, et al. Effect of titrating positive end-expiratory pressure (PEEP) with an esophageal pressure-guided strategy vs an empirical high PEEP-Fio2 strategy on death and days free from mechanical ventilation among patients with acute respiratory distress syndrome: a randomized clinical trial. JAMA. 2019;321(9):846–57.
38. Hata JS, Togashi K, Kumar AB, Hodges LD, Kaiser EF, Tessmann PB, et al. The effect of the pressure-volume curve for positive end-expiratory pressure titration on clinical outcomes in acute respiratory distress syndrome: a systematic review. J Intensive Care Med. 2014;29(6):348–56.
39. Brower RG, Lanken PN, MacIntyre N, Matthay MA, Morris A, Ancukiewicz M, et al. Higher versus lower positive end-expiratory pressures in patients with the acute respiratory distress syndrome. N Engl J Med. 2004;351(4):327–36.
40. Mercat A, Richard JC, Vielle B, Jaber S, Osman D, Diehl JL, et al. Positive end-expiratory pressure setting in adults with acute lung injury and acute respiratory distress syndrome: a randomized controlled trial. JAMA. 2008;299(6):646–55.
41. Rodriguez PO, Bonelli I, Setten M, Attie S, Madorno M, Maskin LP, et al. Transpulmonary pressure and gas exchange during decremental PEEP titration in pulmonary ARDS patients. Respir Care. 2013;58(5):754–63.
42. Pintado MC, de Pablo R, Trascasa M, Milicua JM, Rogero S, Daguerre M, et al. Individualized PEEP setting in subjects with ARDS: a randomized controlled pilot study. Respir Care. 2013;58(9):1416–23.
43. Sahetya SK, Goligher EC, Brower RG. Fifty years of research in ARDS. Setting positive end-expiratory pressure in acute respiratory distress syndrome. Am J Respir Crit Care Med. 2017;195(11):1429–38.
44. Steingrub JS, Tidswell M, Higgins TL. Hemodynamic consequences of heart-lung interactions. J Intensive Care Med. 2003;18(2):92–9.
45. Mitchell JR, Whitelaw WA, Sas R, Smith ER, Tyberg JV, Belenkie I. RV filling modulates LV function by direct ventricular interaction during mechanical ventilation. Am J Physiol Heart Circ Physiol. 2005;289(2):H549–57.
46. Dreyfuss D, Saumon G. Ventilator-induced lung injury: lessons from experimental studies. Am J Respir Crit Care Med. 1998;157(1):294–323.

Mechanical Ventilation in the Trauma Patient

Antonio Joao Gandra d'Almeida, Ricardo Guedes, and Rui Moreno

Thoracic injuries remain a common presentation to medical facilities after a severe trauma injury. Trauma can be classified according to whether the mechanism of injury is penetrating, blunt, or mixed. Penetrating injuries such as penetrating, cutting, and firearm injuries are disruptive to tissue integrity. Blunt injuries can cause damage to organs and structures under the tissue without disrupting the integrity of the tissue, either by concussion or by deceleration. Falling from height, traffic accidents, and occupational accidents are the main mechanisms of blunt injuries.

More common in war scenarios, but also frequently seen in civil accidents, we can see mixed injuries, in which the damage results from a combination of penetrating injuries and blunt ones.

Approximately two-third of the patients have a chest trauma with varying severity from a simple rib fracture to penetrating trauma, road traffic collisions and blunt trauma from tertiary blast injury, penetrating injury of the heart or the major vessels of the mediastinum, or tracheobronchial disruption, and also behind-armor blunt trauma caused by high-impact ammunition or by explosive devices. Conditions common to both mechanisms of injury include hemothorax, pneumothorax, cardiac tamponade, rib fractures (sometimes conditioning flail chest), and aortic lesions (specially aortic dissection). Pulmonary contusion is common in blunt chest trauma but may also occur in association with high-velocity penetrating injuries. The passage of a shock wave through the pulmonary tissue leads to microscopic disruption

A. J. Gandra d'Almeida (✉)
Portuguese Institute of Emergency, Porto, Portugal

R. Guedes
Centro Hospitalar de Sao Joao, Porto, Portugal

R. Moreno
Hospital de San Jose, Centro Hospitalar de Lisboa Central, Facultad de Ciencias Medicas de Lisboa, Facultat de ciencias de saude, Universidade de Beira Interior, Covilha, Portugal

J. Hidalgo et al. (eds.), *Personalized Mechanical Ventilation*,
https://doi.org/10.1007/978-3-031-14138-6_8

at the alveolar-air interface with subsequent inflammation. This results in alveolar hemorrhage and parenchymal damage, which becomes maximal at 24 h, that usually is complicated in the space of days by infection of the pulmonary parenchyma. Blast lung injury is an extreme form of pulmonary contusion and should be borne in mind when lung function deteriorates in the absence of signs of external thoracic injury. As the blast wave passes, there is a rapid expansion of the gas-filled alveoli, leading to secondary explosions within the lung.

Blunt chest trauma is most common in civilian settings, with a 90% incidence, of which less than 10% require surgical intervention of any kind. Mortality is second highest after head injury, which underlines the importance of initial management, usually due to a combination of lesions in other organs and systems, either the brain or the abdomen. Many of these deaths can be prevented by a complete assessment of the patient, repeated a few hours later (secondary evaluation), and prompt diagnosis and treatment of the lesion and of the associated lesions. Many times hidden in the primary assessment (e.g., disinsertion of the Mesos in deceleration injuries). The skin marking of the safety belt is an easy-to-spot sign of the strength of the impact and of the high probability of major lesions.

Although a patent airway is mandatory, it does not ensure per se an adequate ventilation and oxygenation. These vital functions rely upon an intact respiratory center, adequate pulmonary function, and coordinated movement of the diaphragm and chest wall. A number of life-threatening traumatic and medical disease processes may interfere with one or more of these essential processes and lead to respiratory failure. The thorax is a semirigid structure that affords protection to the lungs, heart, and great vessels. Injury to these structures therefore typically requires a significant magnitude of force delivered by either penetrating or blunt injury.

Patients with multiple injuries are known to develop lung injury, which can result in long-term disability or even death. Respiratory failure has been observed in trauma patients for a long time, and some degree of acute respiratory distress syndrome (ARDS) occurs in these patients. ARDS develops as a result of both direct and indirect injury to the lungs. Common causes of ARDS following a direct injury include pneumonia or gastric aspiration. In trauma casualties, direct insults such as pulmonary contusion, inhalation injury, and fat emboli may lead to ARDS. ARDS from indirect lung injury can occur in patients who receive multiple transfusions, who develop septic shock, or in those with severe acute pancreatitis. Also, mechanical ventilation with high tidal volumes can contribute to the development of ARDS in these patients, even in the absence of primary lesion of the pulmonary parenchyma.

The diagnosis of ARDS is typically made in patients who have respiratory failure that requires intubation and mechanical ventilation. The Berlin definition requires all four criteria to be present for the diagnosis of ARDS: (1) Timing: Respiratory symptoms must have begun within one week of a known clinical insult, or the patient must have new or worsening symptoms during the past week. (2) Chest imaging: Bilateral opacities consistent with pulmonary edema must be present on a chest radiograph or computed tomographic scan, which is not fully explained by pleural effusions, lobar collapse, lung collapse, or pulmonary nodules. (3) Origin of edema: The patient's respiratory failure must not be fully explained by cardiac failure or fluid overload. An objective assessment (e.g., echocardiography) to exclude hydrostatic pulmonary edema is required if no risk factors for ARDS are present. (4) Oxygenation: A moderate-to-severe impairment of oxygenation must be present, as defined by the PaO_2/FiO_2 ratio.

Patients suspected of having ARDS on the basis of chest X-ray findings, low PaO_2/FiO_2 ratio, and ventilator settings such as low compliance should have their diagnosis confirmed by following the below guidance. After verifying that the patient is likely to have respiratory failure from either a direct or an indirect pulmonary injury or the need for mechanical ventilation support, then obtain a good-quality anteroposterior upright chest X-ray, look for diffuse infiltrates, consider a chest computer tomography (CT), and ensure that the patient is stable for transport to CT.

Chest injury can lead to hypovolemia secondary to major organ or vessel injury, or to hypoxia and hypercapnia as a result of disruption to the mechanics of ventilation or occlusion (e.g., by coagula or foreign bodies of the intrapulmonary airways). A combination of hypoxia and reduced cardiac output can also occur as a result of cardiac tamponade or tension pneumothorax. If cardiogenic pulmonary edema and/or fluid overload cannot be fully excluded as the cause of or a contributing factor to the patient's respiratory failure, obtain a transthoracic echocardiogram.

Cardiac failure, often due to fluid overload, must be ruled out when considering the diagnosis of ARDS. Several other disease processes can also mimic ARDS. Patients with these conditions will benefit from lung-protective ventilator management but may require disease-specific interventions as well. The diagnosis of ARDS is typically made in patients who have respiratory failure that requires intubation and mechanical ventilation. The Berlin definition requires all four criteria to be present for the diagnosis of ARDS: (1) Timing: Respiratory symptoms must have begun within one week of a known clinical insult, or the patient must have new or worsening symptoms during the past week. (2) Chest imaging: Bilateral opacities consistent with pulmonary edema must be present on a chest radiograph or computed tomographic scan, which is not fully explained by pleural effusions, lobar collapse, lung collapse, or pulmonary nodules. (3) Origin of edema: The patient's respiratory failure must not be fully explained by cardiac failure or fluid overload. An objective assessment (e.g., echocardiography) to exclude hydrostatic pulmonary edema is required if no risk factors for ARDS are present. (4) Oxygenation: A moderate-to-severe impairment of oxygenation must be present, as defined by the PaO_2/FiO_2 ratio.

The mainstay of managing lung injuries is mechanical ventilation, which replaces or assists the function of the respiratory system. Mechanical ventilation may in itself exacerbate the initial injury by direct mechanical damage, induction of surfactant failure, or stimulation of pulmonary and systemic inflammatory cytokines (in other words, what is now globally named ventilator-induced lung injury (VILI) that includes (despite not being limited to) barotrauma, volutrauma, and atelectotrauma. Improved understanding of the pathophysiology of ARDS has led to the development of safer ventilatory practices, unfortunately rarely used outside the ICU. An experienced intensivist should be involved in the care of these patients from the early stages to prevent further deterioration and to minimize secondary damage.

1 Thoracic Trauma

Respiratory distress is a serious problem in individuals with blunt chest trauma. Patients with respiratory distress may breathe with nasal flaring, using accessory muscles, intercostal and subcostal retractions, and signs such as tachypnea. The patient's lungs usually are not equally involved in breathing. Paradoxical respiration can be observed, and immediate diagnosis of flail chest can be made and thereafter rapid intervention can be performed. This happens almost in all cases when the patient presents simultaneous fractures of the anterior and the posterior arcs of the same ribs, which allows the middle part, not supported by the bone, to present a paradoxical movement, expanding in the inspiration and retracting in the expiration.

Tracheobronchial injuries are found in 0.8% of blunt thoracic trauma victims presenting for emergency surgery. The vast majority of these injuries are found within 2.5 cm of the carina and are associated with a high mortality because of the difficulties in maintaining adequate ventilation and oxygenation, as well as delayed diagnosis. Usually, the primary reparation—involving sternotomy—should not be attempted, and the situation is controlled with the insertion and positioning—usually guided by bronchoscopy—of a tube just above the carina during several days in the absence of major bleeding from associated vessels. In the case of a high lesion, without retrosternal compromise, surgical tracheostomy should be attempted if feasible and a trained professional is available.

The management of intrathoracic airway injuries should ideally involve a bronchologist and a thoracic surgeon at an early stage because operative repair will usually be required. However, most trauma surgeons are not cardiothoracic specialists; therefore, adequate risk assessment must be done before embarking any operative procedure. In most of the cases, conservative management frequently becomes the best course of action in carefully selected stable patients. The authors concluded that surgery should be performed in cases of associated esophageal injuries, progressive subcutaneous or mediastinal emphysema, severe dyspnea requiring intubation, difficulty with mechanical ventilation, pneumothorax with air leak through chest drains, or mediastinitis. The remaining cases are likely to do well with conservative medical management. The aim of the initial management should be to improve ventilation and reduce air leak. This can be achieved by placing a cuffed airway device distal to the site of injury typically with the use of a fiber-optic bronchoscope.

1.1 Tension Pneumothorax

Pneumothorax is a clinical entity that is caused by the presence of air between the visceral and the parietal pleura. In short, air is trapped between the lung and the chest wall, because the accumulated air in related side of the lung collapses. Rarely, it can be due to the formation of a major bullae inside the lung parenchyma.

Pneumothorax is the most common life-threatening injury in blunt thoracic trauma. Pneumothorax can be seen in 40–50% of patients with all types of thoracic trauma. Therefore, pneumothorax should not be overlooked in trauma patients. Pneumothorax can be classified as spontaneous and nonspontaneous. We can define spontaneous pneumothorax as nontraumatic pneumothorax, and these are pneumothoraxes that occur without trauma or in the presence of an underlying precipitating factor (usually the presence of multiple large apical bullae in emphysematous patients). Trauma (either blunt or penetrating) is the major cause of nonspontaneous pneumothorax.

Pneumothorax can occur in blunt chest trauma in four mechanisms: (1) alveolar rupture due to increased alveolar pressure, due to high-energy impact; (2) paper bag effect (occurs if epiglottis is closed during sudden pressure increase in tracheobronchial tree); (3) acceleration-deceleration injury; and (4) rib fractures damaging the pleura. In the early period, patients may have chest pain, dyspnea, anxiety, tachypnea, tachycardia, and hyperresonance and decreased respiratory sounds on the pneumothorax side. In the late period, signs such as decreased consciousness, tracheal deviation, hypotension, distension of cervical veins, and cyanosis may be seen. It may happen also in diving accidents, more and more frequent, due to the spontaneous rupture of a bulla or due to high-speed ascension without enough exhalation.

In tension pneumothorax, air enters the pleural space at each inspiration, while the air in the pleural space cannot escape from the pleural space due to the one-way valve mechanism. Due to the continuous accumulation of air in the pleura, the lung collapses, hypoxia becomes severe, and hypotension occurs. It also affects the other lung by sliding to the opposite side and causing cardiovascular collapse due to the effects of direct pressure or by the shifting of the heart to the opposite side, with compromise of the cava vein. In pneumothorax, the patient may have tachypnea and tachycardia, hyperresonance can be obtained in percussion, and tracheal deviation may be seen in late phase. This diagnosis can be hard to make in emergency situations, especially if an associated hemothorax is present. The presence of air in the pleural cavity with mediastinal shift should immediately make us think of tension pneumothorax (although it could also be explained by the collapse of the opposite lung).

Pneumothorax treatment requires a holistic approach including monitoring, resting, oxygen supply, and thoracostomy (usually by tube). Treatment should begin with the principles of ABC approach to the trauma patient. The patient's airway continuity, breathing, and circulation should be monitored repeatedly. Giving 100% oxygen support to the patient increases the absorption of air from the pleural cavity. In very unstable patients, when reasonable doubt exists between cardiac (pericardial) lesions and hemo/pneumothorax approaches and there is no time for other exams, other approaches such as clamshell surgery—easily done on the resuscitation room or in the trauma ICU if care is taken with thoracic vessels, especially the mammary arteries—can be indicated to access and make the primary control of the lesion(s) before a more definitive approach can be done.

The application of positive-pressure ventilation, to support the patient's failing ventilation, will accelerate the buildup of intrapleural pressure exponentially.

Resistance to bagging in experienced hands or raised ventilator peak airway pressures without other explanation (e.g., the patient fighting the ventilator) may be the first indicator of tension pneumothorax in the ventilated patient.

Once recognized, tension pneumothorax is simple to treat. In the awake patient, needle decompression with a large-bore cannula is both simple and effective and aims to convert the tension pneumothorax into a simple pneumothorax. Insertion in the lateral chest is more likely to be successful than the traditional anterior approach due to reduced chest wall thickness and is also more convenient in case of hemo/pneumothoraxes. In the ventilated patient, a simple thoracostomy is the preferred means of treating a tension pneumothorax, before the definitive control of the situation, usually with the placement of a chest tube under aspiration, especially in the case of bronchopleural fistula.

1.2 Open Pneumothorax

Open pneumothorax is an open chest wound that communicates with the pleural cavity. If the chest wound is greater in size than the tracheal diameter, air will preferentially flow through the chest wall rather than the upper airway on inspiration ("sucking chest wound"). An open pneumothorax should be obvious during inspection of the chest and immediately sealed as part of primary survey management. If the patient needs to be intubated and ventilated, it is important to ensure low tidal volume ventilation (6–7 mL/kg of ideal body weight), to prevent volutrauma, and not to seal totally the hole in the chest to avoid a tension pneumothorax. It is easy to have a lost of the inspired gases in a ventilated patient due to escaping through the hole is important to close the hole so well that the patient will very rapidly develop a tension pneumothorax.

1.3 Flail Chest

Flail chest is often caused by blunt trauma to the thorax, such as direct blows, falls from height, and car accidents. Flail chest is usually seen not alone, but with additional injuries like extrathoracic organ injuries, shock, and blood loss. The mortality rate varies between 10 and 20% in patients with such additional injuries.

A flail chest is defined as the fracture of two or more adjacent ribs in two or more places, usually the anterior and the posterior arcs or in less cases the anterior or posterior arcs and the lateral part of the ribs, and leads to segmental loss of continuity with the rest of the thoracic cage. A small flail segment may be difficult to identify because of local muscle spasm and splinting; however, large flail segments are usually obvious. Basically, flail chest occurs when a segment of the chest wall is disconnected from the rest of the chest wall. As the flail segment loses its continuity, the chest wall paradoxically moves in different directions during inspiration and expiration. In the inspiration, the ribs move outward while the flail chest moves inward; in the expiration, the opposite occurs. Tidal volume is reduced and ventilation compromised. Underlying pulmonary contusions add to the insult on the respiratory system and cause hypoxia. Paradoxical chest movement, hypoxia, and respiratory distress characterize a patient with a flail chest. This is called paradoxical motion. Nonetheless, paradoxical movement prevents full expansion of the underlying lung, decreasing minute ventilation. Pain is a contributing factor, preventing the patient from taking full breaths and coughing.

A trauma strong enough to form a flail segment frequently causes parenchymal contusion. As a result of parenchymal contusion, the breathing mechanism is impaired and edema, infection, and even necrosis may occur with pulmonary tissue bleeding. The presence of pulmonary contusion is highly predictive of morbidity. Flail chest is also closely associated with injuries such as hemothorax and pneumothorax. Flail chest may occur as a result of bone fractures as well as separation of the costochondral junction.

These patients should firstly undergo airway-breathing-circulation (ABC) procedures. Frequent monitoring of vital signs is important in all trauma patients. Pulmonary physiotherapy, adequate pain control, endotracheal intubation, mechanical ventilation, and close follow-up should then be performed. Oxygenation is also important in these patients. Usually, high-flow oxygen (15 L/min) and analgesia for painless spontaneous breathing are often sufficient treatment of this condition. Large flail segments with resistant hypoxia may require urgent anesthesia. Intubation/tracheostomy and mechanical ventilation are indicated if the respiratory rate is faster than 35 bpm or less than 8 bpm, if PaO_2 is below 60 mmHg on supplemental oxygen at 50%, if PaCO2 is acutely above 55 mmHg, or if vital capacity is less than 15 mL/kg. For segments larger than 4–6 in, or multiple flail segments, positive-pressure ventilation is the optimal solution. Internal splinting through positive-pressure ventilation not only corrects paradoxical chest movement but also decreases the work of breathing and pain. Prolonged intubation increases morbidity and mortality by increasing the risk of pneumonia. In the last years, early surgery with osteosynthesis of the broken ribs (with the first 24 to 48 hours) has been used increasingly because it is associated with a much lower rate of complications, lower ventilation times, and better outcomes.

2 Cardiac Injury

The diagnosis of blunt cardiac trauma is challenging; visible thoracic lesions might be absent. In addition, clinical signs such as hypotension, hypoxia, or hemodynamic instability might be attributed to other severe injuries with blood loss in trauma patients. Cardiac injury can occur secondary to blunt or penetrating trauma. Defining the severity of blunt cardiac trauma remains challenging; the spectrum ranges from minor "bruises" to penetrating wounds including more than 50% of a chamber and usually needs a fast bedside echocardiogram (nowadays already also outside of the hospital, in the place of the accident) to rule out major lesions.

Blunt cardiac trauma, irrespective of its severity, can most frequently be encountered in male patients between 30 and 50 years of age. It is most commonly caused by the combination of deceleration forces, compression forces, and shearing stress. This triad can frequently be encountered due to road traffic accidents, as could be identified for up to 60.5% of the patients included in this study. Interestingly, cardiac injury due to deceleration forces has been reported after deceleration from velocities of less than 20 mph. Compression forces can result from abdominal and lower extremity trauma as well, often referred to as "hydraulic ram effect."

Blunt cardiac injuries can present as a spectrum ranging from isolated electrocardiogram (ECG) abnormalities to increased troponin I to myocardial rupture, with the right ventricle and interventricular septum being the most frequently involved due to the weaker cardiac wall. Cardiogenic shock may ensue as a result of arrhythmias, structural damage, or impaired ventricular contractility. ECG abnormalities that may indicate cardiac injury include ST segment changes and arrhythmias. These patients should have continuous ECG monitoring. The use of biochemical biomarkers is neither plain sailing. CPK-MB has a high specificity for myocardial infarction, but due to high increases of CPK following trauma, false-positive increases of CPK-MB were found in severely injured patients. In contrast, troponin I and T are highly specific for myocardial injury; normal concentrations strongly indicate the absence of myocardial injury following blunt chest trauma, but even most patients with minor trauma will present an increase in troponin. A repletion of the analysis at 4 h is mandatory.

The relative frequency of injury to the heart is as follows: right ventricle, left ventricle, right atrium, intraventricular septum, left atrium, and least commonly rupture of the intra-atrial septum. Right-heart injury might be missed on an ECG, as the ECG is more sensitive for left ventricular than for right ventricular injuries due to the muscle mass ratio.

A transthoracic and eventually a transesophageal echocardiogram should always be performed and in most cases repeated, especially when there exist pulmonary lesions that are difficult to visualize during the examination. In the advent of cardiogenic shock, consideration should be given to placing an intra-aortic balloon pump to off-load the left ventricle, more and more replaced by VA ECMO, that helps the damaged heart but also the damaged lungs.

Behind-armor blunt trauma (BABT) is a nonpenetrating injury resulting from the deformation of body armor after ballistic impact. It has been shown in animal models that apnea occurring after BABT is a vagally mediated reflex that results in severe hypoxia. The deformation is part of the retardation and energy-absorbing process that captures the projectile. In extreme circumstances, the BABT may result in death, even though the projectile has not perforated the armor. Stress waves are generated and propagate through the body armor and the underlying tissues (including those not in direct contact with the armor); they may be transmitted and/or reflected by the armor components and/or various tissues depending on the speed of sound in the material. A comparison between female and male US police officer BABT injuries suggested that female officers suffer a higher risk of injury.

Supportive ventilation should begin immediately in BABT casualties who are unconscious and apneic or VV (or VA) ECMO in case of life-threatening lesions.

3 Special Cases

3.1 *Primary Blast Lung Injury*

PBLI is defined as "radiological and clinical evidence of acute lung injury occurring within 12 h of exposure and not due to secondary or tertiary injury." This classification does not recognize the significant psychological injury suffered by witnesses and first responders to explosive events, which should perhaps be regarded as a quaternary injury pattern. In reality, the different blast injury mechanisms will rarely exist in isolation and a single casualty will suffer a spectrum of blast injury mechanisms. Secondary blast injury (due to fragmentation, preferentially aiming at the abdomen and thoracic and not at the member, at floor level) predominates in most recent conflicts, especially since some types of blast arms (who does not remember the American Claymore mines in Vietnam war, not officially forbidden by international conventions?) are being increasingly replaced by improvised explosive devices, easy and cheap to make and to use.

Classically, primary blast injury is described as predominantly affecting gas-containing organs such as the larynx, middle ear, and bowel, in addition to the lungs. However, cerebral edema and vascular endothelial injury usually occur, as can life-threatening liver or splenic lacerations, testicular rupture, retroperitoneal bleeding, and muscular compartment syndromes. Thus, exposure to a blast wave can cause a life-threatening primary blast injury syndrome, in which lung injury often predominates.

3.1.1 Abdominal Trauma

Pneumoperitoneum is infrequently seen in blunt trauma with the exception of deceleration lesions, more and more frequent as safety bells are used (that protect the patient from direct injury in the accident but do not protect from deceleration injuries, a major problem nowadays in the brain and in the abdomen), but can be seen with either blunt or penetrating trauma. Stab wounds and gunshot wounds to the chest can traverse the diaphragm and injure bowel. Sometimes, air from thoracic sources such as pneumothorax can cross the diaphragm into the abdomen, resulting in pneumoperitoneum, so the finding of intraperitoneal air or air in both sides of the diaphragm is not pathognomonic for bowel perforation. The goal of the initial evaluation of blunt abdominal trauma is to expeditiously identify patients who require laparotomy and prompt or damage control (primary repair is in many cases just not possible without severe risk) of the intra-abdominal injuries. Unfortunately, victims involved in high-velocity accidents are difficult to assess, especially those associated with closed-head trauma, under the influence of alcohol or drugs and polytrauma. Therefore, diagnostic modalities beyond physical examination are required to identify the injury promptly.

Pneumoretroperitoneum can occur in the presence of pneumomediastinum secondary to barotrauma from mechanical ventilation. It is thought to arise from alveolar rupture into the bronchoalveolar sheath with dissection through the pulmonary interstitium toward and into mediastinum, and then further dissection can occur into the neck superiorly and into the retroperitoneum inferiorly. Frequently, dissection occurs with a subsequent pneumothorax. Air can also leak from the alveolus to the mediastinum via the pores of Kohn. There is a tissue plane that extends anteriorly from the mediastinum to the retroperitoneal space through the sternocostal attachment of the diaphragm. This anterior pathway of infradiaphragmatic extension of air can be erroneously diagnosed as intraperitoneal air, which may lead to unnecessary exploratory laparotomies. The mediastinum also communicates directly with the retroperitoneum by way of the periaortic and periesophageal fascial planes. In this patient, tracking from a pneumomediastinum is the most likely cause of pneumoperitoneum. It is also common in penetration injuries, specially in stabing of the lumbar region.

However, the possibility of a rupture of the diaphragm with deplanement of the abdominal content (liver and bowel at right, stomach, spleen and bowel at left) should be kept always in our mind, because it is not so rare nowadays, in the era of high-impact accidents. The surgical approach is very important, with a thoracic approach allowing the surgeon to directly correct associated pulmonary lesions but making it harder to place the abdominal contents in place without causing lesions, specially torsions or correcting spleen lacerations and the abdominal approach more challenging, because after as time passes and due to edema more difficult to pull out the abdominal content from the thorax, without (surgically) enlarging the primary defect in the diaphragm. It is also more difficult to correct eventual associated lung injuries.

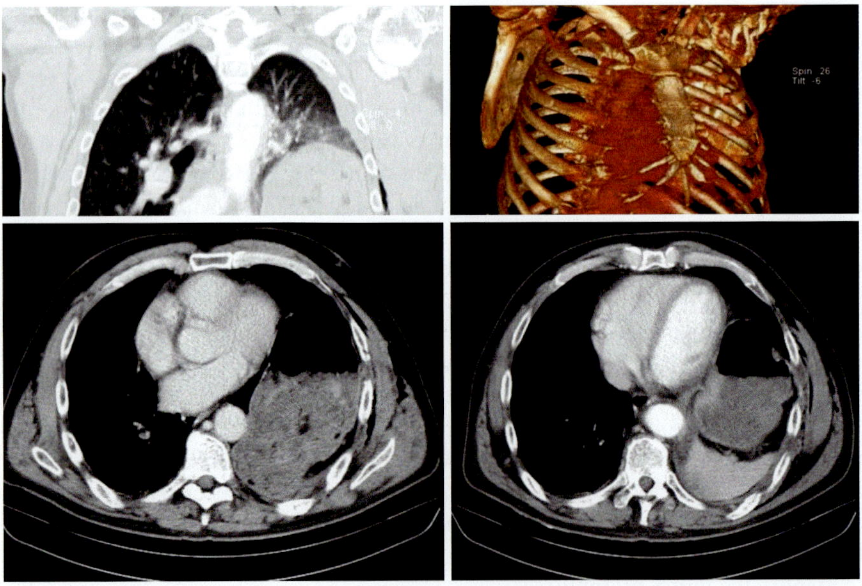

Courtesy of Professor Moreno

3.1.2 Head Trauma

Traumatic brain injury (TBI) is a leading cause of death and disability. In 2013, there were approximately 2.5 million emergency department (ED) visits, 282,000 hospitalizations, and 56,000 deaths related to TBI in the United States.

TBI has traditionally been classified using injury severity scores; the most commonly used is the Glasgow Coma Scale (GCS). A GCS score of 13–15 is considered mild injury, 9–12 is considered moderate injury, and 8 or less is considered severe TBI.

Head injury can result from both relatively minor and high-velocity trauma. Current clinical approaches to the management of TBI center around these concepts of primary and secondary brain injury. Primary brain injury occurs at the time of impact and includes injuries such as subdural or epidural hematoma (this a surgical emergency), cerebral contusions, and diffuse axonal injury (the last one usually due to deacceleration movements at the time of the impact). These brain insults continue to evolve, especially in unstable patients, with hypotension, poor oxygenation, or extreme anemia, and later as a result of the loss of cerebral autoregulation (the capability of the brain to maintain the cerebral perfusion pressure in the presence of low mean arterial pressure of increased intracranial pressure). Likewise, the active prevention and treatment of secondary brain injury are the principal focus of neurointensive care management for patients with severe TBI. Attention should also be always paid to the jugular blood flow, frequently decreased in thoracic lesions, since a decrease in the jugular blood flow will increase the intracranial pressure (ICP). Neuronal cell death as well as cerebral edema and increased ICP can further exacerbate the brain injury. This injury cascade shares many features of the ischemic cascade in acute stroke.

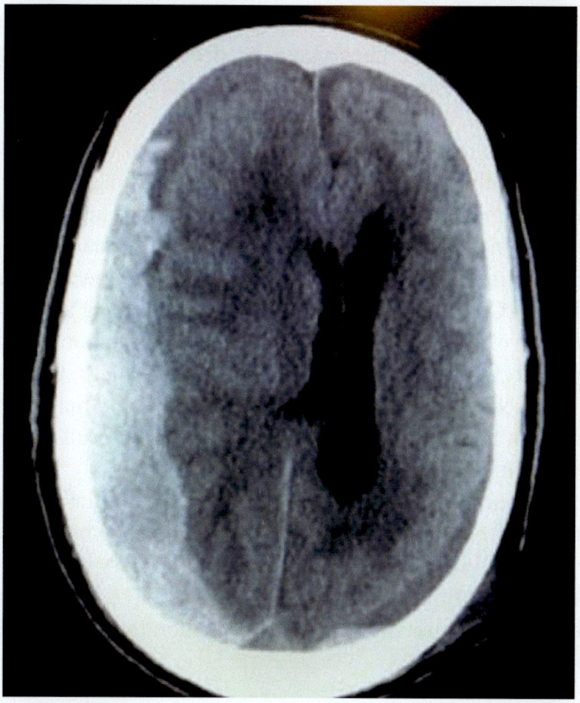

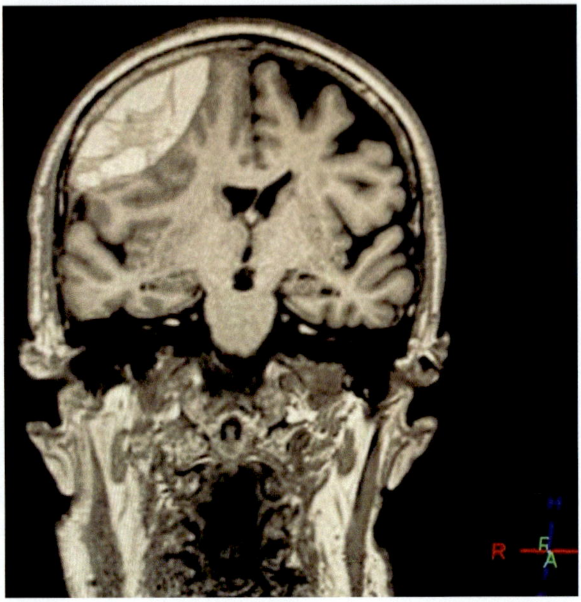

This injury is exacerbated by exogenous factors, which reduce cerebral oxygen supply and raise intracranial pressure. ICP will rise with an increase in volume of any of the cranial contents (blood, brain, cerebrospinal fluid) as the cranium is a rigid box (Monro–Kellie doctrine). When compensatory mechanisms are exhausted, sustained rises in ICP will result in herniation of brain tissue. Clinical signs of impending herniation include significant pupillary asymmetry, unilateral or bilateral fixed and dilated pupils, decorticate or decerebrate posturing, respiratory depression, and the "Cushing triad" of systolic hypertension, bradycardia, and irregular respiration.

$PaCO_2$ is the measure of arterial levels of carbon dioxide levels and heavily depends on the metabolic rate and minute volume of the lung. Exhalation of $PaCO_2$ results in removal of metabolic waste, and, during times of high metabolism, respiratory rate normally increases to lower $PaCO_2$ levels if the patient has the capability to do so. Under normal conditions, $PaCO_2$ is the most powerful determinant of cerebral blood flow (CBF) and, between a range of 20 mmHg and 80 mmHg, CBF is linearly responsive to $PaCO_2$. Cerebral blood flow is important in meeting the brain's metabolic demands. Low $PaCO_2$ (less than 30 mmHg), therefore, results in low CBF due to vasoconstriction of the cerebral vessels and may result in cerebral ischemia, while high $PaCO_2$ levels (above 35 mmHg) can result in cerebral vasodilatation and increasing intracranial pressure (ICP).

When ICP is increased, appropriate management of ventilation is given top priority, and in cases of emergency, hyperventilation management (with a target of 30–35 mmHg of arterial $PaCO_2$) is performed as a temporary measure. Acute hypercarbia may result in elevations in ICP, and hypocarbia may precipitate cerebral ischemia; the use of end-tidal carbon dioxide ($ETCO_2$) monitoring should be considered for all ventilated TBI patients but should always be interpreted with extreme caution, because in some situations it cannot reflect the real $PaCO_2$. Hyperventilation can also increase extracellular lactate and glutamate levels that may contribute to secondary brain injury.

Maintain the $PaCO_2$ at 35–40 mmHg (30–35 mmHg in case of established cerebral hypertension). Cerebral blood flow is often reduced in the first 24 h after head trauma, and hyperventilation should be avoided in this period to prevent further reductions. If hyperventilation is used, jugular venous oxygen saturation (SjO_2) or brain tissue O_2 partial pressure ($BtpO_2$) measurements are recommended to monitor oxygen delivery. Hypoxia should also be avoided and the PaO_2 maintained at >60 mmHg. The use of multimodality monitoring of cerebral oxygenation and metabolism should also be considered when using therapeutic hyperventilation, to monitor its effects and prevent ischemic episodes.

It is important that artificial ventilatory management is to ensure short duration of the procedure (????). While patients with TBI frequently suffer acute hypoxic respiratory failure and require higher levels of positive end-expiratory pressure (PEEP), a theoretical concern has been that elevated intrathoracic pressures will hamper venous return from the brain and worsen ICP. However, a consistent effect on ICP has not been revealed, although patients with severe lung injury did demonstrate a small but statistically significant positive relationship between PEEP and ICP.

3.2 Management of a Patient over Mechanical Ventilator

In order to control respiratory failure, it is necessary to optimize ventilation, maintain oxygenation and ventilation/perfusion ratio, and avoid ventilator-related lung injuries (VILI).

The mainstay of managing lung injuries is mechanical ventilation, which replaces or assists the function of the respiratory system. Invasive mechanical ventilation may be used depending on the severity of pulmonary injuries. However, mechanical ventilation can increase morbidity and mortality. Mechanical ventilation may in itself exacerbate the initial injury by direct mechanical damage, induction of surfactant failure, or stimulation of pulmonary and systemic inflammatory cytokines, a bundle of negative effects usually called ventilator-induced lung injuries (VILI).

To note, if a patient has pneumothorax, it should be corrected first because positive-pressure ventilation can exacerbate pneumothorax. Therefore, invasive ventilation methods should not be used in these patients unless necessary. Early noninvasive ventilation may reduce the need for intubation. Prone position can also be used to help patients with respiratory distress. Rapid mobilization of patients with pulmonary physiotherapy is considered a key factor in preventing thrombosis, embolism, and pulmonary complications such as pneumonia, respiratory failure, and ARDS.

Place the patient on the less invasive and better controllable modality, we should use in those patients and by nonmechanical ventilator experts in volume- or pressure-control ventilation:

1. Tidal volume (VT) should be approximately 6–8 mL/kg using predicted body weight (PBW), see ARDSNet Card, targeting a plateau pressure (PPLAT) of ≤30 cm H2O and a driving pressure lower than 15 cmH_2O, or if using a pressure control mode of ventilation, set the inspiratory pressure to 30–35 cmH_2O and then decrease it gradually to achieve a VT of 6–8 mL/kg. In both cases, plateau pressure should not go over 28–30 cmH_2O.
2. The respiratory rate should be between 10 and 24 and adjust to achieve a pH ≥7.3 (higher rates are associated with the development of auto-PEEP, since expiration time can be insufficient for the needs of the patient).
3. PEEP (minimum 5 cmH_2O) and FiO_2 according to the ARDSNet table to achieve a SpO2 of 88–95% (PaO2 of 55–80 mmHg). Allow the patient's gas exchange to equilibrate for 30 min and then draw an ABG to calculate the patient's P/F ratio.

The management of patients with ARDS should safely support gas exchange without further injuring the patient's lungs. In fact, using a lung-protective ventilator strategy in all intubated patients appears to improve clinical outcomes.

In patients with ALI or ARDS, the goal is to limit barotrauma (PPLAT ≤30 cmH_2O, driving pressure lower than 15 cmH_2O), volutrauma (VT 6–8 mL/kg PBW), and atelectrauma (moderate-to-high PEEP). Goals should include an SpO2 ≥ 88–95% and a pH ≥7.3 (in traumatic brain injury, this pH goal should be met with the PaCO2 maintained at 35–40 mmHg). Always remember that in patients with chest lesions, compliance as measured to the ventilator cannot be reflecting the real compliance of the lungs but the injuries of the chest wall. In this case, the direct measurement of the compliance using an esophageal balloon (that measures the real transpulmonary pressure and not the chest wall pressure) is mandatory in the most critically ill patients to allow a fine-tuning of the ventilator parameters.

Evaluation of ventilation is routinely performed using mechanical parameters and blood gases.

The normal range of $PaCO_2$ is 35–45. However, during artificial ventilation, the appropriate range of $PaCO_2$ varies depending on the condition of the patient. In patients with intracranial pressure elevation or metabolic acidosis due to shock, it is essential to maintain low $PaCO_2$ (never below 30 mmHg in brain trauma patients). In patients with metabolic alkalosis, maintaining higher $PaCO_2$ levels may be indicated, if other lesions are excluded.

A significant absolute reduction in mortality was achieved using the lower tidal volumes and maintaining driving pressure lower than 15 cmH_2O and plateau pressures less than 30 cmH_2O. However, these protective ventilation strategies sometimes frequently result in hypercapnia and respiratory acidosis, usually due to an incorrect regulation of the respiratory frequency.

One-lung-independent lung ventilation (OL-ILV) is a technique that allows ventilation of one lung while the other main bronchus is artificially blocked to isolate fluid (i.e., blood) or secretions, avoiding contamination of normal lung alveoli and improving gas exchange. OL-ILV can be facilitated by deliberate left or right main bronchus selective intubation with a normal endotracheal tube, use of a DLEBT, or placement of a bronchial blocker (easily replaced in emergency conditions by an urinary cathether with the balloon inflated at the entrance of the bronchus of interest).

Independent lung ventilation (TL-ILV), synchronous or asynchronous, allows different ventilatory parameters and ventilatory modes to be applied to each lung. Separate ventilators are used for each lung. Synchronous TL-ILV maintains the same respiratory rate for both lungs and prevents the swinging of the mediastinum due to different inspiration and expiration times, but the flow rates, tidal volumes, and positive end-expiratory pressure are set separately. Asynchronous TL-ILV must use two separate ventilators to deliver different modes as well as different ventilator settings, does not require a special connection between the two ventilators (what is not available in most cases), and seems not to be deleterious.

4 ECMO Strategies

The goal of extracorporeal membrane oxygenation (ECMO) is to support gas exchange while allowing a reduction in the intensity of mechanical ventilation. Veno-venous or veno-arterial catheters are utilized to remove blood from the patient and circulate it through an artificial lung back to the patient.

Early consideration for veno-venous extracorporeal life support (vvECLS) is vital in patients who are failing attempts at lung-protective ventilation and do not have contraindications for the technique. If the gas exchange and perfusion goals are not met after 12 h of lung-protective ventilation and the patient has been paralyzed and correctly proned for at least 16–18 h a day, then extracorporeal support should be considered. Additionally, transport of patients who are supported with vvECLS may be safer and easier if an extracorporeal transport team is available. The trauma patient is particularly ingrate to the use of these techniques, because usually they need full anticoagulation, which can be challenging if the cause is trauma (in particular brain trauma).

References

1. https://doi.org/10.1513/AnnalsATS.201704-340OT
2. http://www.ijcasereportsandimages.com/archive/2011/012-2011-ijcri/006-12-2011-ahmad/ijcri-00612201166-ahmad-full-text.php#ref8
3. Bastos R, Calhoon JH, Baisden CE. Flail chest and pulmonary contusion. Semin Thorac Cardiovasc Surg. 2008;20:39–45.
4. Borman JB, Aharonson-Daniel L, Savitsky B. Unilateral flail chest is seldom a lethal injury. Emerg Med J. 2006;23:903–5.
5. Naidoo K, Hanbali L, Bates P. The natural history of flail chest injuries. Chin J Traumatol. 2017;20:293–6.

6. Dehghan N, de Mestral C, McKee MD. Flail chest injuries: a review of outcomes and treatment practices from the National Trauma Data Bank. J Trauma Acute Care Surg. 2014;76:462–8.
7. Clark GC, Schecter WP, Trunkey DD. Variables affecting outcome in blunt chest trauma: flail chest vs. pulmonary contusion. J Trauma. 1988;28:298–304.
8. Beal SL, Oreskovich MR. Long-term disability associated with flail chest injury. Am J Surg. 1985;150:324–6.
9. Wilson H, Ellsmere J, Tallon J. Occult pneumothorax in the blunt trauma patient: tube thoracostomy or observation? Injury. 2009;40:928–31.
10. Sharma A, Jindal P. Principles of diagnosis and management of traumatic pneumothorax. J Emerg Trauma Shock. 2008;1:34–41.
11. Berlot G, Massarutti D, Carchietti E. Treatment of acute pneumothorax in the field. In: Gullo A, editor. Anaesthesia, pain, intensive care and emergency medicine—A.P.I.C.E. Milan: Springer; 2005. p. 683–91.
12. Arshad H, Young M, Adurty R. Acute pneumothorax. Crit Care Nurs Q. 2016;39:176–89.
13. Driscoll P, Gwinnutt C, Goodall O. Thoracic trauma. In: Driscoll PA, Gwinnutt CL, Jimmerson CL, editors. Trauma resuscitation. London: Macmillan Education UK; 1993. p. 67–101.
14. Leixeira-Dias F, Dodd B, Torres Marques A, Lach L, Walley S, Proud WG, Goldrein HT, Esmail S, et al. A review of wound ballistics literature: the human body and injury processes. In: Leixeira-Dias F, Dodd B, Torres Marques A, Lach L, Walley S, editors. Security and use of innovative technologies against terrorism LWAG light-weight armour for defence & security; 18–19 May 2009. Aveiro: Universidade de Aveiro; 2009. p. 65–82.
15. Gotts PL, Kelly PM, van Bree JLMJ, van der Heiden N. Behind armour blunt trauma analysis of compression waves. In: Gotts PL, Kelly PM, editors. Personal armour systems symposium 1998 (PASS98). Defence Clothing and Textiles Agency, Science and Technology Division, UK MoD: Colchester; 1998. p. 433–40.
16. Crewther IR, Cannon L, Tam W. The development of a physical model of non-penetrating ballistic injury. In: Crewther IR, editor. 19th international symposium of ballistics; 7–11 May. Switzerland: Interlaken; 2001.
17. Stuhmiller JH, Shen WS, Niu E. Modeling for military operational medicine scientific and technical objectives. San Diego: Jaycor; 2003.
18. Cannon L. Behind armour blunt trauma—an emerging problem. J R Army Med Corps. 2001;147(1):87–96.
19. van Bree JLMJ, Bir CA, Wilhelm M. Female body armor assessment: current methods and future techniques. In: van Bree JLMJ, editor. Personal armour systems symposium 2004 (PASS2004). The Hague: TNO Prins Maurits Laboratory; 2004. p. 139–50.
20. Wilson LB. Dispersion of bullet energy in relation to wound effects. Mil Surg. 1921;XLIX:241–51.
21. Shen W, Niu Y, Bykanova L, et al. Characterizing the interaction among bullet, body armor, and human and surrogate targets. J Biomech Eng. 2010;132:1–11.
22. Mabry RL, Holcomb JB, Baker AM, et al. United States army rangers in Somalia: an analysis of combat casualties on an urban battlefield. J Trauma. 2000;49:515–29.
23. Thomas GE. Fatal .45–70 rifle wounding of a policeman wearing a bulletproof vest. J Forensic Sci. 1982;27:445–9.
24. Prather RN, Swann CL, Hawkins CE. Technical report eb-tr-77055. Backface signatures of soft body armors and the associated trauma effects. Chemical Systems Laboratory, Aberdeen Proving Ground Maryland: Department of the Army, 1977.
25. Montanarelli N, Hawkins CE, Goldfarb MA, et al. Technical report lwl-tr-30b73. Protective garments for public officials. US Army Land Warfare Laboratory, Aberdeen Proving Ground, Maryland: Department of the Army, 1973.
26. Powell MA, McMahon D, Peitzman AB. Thoracic injury. In: Peitzman AB, Rhodes M, Schuab CW, Yealy DM, editors. The trauma manual. Philadelphia: Lippincott Williams & Wilkins.

27. O'Connor RE, Levine BJ. Airway management in the trauma setting. In: Ferrera PC, Colucciello SA, Marx JA, Verdile VP, Gibbs MA, editors. Trauma management: an emergency medicine approach. St. Louis: Mosby; 2001. p. 52–74.
28. Rosen CL, Wolfe RE. Blunt chest trauma. In: Ferrera PC, Colucciello SA, Marx JA, Verdile VP, Gibbs MA, editors. Trauma management: an emergency medicine approach. St. Louis: Mosby; 2001. p. 232–58.
29. Sawyer MAJ. Blunt chest trauma. eMed J[serialonline]. 2004. http://www.emedicine.com/med/topic3658.htm. Accessed 15 Sept 2004.

Mechanical Ventilation in the Obese Patient

Jorge Hidalgo, Jorge E. Sinclair De Frías, and Allyson Hidalgo

1 Introduction

Several potential problems associated with obesity are essential to be familiar with as an intensivist. Understanding that obesity alters the anatomy and pulmonary physiology like reduced functional residual capacity. Patients can present with an early desaturation with apnea, airway obstruction using the face mask, possible difficulty with intubation if the patient has a large tongue, redundant folds of oropharyngeal tissue, and short and thick neck; also, decreased chest wall compliance (restrictive lung defect), increased degree of airway closure showing as hypoxemia, and surgical airways such as a tracheostomy or cricothyrotomy can be difficult and dangerous to be handled because of difficulty in identifying the various anatomical structures and increased risk of regurgitation and aspiration. As known, obesity predisposes to obstructive sleep apnea. We can say that adipocytes are far more than lipid storage vessels [1, 2]. Adipocytes are responsible for adipokine secretion and contribute to linked abnormalities such as insulin resistance and metabolic syndrome. Adipocytes also attract and activate inflammatory cells with multisystemic effects, vascular and cardiac remodeling, airway inflammation, and altered microvascular flow patterns. As an intensivist, we need to be aware of the current best practices in managing the airway and mechanical ventilation strategies of patients with obesity [1–3].

J. Hidalgo (✉)
Critical Care Division, Belize Healthcare Partners, Belize, Belize

J. E. Sinclair De Frías
Faculty of Medicine, University of Panama, Panama City, Panama

A. Hidalgo
Biochemistry, Arizona State University, Phoenix, AZ, USA

J. Hidalgo et al. (eds.), *Personalized Mechanical Ventilation*,
https://doi.org/10.1007/978-3-031-14138-6_9

2 Definition

Obesity is the increase of the body adipose tissue and is related with an increased incidence of noncommunicable diseases such as coronary artery disease, hyperlipidemia, and diabetes among others; the World Health Organization defined adults' healthy BMI to be in the range of 18.5–24.9, overweight is defined as BMI of 25–29.9, and we define obesity when the body mass index (BMI) is more than 30 kg m^2; morbid obesity is defined by a BMI of more than 35 or <40 kg m^2; extreme obesity, super-obesity, super-super-obesity, etc. are terms for describing higher degrees of morbid obesity [4].

3 Pathophysiology Ventilation Aspects

We need to take into consideration several pathophysiology aspects when we are planning to place an obese patient on mechanical ventilation:

Lung volume: There can be a reduction in the functional residual capacity (FCR) and an increase in the intra-abdominal pressure, the diaphragm can be passively pushed cranially, a decrease in the thoracic and pulmonary compliance can be caused, and there can be increased possibility of atelectasis in the dependent pulmonary areas. Respiratory system compliance is markedly reduced, due to increased chest wall mass and limited diaphragmatic excursion, and FEV1/FVC is preserved.

The alveolar-arterial oxygen difference is also increased, suggestive of V-P mismatch.

Airway: There can be an increase in the resistance (but typically after normalization to the functional lung volume), increase in the work of breathing (increased displacement of tissue during breathing both in the abdomen and chest wall), and increased airway resistance because of a smaller airway dimension, and we can see an increased incidence in asthma and increased risk factors for difficult mask ventilation.

Ventilatory control: We will see an impaired gas exchange, reduced ventilatory response to hypercapnia and hypoxia, and, in case of obesity, hypoventilation syndrome. There will also be an increase in the breathing rate.

Pulmonary circulation: Postcapillary pulmonary hypertension is associated with cardiac dysfunction. Oxygen consumption is increased, and an unusually high proportion of this consumption is spent on the work of breathing event at rest and an increased carbon dioxide production. Furthermore, it is essential to look for comorbidities like obstructive apnea syndrome and obesity hypoventilation syndrome that are more commonly see in obese population (Table 1) [5–7].

The assessment:

In the acute management of an obese patient, there are some issues we need to take into account as follows:

Table 1 Comorbidities like obstructive apnea syndrome and obesity hypoventilation syndrome

Obstructive sleep apnea	Obesity hypoventilation syndrome
Obstructive sleep apnea (OSA) is a sleep disorder that involves cessation or significant decrease in airflow in the presence of breathing effort. It is the most common type of sleep-disordered breathing and is characterized by recurrent episodes of upper airway collapse during sleep. These episodes are associated with recurrent oxyhemoglobin desaturations and arousal from sleep	Obesity hypoventilation syndrome (OHS) refers to the appearance of awake hypercapnia ($PaCO_2$ >45 mmHg) in the obese patient (BMI >30 kg/m^2) after other causes that could account for awake hypoventilation, such as lung or neuromuscular disease, have been excluded
	OHS: A great mimic in the immediate postoperative period. Can have a myriad of presentations like arrhythmias, hypotension, and obtunded sensorium. We need to have a high index of suspicion

1. Transport and positioning
2. Procedural difficulties
   (a) Vascular access
   (b) Tracheal intubation
3. Monitoring problems
4. Difficult airway maintenance
5. Impaired ventilation
6. Disordered gas exchange
7. Altered pharmacokinetics
8. Hemodynamic instability
9. Aspiration risk

4 Intubation Consideration

The main challenges for ICU clinicians are to consider the pulmonary pathophysiological specificities of the obese patient to optimize airway management.

Hence, we need to anticipate and consider all obese as difficult airway and difficult mask ventilation management. It is a general recommendation to preoxygenate with a 100% FiO_2, continuous positive pressure, or noninvasive positive-pressure ventilation. In addition, we also need to be prepared with fluids and vasoactive drugs in the event of hemodynamic instability. We need to take into consideration different scores; review the Mallampati, if the patients have a history of obstructive apnea syndrome; check cervical mobility and mouth opening, if the patient is in a coma; check the level of hypoxemia, if there are other associated problems that can make the intubation process more complicated, like the lack of teeth, snoring, beard, and associated congenital disease; and check the availability of equipment for the management of a difficult airway. We can also accommodate the patient in a sitting or semi-sitting position during preoxygenation, may reduce positional flow limitation and air trapping, reduce the possibility of atelectasis formation, and make a decision on the type of laryngoscope; whenever possible, the recommendation is to use video laryngoscopy; however, in the absence of additional risk factors or if the video laryngoscope is not available, we need to use direct laryngoscopy [8, 9] (see Tables 2, 3, and 4).

Table 2 Mechanical ventilation in the obese patient

Mechanical ventilation in the obese patient
Consider all obese patients as having **high-risk airway** and assess additional risk factors for difficult intubation and mask ventilation: Mallampati III–IV, obstructive apnea syndrome, reduced cervical mobility, mouth opening limitations, increased size of pharyngeal and glossal soft tissues, decreased thyromental distance, COMA, hypoxemia, skill of the operator, beard, snoring, associated congenital disease
Check the availability of equipment for the management of a difficult airway
Preoxygenation: Preoxygenate with a FiO_2 at 100%, continuous positive pressure on noninvasive ventilation. High-flow oxygen and in a semi-sitting position. Be prepared with iv fluids and vasoactive drugs in case of hemodynamic instability
For a tracheal intubation: Laryngoscopy: video laryngoscopy is recommended; however, in the absence of an additional risk factor or if video laryngoscope is not available, we need to be prepared for a traditional direct laryngoscopy
Mechanical ventilation settings
1. Low-volume ventilation
2. Moderate-to-high PEEP
3. Recruitment maneuvers
Extubation
Weaning test: According to your hospital protocol
You might consider for all obese patients: preventative noninvasive ventilation and you can alternate with high-flow nasal cannula oxygen

Table 3 Mechanical ventilation in the critically ill obese patient challenges

Mechanical ventilation in the critically ill obese patient: challenges	
Small mouth opening	↓ FRC
Short thyromental distance	Increased intrapulmonary shunt
↑ Neck circumference	↓ Chest wall and lung compliances
↓ Neck mobility	↑ Airway resistances
Large breast and tongue	↑ Mechanical pressure
Poor view with direct laryngoscopy	↑ Metabolic demands
Short laryngoscope handle	↑ Intra-abdominal pressure
Difficult to bag/mask ventilation	↓ Diaphragmatic excursion
Unfavorable conformation and positioning of the larynx	Airway compression through increased airway fat deposits, and placing the patient with obesity recumbent may lead to sudden death
• It is very important to encourage upright positioning and avoid supine positioning	
• The main mechanism of gas exchange impairment is, therefore, shunt (atelectasis) in patients with obesity	

Table 4 Factors affecting mechanical ventilation in obese patients

Factors affecting mechanical ventilation in obese patients
The supine position reduces lung volumes and decreases respiratory compliance, especially in obese patients
Chest wall compliance decreases in obese patients since the increased abdominal girth pushes against the diaphragm
Anesthesia reduces functional residual capacity (FRC) to approximately half of the preinduction value in obese patients, promoting atelectasis

5 Obesity Paradox

The etiologies for this presumed paradox are not clear. Leptin, secreted from adipose tissue, augmented the immune response and improved bacterial clearance in animals. A critically ill septic patient who survived from sepsis had threefold higher plasma concentrations of leptin compared with those who died. This is not a real phenomenon but rather a reflection of a selection bias with more severely ill patients, those with inflammation, prolonged ICU stay, and preexisting comorbidities, such as malignant diseases having a lower BMI and expectedly a worse outcome. BMI is the associated comorbidity that determines the potential for a better or worse outcome.

Despite the increasing incidence of cardiovascular diseases and DMII in the obese population, we see that those with a higher BMI may survive longer when compared with those with lower BMI and thus the term "obesity paradox" [10].

6 The Ventilator and Settings

Mechanical ventilation for an obese patient is a challenge. We start with a lung-protective strategy approach with a tidal volume 4–6 mL/kg according to the predictive body weight (PBW) in a patient with an ARDS. And in non-ARDS patients, adopt a volume-controlled approach, with low-moderate PEEP adjusted according to the recommendation of the ARDSnet of low-PEEP strategy. And we need to titrate the FIO2 according to the oxygenation goals gradually.

At a minimum, the recommended oxygenation goals are with PEEP, to keep PaO_2 at 55–80 mmHg or peripheral oxygen saturation of 88–92% in both ARDS and non-ARDS. Also, the respiratory rate is calculated to maintain a pH >7.25 in the non-ARDS and ARDS patients and tolerate mild hypercapnia in the ARDS group of patients. The recruitment maneuvers are not routinely recommended. We need to avoid hyperoxia, and if we experience a desaturation, the recommendation is to prioritize FiO_2 adjustments over PEEP.

Plateau targets are critical and should be maintained below $27\ cmH_2O + (IAP - 13)/2$ in the ARDS group patients and $20\ cmH_2O + (IAP - 13)/2$ in the non-ARDS group. The recruitment maneuvers, only as rescue, stepwise increase airway pressure. Having in mind a prone position that is safe in ARDS obese patients and ECMO is also an option in some selected ARDS cases [11, 12].

7 Rescue Therapies

Generally, the use of recruitment maneuvers as part of the standard ventilatory management of obese patients is not a routine consideration, and the use remains a decision based on an individual risk/benefit assessment. It is rather a rescue tool in case of refractory gas exchange impairment to be performed with gradual changes in the ventilator settings, such as stepwise increases in PEEP and/or inspiratory pressures. Prone positioning has an established role as rescue therapy in ARDS patients, and its feasibility, safety, and effectiveness have also been shown in obese patients. By moving from a supine to a prone position, we can reduce dependent edema, increase lung volumes (from reduced atelectasis), and improve secretion clearance approach:

- Apply soft pads, secure all tubes/lines, place pillows on chest, and wrap with sheets; using a team (six or more skilled people), rotate the patient as a unit; supinate once per day for 16 h.

When these conventional rescue therapies fail, extracorporeal membrane oxygenation should be considered. The use of neuromuscular blocking agents and opioids should be limited in obese patients; in both cases, they prefer medication with a short-action molecule and with effective antidotes. At the moment of extubation, noninvasive ventilatory support can be considered in selected patients.

The use of mechanical ventilation in the obese group of patients presents with unique challenges, and the understanding of the different physiological aspects related with this group of patients is critical. Teamwork is the key to optimizing mechanical ventilation to aim for better clinical outcomes [13–15].

8 Conclusion

- Obese patients admitted to the intensive care unit are at risk to develop several complications with significant increase in morbidity and mortality. There is also increased risk for difficult intubation and difficult mask ventilation.
- The airway management of an obese patient needs to be approached as a high-risk case, hence the reason to have a protocol for the management of a difficult airway in order to prevent the complication related to the intubation like severe hypoxia, hemodynamic instability, and cardiac arrest.
- A semi-sitting position and preoxygenation should be optimized using positive-pressure ventilation (CPAP or NIV).
- Lung protection ventilation needs to be applied, with individualized PEEP and individualized rescue maneuvers. When ARDS is confirmed and we see refractory hypoxemia, a prone position as a rescue strategy is considered a safe procedure, which permits respiratory mechanic improvements and oxygenation.

Obstructive-apnea syndrome and obesity-hypoventilation syndrome should be investigated to plan treatment accordingly.

- We need to develop an airway and ventilation management algorithm in the obese patient in the intensive care unit.

References

1. De Jong A, Chanques G, et al. Mechanical ventilation in obese ICU patient: from intubation to extubation. Crit Care. 2017;21:63. https://doi.org/10.1186/s13054-017-1641-1. open access.
2. Ball L, Pelosi P. How I ventilate the obese patient. Crit Care. 2019;23:176. https://doi.org/10.1186/s13054-019-2466-x.
3. De Jong A, Wrigge H, et al. How to ventilate obese patients in ICU. Intensive Care Med. 2020;46:2423–35.
4. Schetz M, De Jong A, Deane AM, et al. Obesity in the critically ill: a narrative review. Intensive Care Med. 2019;45(6):757–69.
5. Pépin JL, Timsit JF, Tamisier R, et al. Prevention and care of respiratory failure in obese patients. Lancet Respir Med. 2016;4(5):407–18.
6. Kress JP, Pohlman AS, Alverdy J, Hall JB. The impact of morbid obesity on oxygen cost of breathing (VO(2RESP)) at rest. Am J Respir Crit Care Med. 1999;160:883–6.
7. Global BMI Mortality Collaboration, Di Angelantonio E, Bhupathiraju S, Wormser D, Gao P, Kaptoge S, de Gonzalez AB, Cairns BJ, Huxley R, Jackson C, Joshy G, Lewington S, Manson JE, Murphy N, Patel AV, Samet JM, Woodward M, Zheng W, Zhou M, Bansal N, Barricarte A, Carter B, Cerhan JR, Smith GD, Fang X, Franco OH, Green J, Halsey J, Hildebrand JS, Jung KJ, Korda RJ, McLerran DF, Moore SC, O'Keeffe LM, Paige E, Ramond A, Reeves GK, Rolland B, Sacerdote C, Sattar N, Sofianopoulou E, Stevens J, Thun M, Ueshima H, Yang L, Yun YD, Willeit P, Banks E, Beral V, Chen Z, Gapstur SM, Gunter MJ, Hartge P, Jee SH, Lam TH, Peto R, Potter JD, Willett WC, Thompson SG, Danesh J, Hu FB. Body-mass index and all-cause mortality: individual-participant-data meta-analysis of 239 prospective studies in four continents. Lancet. 2016;388:776–86.
8. Pepin J, Borel JC, Janssens JP. Obesity hypoventilation syndrome: an underdiagnosed and undertreated condition. Am J Respir Crit Care Med. 2012;186:1205–7.
9. Chlif M, Keochkerian D, Choquet D, Vaidie A, Ahmaidi S. Effects of obesity on breathing pattern, ventilatory neural drive and mechanics. Respir Physiol Neurobiol. 2009;168:198–202.
10. Zhi G, Xin W, Ying W, Guohong X, Shuying L. "Obesity Paradox" in acute respiratory distress syndrome: a systematic review and meta-analysis. PLoS One. 2016;11:e0163677.
11. Futier E, Constantin JM, Pelosi P, et al. Noninvasive ventilation and alveolar recruitment maneuver improve respiratory function during and after intubation of morbidly obese patients: a randomized controlled study. Anesthesiology. 2011;114(6):1354–63.
12. Ball L, Hemmes SNT, Serpa Neto A, et al. Intraoperative ventilation settings and their associations with postoperative pulmonary complications in obese patients. Br J Anaesth. 2018;121(4):899–908.
13. Serpa Neto A, Deliberato RO, Johnson AEW, et al. Mechanical power of ventilation is associated with mortality in critically ill patients: an analysis of patients in two observational cohorts. Intensive Care Med. 2018;44(11):1914–22.
14. De Jong A, Molinari N, Sebbane M, et al. Feasibility and effectiveness of prone position in morbidly obese patients with ARDS: a case-control clinical study. Chest. 2013;143(6):1554–61.
15. Bazurro S, Ball L, Pelosi P. Perioperative management of obese patient. Curr Opin Crit Care. 2018;24(6):560–7.

Postoperative Mechanical Ventilation: Fast Track

Jorge E. Sinclair Ávila, Jorge E. Sinclair De Frías, Juan P. Herrera Berríos, and Allyson Hidalgo

1 Introduction

Early rapid extubation, also known as fast-track extubation (FTE), following surgical procedures has grown substantially in recent decades. There is a vast proportion of postoperative patients who might benefit from this emerging approach including, but not limited to, patients undergoing cardiac surgery, orthotopic liver transplantation, or intracranial hematoma evacuation [1, 2].

Indeed, data from multiple RCTs show that fortunately, 75% of postoperative patients subjected to mechanical ventilation will meet the criteria for prompt discontinuation of mechanical ventilation within the first 2–8 h post-ICU admission. This patient population may be directly transitioned from the OR to a regular ward [2]. This translates not only to improved pulmonary physiology (bypassing the deleterious effects of positive-pressure ventilation) but also to the rapid systemic clearance of opioid medications such as fentanyl. Moreover, with the recent advent of short-half-life anesthetics, it is safe to say that a trend exists towards earlier and faster extubation times [3].

J. E. Sinclair Ávila (✉)
Punta Pacific Hospital/Johns Hopkins Medicine, Panama City, Panama

J. E. Sinclair De Frías
Department of Physiology, Faculty of Medicine, University of Panama, Panama City, Panama

J. P. Herrera Berríos
Department of Neurological Surgery, Complejo Hospitalario Dr. Arnulfo Arias Madrid, Caja de Seguro Social, Panama City, Panama

A. Hidalgo
Biochemistry, Arizona State University, Phoenix, AZ, USA

J. Hidalgo et al. (eds.), *Personalized Mechanical Ventilation*,
https://doi.org/10.1007/978-3-031-14138-6_10

Specifically, recent data highlights FTE as a highly effective strategy given that 71% of posthepatic transplant patients are successfully extubated in the 12 h posterior to ICU admission [2].

FTE improves patient outcomes via different mechanisms including [4]:

- Reduced ventilator-associated morbidity and mortality
- Reduced number of in-hospital days
- Reducing excessive use of hypnotic drugs and deep sedation that are usually warranted for maintenance of patient-ventilator synchrony
- Allowing for early mobilization of patients and therefore preventing physical deconditioning and loss of function associated with prolonged ICU stays
- Decreased in-hospital medical costs without compromising patient satisfaction

2 Definitions: Is Fast Track Just Accelerated Weaning?

Weaning is the stepwise process of discontinuing ventilatory support. This process comprises around 40% of total ventilatory time in a given clinical scenario [5]. Failure to initiate prompt weaning may lead to severe pulmonary complications such as ventilator-associated pneumonia (VAP), ventilator-induced lung injury (VILI), or even ventilator-induced diaphragmatic dysfunction (VIDD).

On the contrary, FTE implies early and rapid extubation immediately post-surgery, based on the assessment of the integrity of the patient's own respiratory drive and capacity to maintain a permeable airway (as measured by a successful spontaneous breathing trial [SBT]).

3 Primum Non Nocere

Clinicians must, however, weigh the benefits of early-onset extubation against the possible risks associated with conducting a premature SBT. While this technique is not exempted from complications itself, appropriate patient selection is key. Moreover, one must prepare for extubation long before the endotracheal tube is in position, the rationale being not to keep patients mechanically ventilated unless deemed absolutely necessary (i.e., a failed SBT post-op).

4 Predictors and Criteria for Weaning and Extubation

Predictors and criteria are best thought of as a continuum. They must be employed in an organized and synchronous manner in order to guarantee the best possible outcome for patients at the moment of intended extubation [6]. This leads to the confection of a procedural guideline with the intention of elevating extubation success rates in these patients.

Subjective predictive values may be insufficient and for this reason have been complemented [7] or replaced [8] by objective clinical assessments that serve as surrogate markers for extubation. These include:

- Heart rate variability
- Sleep quality
- Hand squeezing strength
- Diaphragmatic dysfunction
- Oxidative stress markers

De-escalation of ventilation, including weaning and voluntary or involuntary extubation, entails several physiological changes in regard to hemodynamics and the neural circuitry connected to the medullary respiratory center.

Two prospective observational studies, one of them by Arcentales et al. [9], demonstrated that the presence of reduced heart rate variability during the spontaneous breathing test led to extubation failure. Likewise, poor sleep quality, associated fatigue and diaphragmatic weakness, and poor hand grip strength were all predictors of extubation failure [10–12]. Other negative prognostic measures were the presence of oxidative stress marker levels. Worthy of note is that the markers presented are much more in line with patients who have been on prolonged ventilatory support or those with longer than 48 h on the ventilator.

This all serves to highlight the importance of postulating an indication for early and rapid extubation (namely, the fast-track approach) especially in surgical patients who naturally meet or fulfill the established extubation criteria.

4.1 Criteria for Weaning and Extubation

The International Consensus Conference of 2005 proposed a set of criteria that are useful to consider when deciding whether extubation is feasible. These are not to be used as an imperative checklist, but rather as subjective and objective recommendations that may lead to better outcomes [13]. This is illustrated by the fact that some patients only fulfill a few criteria, yet also have successful results [6].

Subjective Criteria

- Preserved coughing
- Absence of neuromuscular blockade
- Absence of continuous sedation infusions
- No excess of tracheobronchial secretions
- Preserved mentation
- Reversal of the underlying cause that led to the patient being mechanically ventilated in the first place

Objective Criteria

- Hemodynamic stability
- Heart rate <140x'
- No clinical findings suggesting myocardial ischemia
- Hemoglobin >8 g/dL
- Systolic BP: 90–160 mmHg
- Normothermia
- Absence of vasopressor or inotropic support or minimal support

Adequate Oxygenation Criteria

- Tidal volume >5 mL/kg
- Vital capacity >10 mL/kg
- Proper inspiratory effort
- Respiratory rate $\leq$35/min
- $PaO_2 \geq 60$ and $PaCO_2 \leq 60$ mmHg
- Positive end-expiratory pressure $\leq$8 cmH_2O
- No significant respiratory acidosis (pH $\geq$7.30)
- Maximal inspiratory pressure (MIP) ≤ -20 to -25 cmH_2O
- O_2 saturation >90% on $FiO_2 \leq 0.4$ (or $PaO_2/FiO_2 \geq 200$)
- Rapid shallow breathing index (respiratory frequency/tidal volume) <105

As mentioned, not every single patient fulfills 2 or more absolute criteria. Moreover, this clinical framework supposes a rigid (as opposed to flexible) approach towards extubation and could lead to detrimental outcomes by prolonging ventilation in a patient who may not require it.

At this point, it remains a fact that the amount of time a patient spends inside the ICU while on mechanical ventilation is directly proportional to the odds of developing complications associated to the ventilator itself (namely VAP, VILI, VIDD). Simply put, extubation within the first 8 h post-op leads to improved patient outcomes by means of reduced time on the ventilator, reduced ICU time, and consecutive decrease in costs [4] for both patients and institutions.

An important concept to have in mind is that the postoperative patient cohort has better odds at successful extubation, granted that there were no underlying respiratory comorbidities pre-intubation. Extubation must not be delayed in these patients.

When compared to patients who have undergone more than 48 h of MV, most surgical patients have relatively short operating times which, in turn, leads to less sedation infused and therefore are more likely to fulfill subjective and/or objective criteria [3].

This clinical scenario allows for a very straightforward and practical approach by ensuring proper ventilation via any of the following techniques:

- T-piece trial, in which only supplemental oxygen is supplied through a T-piece connected to an endotracheal tube
- Continuous positive airway pressure (CPAP) trial using a CPAP level equal to the previous positive end-expiratory pressure (PEEP) level
- Invasive ventilation with low level of pressure support (5–8 cmH_2O) or automatic tube compensation

There is no recent evidence to suggest the superiority of one technique over the other [14]. A Cochrane systematic review demonstrated that there is no significant difference in mortality and extubation failure when comparing the T-piece trial with the pressure support trial, with a low level of evidence. However, with a moderate level of evidence, it was found that the pressure support trial was superior to the T-tube trial (STT) in patients considered to be under simple weaning [15].

Over the last four decades, it has been demonstrated that with the use of the fast-track technique, up to 71% of patients undergoing both liver and cardiovascular transplantation have been extubated within the first 8 h postoperatively as long as it is not life threatening or there are no contraindications due to severe comorbidities [2].

Recently, a meta-analyses conducted by Van Mastright et al. [4] showed that patients undergoing fast-track extubation lead to a decrease in both ICU and hospital stays in patients undergoing coronary artery bypass grafting (CABG). A total of 27 studies that were analyzed concluded that early extubation led to positive results both medically and in terms of hospital costs [4].

In a 2015 study, Hashemian et al. used the ultra-fast-track extubation technique in patients undergoing cardiac transplantation with excellent results, with ICU stay times being much shorter than those undergoing late extubation, with both methods having excellent results in mortality and morbidity [16].

In another study performed in patients with orthotopic liver transplantation and under the approval of the bioethics committee, Villar Dolores et al. [2] performed a one-year follow-up analysis from October 2019 to October 2020 in which 76 patients were admitted to ICU; 31 were excluded and 45 were analyzed. Of the patients who entered the study, 71% were extubated within the first 12 h with an average of 7.5 h. The limitation of the study was the sample size (45 patients), but considering the type of transplantation, it is considered a positive analysis for fast-track extubation in transplanted patients [2].

5 Conclusion

Growing evidence supports the importance of fast-tracking by either the ultra-rapid or the rapid method within the first 8 h postoperatively or immediately after surgery by reducing comorbidity, death, and associated complications. With fast-track, it can be affirmed that the incidence of ventilator-associated medical complications is reduced, among which ventilator-associated pneumonia, ventilator-induced lung injury (VILI), volutrauma, barotrauma, and biotrauma are common. With this method, it has been possible to reduce the excessive and continuous use of opioid drugs that manage to impregnate the adipose tissue and subsequently dilate the extubation process, not without mentioning a long list of possible cardiovascular and hemodynamic complications that can be avoided [3].

Finally, it has been possible to reduce the costs of intrahospital stay and stay in intensive care units, in some cases even avoiding admission to intensive care if the postoperative patient remains stable in the post-anesthesia care unit (PACU) [4].

References

1. González-Cordero G, Garduño-Chávez BI, Palacios-Ríos D, et al. Fast-track extubation in patients after intracranial hematoma surgery. Exp Ther Med. 2020;19(4):2563–9. https://doi.org/10.3892/etm.2020.8507. Epub 2020 Feb 10. PMID: 32256735; PMCID: PMC7098210.
2. Villar D, Carmon S, Lowman P, Santos C. Fast-track extubation for liver transplant patients admitted to ICU postoperatively. Crit Care Med. 2022;50(1):606. https://doi.org/10.1097/01.ccm.0000811172.56986.4e.
3. Rosow C. Remifentanil: a unique opioid analgesic. Anesthesiology. 1993;79(5):875–6. PMID: 7902031.
4. van Mastrigt GA, Maessen JG, Heijmans J, et al. Does fast-track treatment lead to a decrease of intensive care unit and hospital length of stay in coronary artery bypass patients? A meta-regression of randomized clinical trials. Crit Care Med. 2006;34(6):1624–34. https://doi.org/10.1097/01.CCM.0000217963.87227.7B. PMID: 16614584.
5. Esteban A, Ferguson ND, Meade MO, et al. Evolution of mechanical ventilation in response to clinical research. Am J Respir Crit Care Med. 2008;177(2):170–7. https://doi.org/10.1164/rccm.200706-893OC. Epub 2007 Oct 25. PMID: 17962636.
6. Boles JM, Bion J, Connors A, Herridge M, et al. Weaning from mechanical ventilation. Eur Respir J. 2007;29(5):1033–56. https://doi.org/10.1183/09031936.00010206. PMID: 17470624.
7. Esteban A, Frutos F, Tobin MJ, et al. A comparison of four methods of weaning patients from mechanical ventilation. Spanish Lung Failure Collaborative Group. N Engl J Med. 1995;332(6):345–50. https://doi.org/10.1056/NEJM199502093320601. PMID: 7823995.
8. Ely EW, Baker AM, Dunagan DP, et al. Effect on the duration of mechanical ventilation of identifying patients capable of breathing spontaneously. N Engl J Med. 1996;335(25):1864–9. https://doi.org/10.1056/NEJM199612193352502. PMID: 8948561.
9. Arcentales A, Caminal P, Diaz I, Benito S, Giraldo BF. Classification of patients undergoing weaning from mechanical ventilation using the coherence between heart rate variability and respiratory flow signal. Physiol Meas. 2015;36(7):1439–52. https://doi.org/10.1088/0967-3334/36/7/1439. Epub 2015 May 28. PMID: 26020593.
10. Chen CJ, Hsu LN, McHugh G, Campbell M, Tzeng YL. Predictors of sleep quality and successful weaning from mechanical ventilation among patients in respiratory care centers. J Nurs Res. 2015;23(1):65–74. https://doi.org/10.1097/jnr.0000000000000066. PMID: 25668737.
11. Hermans G, Bernard DJ, Bruyninckx F, et al. Clinical review: critical illness polyneuropathy and myopathy. Crit Care. 2008;12:238–47.
12. DiNino E, Gartman EJ, Sethi JM, McCool FD. Diaphragm ultrasound as a predictor of successful extubation from mechanical ventilation. Thorax. 2014;69(5):423–7. https://doi.org/10.1136/thoraxjnl-2013-204111. Epub 2013 Dec 23. PMID: 24365607.
13. Peñuelas Ó, Thille AW, Esteban A. Discontinuation of ventilatory support: new solutions to old dilemmas. Curr Opin Crit Care. 2015;21(1):74–81. https://doi.org/10.1097/MCC.0000000000000169. PMID: 25546535.
14. Bailey CR, Jones RM, Kelleher AA. The role of continuous positive airway pressure during weaning from mechanical ventilation in cardiac surgical patients. Anaesthesia. 1995;50(8):677–81. https://doi.org/10.1111/j.1365-2044.1995.tb06092.x. PMID: 7645695.
15. Ladeira MT, Vital FM, Andriolo RB, Andriolo BN, Atallah AN, Peccin MS. Pressure support versus T-tube for weaning from mechanical ventilation in adults. Cochrane Database Syst Rev. 2014;2014(5):CD006056. https://doi.org/10.1002/14651858.CD006056.pub2. PMID: 24865303; PMCID: PMC6492521.
16. Kianfar AA, Ahmadi ZH, Mirhossein SM, et al. Ultra fast-track extubation in heart transplant surgery patients. Int J Crit Illn Inj Sci. 2015;5(2):89–92. https://doi.org/10.4103/2229-5151.158394.

Mechanical Ventilation in COVID

Javier Perez-Fernandez, Enrique Puig, Jaskaran Kaur Purewal, and Paola Perez

For the first time since the late 1950s, during the polio epidemic, the world, in its entirety, has confronted a shortage of elements for respiratory support, creating anxiety and raising controversy among the population, public criticism, and government crisis [1–3]. More than one million people have received mechanical ventilation throughout the pandemic [4]. Patients receiving this form of treatment have had a reported mortality between 40 and 90% [5–7].

Amid the variety of management strategies described and recommended, clinicians worldwide have experienced confusion resulting from the lack of uniformity in the recommendations and frustration caused by the conflicting results appearing in the literature as well as the noise generated by the media. From the "classic" ARDS-protective lung strategies to a more liberal approach and a variety of recommendations including treatments such as proning, ECMO, or nitric oxide among others, different ventilatory approaches have attempted to find the "right ventilator node" for COVID-ARDS (C-ARDS) patients.

The phrase "avoid intubation at all costs" when referring to patients with COVID was a favorite to news and social media for some time [8]. That was in great part favored by the high mortality reflected in the first publications of COVID and respiratory failure [9]. It is obvious for the clinicians that patients requiring respiratory assistance, especially invasive mechanical ventilation, have greater mortality than

J. Perez-Fernandez (✉)
Baptist Hospital of Miami, Critical Care Services, Miami, FL, USA

E. Puig
West Kendall Baptist Hospital, Critical Care Services, Miami, FL, USA

J. K. Purewal
Larkin Community Hospital, Palm Springs Campus, Hialeah, FL, USA

P. Perez
University of Virginia, School of Medicine, Charlottesville, VA, USA

J. Hidalgo et al. (eds.), *Personalized Mechanical Ventilation*,
https://doi.org/10.1007/978-3-031-14138-6_11

those with the same condition but certainly less severe forms. This fact was never adequately represented in the media reports, causing confusion for the nonclinical population. Many studies have been published attempting to identify risk factors associated with higher mortality in COVID-19 ventilated patients. However, non-patient-related factors are likely to be involved in such incremental death rate: patients included in those reports were sometimes left in the hands of non-experienced management teams, the heterogenicity of diseases and baseline conditions, and the use of basic ventilatory equipment that in some cases was "too basic" to support complicated respiratory dynamics frequently seen in C-ARDS.

Additionally, clinicians managing these patients were subject to stress motivated by many factors. The fight against an unknown enemy, the scarceness of equipment and personnel, the media attention, and the increasing pressure produced by misinformation were the perfect ingredients for the boiling scenario encountered by the healthcare professionals. Scientific literature was flooded by frequent and changing reports many times in response to emergent public request and pressure by politicians and administrations, searching for an answer to the unknown. Recommendations regarding the management of ventilated patients as well as protocols and guidelines were continuously present in journals as well as in the press and media communication platforms.

With this amount of varied and sometimes conflicting information, the management of patients with COVID-19 and respiratory failure has become challenging to say the least. We understand the rapidly changing environment that surrounds COVID-19. Therefore, we predict that some or more of the aspects and recommendations reflected in this chapter might evolve soon after publication. Nonetheless, we will attempt to describe the accepted principles based on research and trials and utilize the best rigor in selecting the terms for discussion. We will tour the recommendations in the ventilatory management of patients with COVID-19 based on what clinicians have learnt and on the current proven evidence at the time of preparation of this chapter.

1 Airway Management

Intubation has always been the last resource for critically ill patients in respiratory failure. However, elective or planned airway management has been preferred to emergency intubation. The latter was associated with complications at the time of intubation and late post-intubation hypoxemia in patients with COVID-19 [10].

In the times of the COVID-19, management of the airway has become more than ever a terrain for the intervention of experienced operators. The virus is easily aerosolized, and cough and secretions can be a mechanism of spread during the process of intubation [11]. Management of the airway is preferred in a controlled setting, with personnel wearing high-protection equipment, such as N95 or PAR-2 equivalent, and the patient conveniently sedated and paralyzed. Rapid sequence intubation has been proposed as the mode of intervention in these patients [12]. The room should be emptied of nonessential personnel and maneuvers, and airway attempts should be minimized to decrease the risk of exposure.

2 When to Intubate?

Timing of intubation in relation to COVID-19 has been controversial, variable, and challenging throughout the pandemic. Initial reports from China demonstrated severe respiratory failure associated with significant morbidity and mortality affecting a large portion of the population [9]. This imposed a dilemma from a resource utilization and infection control standpoint, and subsequently late intubation was favored. Only patients that were severely hypoxemic and clinically deteriorating were subject to mechanical ventilation, action this, occurring at a late phase of the disease after exhaustion of alternatives [13]. At the very same time, some reports indicated that the use of noninvasive ventilation and high-flow nasal cannula, besides not being clinically effective, created an unnecessary exposure to healthcare professionals and other patients, exposing them to aerosolized viral particles [14].

Studies continued to show mixed results regarding benefits in early versus late intubation. A retrospective study published in 2020 showed that late intubation (>1.27 days) had a worse prognosis compared to early intubation (<1.27 days) due to prolonged ICU stay and longer duration of mechanical ventilation [15]. However, a systematic review of meta-analysis showed no difference in mortality or duration of mechanical ventilation with relation to timing of intubation [16]. Nonetheless, the current opinion, at the moment of this publication, favors early intervention to avoid further damage and respiratory exhaustion in these patients.

A plausible mechanism to explain the damage inflicted by delayed intubation could be SIVI or self-inflected ventilation injury [17]. The injury is explained by repeated negative intrathoracic pressures and high respiratory drive producing fatigue of the tissues [18]. If noninvasive ventilation is applied, this damage could be enhanced [19, 20]. Thus, controlled ventilation, with fixed volumes and pressures, could be the only mechanism of management.

If patients do not undergo early intubation, this process could become irreversible requiring, then, higher pressures and PEEP levels to achieve effective ventilation [15].

3 Mechanical Ventilation: General Considerations

ARDS is a syndrome characterized by the development of hypoxemia in the setting of an inciting event, leading to increased pulmonary vascular permeability, loss of lung volume, and loss of lung compliance. While COVID-19 pneumonia largely encompasses most of the components of the Berlin criteria, we continue to learn more about the virus and its distinguishing features that differentiate it from typical ARDS [21]. As this concept was evolving, clinicians deviated from the lung-protective ventilation management strategy as they found it not as effective in the treatment of COVID-19 [22].

Two phenotypes have been described in patients with COVID-19 pneumonia, L (type 1) and H (type 2). The L phenotype is associated with severe hypoxemia in the setting of normal pulmonary compliance (>50 mL/cm H_2O); hypoxemia results from impaired V/Q mismatch due to the dysregulation of the hypoxic vasoconstriction mechanism. Overall, lung volumes remain unchanged and respond minimally to recruitment maneuvers. The likely pathogenic insult is caused by the virus and its direct effect on the lung parenchyma causing interstitial edema, damaging the elastic recoil and inducing vasoplegia, ultimately leading to increased minute ventilation and hypoxemia. A recent study described that ventilated C-ARDS patients showed improvement in arterial oxygenation with high PEEP strategies, but no change in compliance and no change in $PaCO_2$, hence postulating this as secondary to hyperinflation and overdistention of the alveoli [23]. In this scenario, the protective lung ventilation settings (low tidal volume and high PEEP model) classically used in ARDS as defined in the Berlin criteria might not be as effective and require some adjustments. In the setting of constrained lung with impaired VQ relation, the application of high PEEP levels could decrease lung compliances even more and exercise strain on the right heart, therefore promoting hemodynamic instability. Conversely for this group of patients, liberation of the tidal volume and application of more conservative levels of PEEP have been associated with better outcomes [17, 18].

As the disease progresses, H phenotype is more dominant. Interstitial edema worsens, causing decreased lung volumes. This phase can be seen in about one-third of COVID-19 patients and is characterized by severe hypoxemia with compliance <40 mL/cmH_2O and high elastance, elements that are more consistent with the standard definition of ARDS. In this stage, patients might require high levels of PEEP, recruitment maneuvers, and proning all aimed to increase alveolar recruitment [19, 24].

Mechanical ventilation in these patients has been a challenge due to the severity of respiratory dysfunction. Low lung compliance and high airway pressures contribute to increased incidence of ventilator-induced lung injury and barotrauma [25]. Current recommendations for mechanical ventilation based on the Surviving Sepsis Campaign continue to adhere to lung-protective ventilation strategies. Low tidal volumes (V_T 4–8 mL/kg of predicted body weight) to maintain driving pressures <15 cmH_2O and plateau pressures <30 cmH_2O reduced airway pressures and limited complications of barotrauma [26]. High driving pressures have been associated with increased mortality and should be avoided [27]. Neuromuscular blocking agent boluses, or even continuous infusion, are recommended to aid in ventilation goals and to facilitate patient-ventilator synchrony [28]. Staircase recruitment maneuvers, which can be safely used in non-COVID ARDS patients, are not recommended due to the increased risk of barotrauma.

There is a phenotypic response to PEEP associated with C-ARDS that requires attention. Early in the disease course, there remains potential response to PEEP and typical recruitment maneuvers to aid in oxygenation [23]. Overall, high PEEP strategies need to be individualized towards the patient's response, which may be due to their phenotypic presentation of C-ARDS. Using this clinical guidance might help in the consideration of PEEP and other maneuvers such as proning. However, even in patients that were responsive to high PEEP, evidenced by improvement in arterial oxygenation, no changes in lung compliance or $PaCO_2$ were noted [23]. This brings into question the overall significance of PEEP in the treatment of these patients. Some studies have suggested that conservative levels of PEEP could be associated with improved outcomes [19, 24].

The recognition of various phenotypes with C-ARDS challenged the prior conventional treatment for ARDS and highlights the need to individualized mechanical ventilation treatment according to each patient's needs.

4 Prone Position

Prone positioning improves oxygenation by matching ventilation-perfusion in a heterogenous lung parenchyma with nonhomogeneous expansion, in the ventral to dorsal direction. Turning the body favors the displacement of pressure and thus volumes, from the dorsal to ventral lung, in a more homogeneous distribution. Prone ventilation has shown to increase lung volumes, decrease atelectatic lung, and improve oxygenation through alveolar recruitment. It has been frequently used in mechanically ventilated patients with ARDS, and while initial trials showed conflicting evidence, a clear mortality benefit was demonstrated when used early, with appropriate lung-protective strategies, in the PROSEVA trial [29].

Unsurprisingly, proning continued to be an intervention used to improve oxygenation in mechanically ventilated C-ARDS patients. A recent study demonstrated that in a similar fashion to "general" ARDS patients, most C-ARDS patients showed better ventilation and perfusion matching and thereby improved oxygenation, noted by increased PaO_2/FiO_2 ratio in the prone position [30]. However, they also noted a subsection of patients that did not improve oxygenation, had higher driving pressures, and had higher ventilator ratios, perhaps because of more severe disease; these patients had a higher mortality. Unlike typical ARDS, the lung compliance did not change with proning. This raises the question on whether the phenotype could determine the response to different maneuvers [19, 24]. Patients with type L pneumonia have low elastance, normal compliance, and low oxygen recruitability: therefore, these patients may not respond as well to proning [24]. In these patients, proning facilitates pulmonary blood flow rather than the recruitment of alveoli; it is used as a rescue maneuver. Currently, there are no strong recommendations for prone ventilation in mechanically ventilated COVID-19 patients with ARDS [26]. However, based on the results of the large trial in non-COVID patients and the observational data collected during the pandemic, proning ventilation might continue being offered along protective lung strategies in patients with C-ARDS. This indication should be individualized and considered upon assessment of the singular patient and the phenotype of the lung damage presented. It is also important to consider that while proning is a relatively effective and cheap maneuver, it does require experienced personnel to aid in repositioning the patients to avoid device displacement and to avoid development of pressure ulcers. Furthermore, patients often require frequent monitoring due to the risk for hemodynamic instability, the increased use of sedatives and neuromuscular blocking agents, as well as the need for position changes. Proning requires significant resources, which can be a challenge for the healthcare system and has been an even greater stress amidst a pandemic. Institutions that use proning as a treatment tool for patients with C-ARDS have shown success in the designation of dedicated proning teams, which have been able to meet the demands for the rotational maneuvers required for these patients in a timely manner [31].

Prior to the pandemic, there has been limited research into the utility of proning in the non-intubated patient. Due to the resource constraints and the overwhelming number of people affected by the disease, awake proning has been encouraged in practice. Small observational studies done in several countries have shown improved oxygenation in non-intubated COVID patients [32–34]. One randomized control trial on 125 patients showed an improved 28-day mortality benefit when awake prone position was instituted within 24 h of initiation of high-flow nasal cannula treatment [35]. Larger randomized clinical trials are needed for further evaluation on its benefit. Currently, no sufficient evidence supports its efficacy and it continues to be a subject of discussion.

5 Recruitment Maneuvers

As previously discussed, C-ARDS does not appear to behave as the "classic" ARDS. This begs the question: Do treatment techniques studied under "classic" ARDS deserve a second look? One of the many strategies that come to mind is the implementation of recruitment maneuvers. These tactics are not identified by any one particular method, but rather as a group of parameter adjustments made on mechanically ventilated patients to improve oxygenation. Within this group, there lies a "sigh" approach, delivering breaths at a specified interval with increased pressure/volume versus a "staircase" approach with incremental increases in PEEP [36, 37]. There does not appear to be a consensus in terms of preference for which method is superior.

Studies supporting these maneuvers in ARDS show improvement in oxygenation, although they remain inconclusive in terms of mortality benefit. The consequences of increasing airway pressures must also be considered. There is a risk of hemodynamic compromise especially in this already very critically ill group as well as further barotrauma. Although the true incidence of airway injury is unclear, including pneumomediastinum and pneumothorax, it does appear to be a major concern with each increasing wave of C-ARDS patients.

Just as in the "classic" ARDS patients, it remains unclear if recruitment maneuvers have a positive effect on the C-ARDS patients. Following the current NIH COVID-19 Treatment Guidelines, it is recommended "using recruitment maneuvers rather than not using" them (grade recommendation IIa). They also recommend against using "staircase" approach as there appears to be a signal of increased mortality in the reviewed literature (grade recommendation IIa) [38]. While there remains a need for additional studies, we recommend directing the treatment in an individualized manner tailored to every patient's characteristic and status.

6 Rescue Maneuvers

The efficacy of rescue maneuvers depends largely on the pathophysiology of the C-ARDS phenotype, and they require individual consideration. In type I COVID pneumonia, hypoxemia is due to vascular dysregulation and V/Q mismatch. Therefore, the utility of agents such as nitric oxide and pulmonary vasodilators may not be as effective [19]. While these agents may have some utility in type 2 COVID pneumonia patients, especially in those who also suffer from a component of pulmonary hypertension, its routine use is not currently recommended [26].

ECMO has been used historically used in ARDS patients with refractory hypoxemia despite maximal optimization of ventilator settings and other less invasive maneuvers. No clear literature review or randomized trial has been conducted to determine the effects of ECMO support in COVID patients; however, a small study demonstrated that 90-day mortality was worse in patients supported by ECMO [39]. As the rationale behind those results was not clear, further evaluation is required to determine the benefit of ECMO as a general treatment option for patients with C-ARDS and refractory hypoxemia despite maximized mechanical ventilation. Currently, ECMO is not routinely recommended as a rescue therapy. Individual selection of candidates must be carefully performed, and it is certainly limited by its extensive resource utilization required [26].

7 Sedation and Neuromuscular Blockade (NMB)

Current sedation practice is ultimately based on the Society of Critical Care Medicine's PADIS guidelines [40]. The general recommendations are focused on multidisciplinary sedation protocols with special attention on assessing and maintaining light sedation while also focusing on analgesic-based sedative agents as a first choice. Neuromuscular blockade and its mortality benefit continue to be a topic of study. ACURASYS trial showed 90-day mortality benefit with early (within 48 hours) NMB [41]. However, the more recent follow-up trial, the ROSE trial, showed that there was no mortality benefit between light sedation with neuromuscular blockade and early deep sedation and noted deep sedatives causing some ventilator asynchrony [42].

Despite prior practice, intubated COVID-19 patients generally received longer duration of sedation, with many of them also receiving more benzodiazepines in comparison to their non-COVID counterparts. In a recent study, mobilization, spontaneous breathing/awakening trials, and avoidance of benzodiazepines occurred significantly less often [43]. A large portion of the patients in the study showed neurological dysfunction with 50% developing delirium and 80% found in a coma. The prolonged and deeper sedation needs are likely multifactorial due in part to insufficient personnel resources and in part to patient clinical conditions as well as the clinical goal of decreasing patient-ventilator asynchrony as well as allowing for prone ventilation.

Overall, it is important to adhere to current guidelines and maintain the standard of practice to prevent adverse neurological events in patients.

8 Conclusions

Much is to be learnt yet in regard to mechanical ventilation for C-ARDS. The phenotype differences mark clinical and radiologic differentiation in the different stages of the disease and might influence the response of the lungs to ventilation parameters. Clinicians must evaluate every patient and act upon experience and careful observation and procced to management based on clinical response from each individual patient. Adherence to protocols and standardization of care, including mechanical ventilation methods, is suggested as best practice to avoid variations of care and mismanagement.

In addition, literature review and adapting methods described in some articles must be carefully observed and considered in the context of each patient, avoiding adapting absolute concepts without the necessary individual evaluation. In the rapidly changing environment of COVID-19, clinicians must exercise the best judgment and use their experience as well as their colleagues' experience in establishing the best ventilatory strategies to treat patients with C-ARDS.

References

1. McMahon DE, Peters GA, Ivers LC, Freeman EE. Global resource shortages during COVID-19: bad news for low-income countries. PLoS Negl Trop Dis. 2020;14:e0008412. https://doi.org/10.1371/journal.pntd.0008412.
2. Goodman S, Chokshi N. How the world ran out of everything. NY Times. 2021. Updated 22 Oct 2021.
3. Schultz MJ, Serpa Neto A, Paulus F. Battling COVID-19 related mortality: from a fight for ventilators to a cry for oxygen. Lancet. 2021;9(9):939–41.

4. Centers for Disease Control and Prevention. National Center for Health Statistics. Accessed online 15 Dec 2021.
5. Auld S, Caridi-Scheibe M, Blum JM, the Emory COVID-19 Quality and Clinical Research Collaborative. ICU and ventilator mortality among critically ill adults with coronavirus disease 2019. Crit Care Med. 2020;48(9):e799–804. https://doi.org/10.1097/CCm.0000000000004457.
6. Richardson S, Hirsch JS, Narasimhan M, et al. Presenting characteristics, comorbidities, and outcomes among 5700 patients hospitalized with COVID-19 in the New York City area. JAMA. 2020;323(20):2052–9. https://doi.org/10.1001/jama.2020.6775.
7. Nicholson JN, Wooster L, Sigurslid HH, et al. Estimating risk of mechanical ventilation and in-hospital mortality among adult COVID-19 patients admitted to Mass General Brigham: the VICE and DICE scores. EClinicalMedicine. 2021;33:100765. https://doi.org/10.1016/j.eclinm.2021.100765.
8. Ducharme J. Why ventilators might not be working as well for COVID-19 patients as doctors hoped. Time magazine. 2020. Accessed online.
9. Yang X, Yu Y, Xu J, et al. Clinical course and outcomes of critically ill patients with SARS-CoV-2 pneumonia in Wuhan, China: a single-centered, retrospective, observational study. Lancet Respir Med. 2020;8:475–81; (published online Feb 21). https://doi.org/10.1016/S2213-2600(20)30079-5.
10. Nauka P, Chen J, Shiloh A, Eisen L, Fein D. Practice, outcomes, and complications of emergent endotracheal intubation by critical care practitioners during the COVID-19 pandemic. Chest. 2021;160:2112. https://doi.org/10.1016/j.chest.2021.06.008.
11. Orser BA. Recommendations for endotracheal intubation of COVID-19 patients. Anesth Analg. 2020;130(5):1109–10. https://doi.org/10.1213/ANE.0000000000004803.
12. Tran K, Cimon K, Severn M, Pessoa-Silva CL, Conly J. Aerosol generating procedures and risk of transmission of acute respiratory infections to healthcare workers: a systematic review. PLoS One. 2012;7:e35797. https://doi.org/10.1371/journal.pone.0035797.
13. Tobin MJ, Laghi F, Jubran A. Caution about early intubation and mechanical ventilation in COVID-19. Ann Intensive Care. 2020;10:78. https://doi.org/10.1186/s13613-020-00692-6.
14. Intensive Care Society. 2020. Use of continuous positive airway pressure (CPAP) for COVID-19 positive patients. www.ics.ac.uk
15. Pandya A, Kaur N, Sacher D, O'Corragain O, Salerno D, Desai P, et al. Ventilatory mechanics in early vs late intubation in a cohort of coronavirus disease 2019 patients with ARDS. Chest. 2021;159(2):653–6. https://doi.org/10.1016/j.chest.2020.08.2084.
16. Papoutsi E, Giannakoulis V, Xourgia E, Routsi C, Kotanidou A, Siempos I. Effect of timing of intubation on clinical outcomes of critically ill patients with COVID-19: a systematic review and meta-analysis of non-randomized cohort studies. Crit Care. 2021;25(1):121. https://doi.org/10.1186/s13054-021-03540-6.
17. Grieco DL, Menga LS, Eleuteri D, Antonelli M. Patient self- inflicted lung injury: implications for acute hypoxaemic respiratory failure and ARDS patients on non-invasive support. Minerva Anaestesiol. 2019;85:1014–23. https://doi.org/10.23736/s0375-9393.19.13418-9.
18. Gattinoni L, Marini JJ, Camporota L. The respiratory drive: an overlooked tile of COVID-19 pathophysiology. Am J Respir Crit Care Med. 2020;202(8):1079–80.
19. Gattinoni L, Chiumello D, Rossi S. COVID-19 pneumonia: ARDS or not? Crit Care. 2020;24(1):154. https://doi.org/10.1186/s13054-020-02880-z.
20. Weaver L, Das A, Saffaran S, et al. High risk of patient self-inflicted lung injury in COVID-19 with frequently encountered spontaneous breathing patterns: a computational modelling study. Ann Intensive Care. 2021;11:109. https://doi.org/10.1186/s13613-021-00904-7.
21. Panwar R, Madotto F, Laffey J, van Haren F. Compliance phenotypes in early acute respiratory distress syndrome before the COVID-19 pandemic. Am J Respir Crit Care Med. 2020;202(9):1244–52. https://doi.org/10.1164/rccm.202005-2046oc.
22. Gattinoni L, Marini J. Isn't it time to abandon ARDS? The COVID-19 lesson. Crit Care. 2021;25(1):326. https://doi.org/10.1186/s13054-021-03748-6.

23. Protti A, Santini A, Pennati F, Chiurazzi C, Cressoni M, Ferrari M, et al. Lung response to a higher positive end-expiratory pressure in mechanically ventilated patients with COVID-19. Chest. 2021;161:979. https://doi.org/10.1016/j.chest.2021.10.012.
24. Gattinoni L, Chiumello D, Caironi P, Busana M, Romitti F, Brazzi L, Camporota L. COVID-19 pneumonia: different respiratory treatments for different phenotypes? Intensive Care Med. 2020;46(6):1099–102. https://doi.org/10.1007/s00134-020-06033-2.
25. Maslove D, Sibley S, Boyd J, Goligher E, Munshi L, Bogoch I, Rochwerg B. Complications of critical COVID-19: diagnostic and therapeutic considerations for the mechanically ventilated patient. Chest. 2022;161(4):989–98. https://doi.org/10.1016/j.chest.2021.10.011.
26. Alhazzani W, Evans L, Alshamsi F, Møller M, Ostermann M, Prescott H, et al. Surviving sepsis campaign guidelines on the management of adults with coronavirus disease 2019 (COVID-19) in the ICU: first update. Crit Care Med. 2021;49(3):e219–34. https://doi.org/10.1097/ccm.0000000000004899.
27. Boscolo A, Sella N, Lorenzoni G, et al. Static compliance and driving pressure are associated with ICU mortality in intubated COVID-19 ARDS. Crit Care. 2021;25:263. https://doi.org/10.1186/s13054-021-03667-6.
28. Courcelle R, Gaudry S, Serck N, et al. Neuromuscular blocking agents (NMBA) for COVID-19 acute respiratory distress syndrome: a multicenter observational study. Crit Care. 2020;24:446.
29. Guérin C, Reignier J, Richard J, Beuret P, Gacouin A, Boulain T, et al. Prone positioning in severe acute respiratory distress syndrome. N Engl J Med. 2013;368(23):2159–68. https://doi.org/10.1056/nejmoa1214103.
30. Langer T, Brioni M, Guzzardella A, Carlesso E, Cabrini L, Castelli G, et al. Prone position in intubated, mechanically ventilated patients with COVID-19: a multi-centric study of more than 1000 patients. Crit Care. 2021;25(1):128. https://doi.org/10.1186/s13054-021-03552-2.
31. Wells C, Zhang Z, Huelskamp S, Hughes E, Aguila D, Sevillano M, Garrett L, Acquah S, Chan C, Kohli-Seth R. Prone team: a large-scale prone position initiative during COVID-19 pandemic. J Nurs Adm. 2021;51(4):E13–7. https://doi.org/10.1097/NNA.0000000000001003. PMID: 33734184.
32. Sarma A, Calfee C. Prone positioning in awake, nonintubated patients with COVID-19. JAMA Intern Med. 2020;180(11):1539. https://doi.org/10.1001/jamainternmed.2020.3027.
33. Rosén J, von Oelreich E, Fors D, et al. Awake prone positioning in patients with hypoxemic respiratory failure due to COVID-19: the PROFLO multicenter randomized clinical trial. Crit Care. 2021;25:209. https://doi.org/10.1186/s13054-021-03602-9.
34. Sztajnbok J, Maselli-Schoueri JH, Cunha de Resende Brasil LM, Farias de Sousa L, Cordeiro CM, Sansão Borges LM, Malaque CMSA. Prone positioning to improve oxygenation and relieve respiratory symptoms in awake, spontaneously breathing non-intubated patients with COVID-19 pneumonia. Respir Med Case Rep. 2020;30:101096. https://doi.org/10.1016/j.rmcr.2020.101096. Epub 2020 May 19. PMID: 32455107; PMCID: PMC7236748.
35. Kaur R, Vines D, Mirza S, Elshafei A, Jackson J, Harnois L, et al. Early versus late awake prone positioning in non-intubated patients with COVID-19. Crit Care. 2021;25(1):340. https://doi.org/10.1186/s13054-021-03761-9.
36. Santos RS, Silva PL, Pelosi P, Rocco PR. Recruitment maneuvers in acute respiratory distress syndrome: the safe way is the best way. World J Crit Care Med. 2015;4(4):278–86. Published 2015 Nov 4. https://doi.org/10.5492/wjccm.v4.i4.278.
37. Cammarota G, Simonte R, De Robertis E. PEEP-induced alveolar recruitment in patients with COVID-19 pneumonia: take the right time! Crit Care. 2021;25:163. https://doi.org/10.1186/s13054-021-03573-x.
38. COVID-19 Treatment Guidelines Panel. Coronavirus disease 2019 (COVID-19) treatment guidelines. National Institutes of Health. https://www.covid19treatmentguidelines.nih.gov/.
39. Barbaro R, MacLaren G, Boonstra P, Combes A, Agerstrand C, Annich G, et al. Extracorporeal membrane oxygenation for COVID-19: evolving outcomes from the international extracorporeal life support organization registry. Lancet. 2021;398(10307):1230–8. https://doi.org/10.1016/s0140-6736(21)01960-7.

40. Devlin J, Skrobik Y, Gélinas C, Needham D, Slooter A, Pandharipande P, et al. Clinical practice guidelines for the prevention and management of pain, agitation/sedation, delirium, immobility, and sleep disruption in adult patients in the ICU. Crit Care Med. 2018;46(9):e825–73. https://doi.org/10.1097/ccm.0000000000003299.
41. Papazian L, Forel J, Gacouin A, Penot-Ragon C, Perrin G, Loundou A, et al. Neuromuscular blockers in early acute respiratory distress syndrome. N Engl J Med. 2010;363(12):1107–16. https://doi.org/10.1056/nejmoa1005372.
42. Early neuromuscular blockade in the acute respiratory distress syndrome. N Engl J Med. 2019;380(21):1997–2008. https://doi.org/10.1056/nejmoa1901686.
43. Pun B, Badenes R, Heras La Calle G, Orun O, Chen W, Raman R, et al. Prevalence and risk factors for delirium in critically ill patients with COVID-19 (COVID-D): a multicentre cohort study. Lancet Respir Med. 2021;9(3):239–50.

Prone Position During Mechanical Ventilation

Orlando Pérez-Nieto, Carlos Sánchez, and Eder Zamarrón

1 Introduction

Because the mechanisms of hypoxemia in acute respiratory distress syndrome (ARDS) are usually several, the strategies proposed to improve oxygenation are multiple; most of them focus on increasing transpulmonary pressure (Ptp) through increased pressure airway, particularly with elevated levels of positive end-expiratory pressure (PEEP). One of the ways to increase Ptp in patients with ARDS that do not require modifying the ventilator parameters is to apply the prone position, which has shown encouraging results during the last decade [1].

2 Pathophysiological Implications of the Prone Position in IMV and ARDS

The prone position in patients under invasive mechanical ventilation (IMV) has been widely studied and used for the treatment of ARDS patients for more than 45 years. This posture has shown beneficial effects on gas exchange and ventilatory mechanics compared to the supine position. In the supine posture, the most dependent alveoli are small due to lung compression from the heart and abdominal

O. Pérez-Nieto
Hospital General San Juan del Río, Querétaro, Mexico

C. Sánchez (✉)
Hospital General IESS, Quevedo, Ecuador

E. Zamarrón
Hospital Regional #6 IMSS, Madero City, Tamaulipas, Mexico

J. Hidalgo et al. (eds.), *Personalized Mechanical Ventilation*,
https://doi.org/10.1007/978-3-031-14138-6_12

contents as compared with the prone posture. During inspiration, the distribution of local ventilation is more uniform in the prone posture because the alveolar volumes are more uniform [2].

Gas exchange is markedly improved in the prone position. The alveolar opening of the dependent zones increases the contact area of the alveolar-capillary membrane, favoring the diffusion of O_2 and CO_2. The increase in airy areas manifests clinically as a reduction in atelectasis and microatelectasis. Blood perfusion is also increased at the level of the pulmonary capillaries because the posterobasal areas of the lungs are the ones with the highest capillarity and blood flow; this flow contacts recruited alveoli, reducing short circuits and optimizing the ventilation/perfusion index (V/Q) [2].

3 The Evidence for the Prone Position in ARDS and IMV

The prospective, randomized, controlled, multicenter PROSEVA study demonstrated that the prone position is a strategy that improves outcomes in patients with moderate-severe ARDS when combined with low VT. Patients with a fraction of inspired oxygen (FiO_2) of less than 150 mmHg, an FiO_2 of at least 0.6, a positive end-expiratory pressure of at least 5 cmH_2O, and a tidal volume close to 6 mL were included in this study per kilogram of predicted body weight. When the prone position was applied for more than 16 continuous hours per day, it was associated with lower mortality at 28 and 90 days versus the supine position [HR 0.44 (95% CI, 0.29–0.67)] [3]. From this study, it is formally recommended to pronate patients with moderate-to-severe ARDS under IMV who do not respond favorably, and increased PEEP or neuromuscular paralysis in this position may be considered, which could contribute to improved survival [4].

In patients with COVID-19 under IMV, it may be recommended to start this position <48 h after intubation and with a PaO_2/FiO_2 ratio <200, since early pronation was associated with lower mortality compared to those who prone after intubation for 48 h in a 68-site multicenter cohort (hazard ratio, 0.84; 95% CI, 0.73–0.97) [5]. A meta-analysis that included 5 randomized controlled trials showed in favor of the prone position with respect to a decrease in mortality in patients with ARDS [($P = 0.04$, 95% CI Risk Ratio 0.74 (0.56–0.99)] [6]. The COVID-19 pandemic made the use of the prone position popular earlier [7], although the evidence regarding the survival benefit in this type of patient is still inconclusive [8, 9].

The proposed criteria for classifying a patient with ARDS as a prone responder are >20 mmHg increase in arterial partial pressure of oxygen (PaO_2), >10% increase in the ratio of arterial partial pressure of oxygen over FiO2 (PaO_2/FiO_2), and a decrease in arterial carbon dioxide pressure ($paCO_2$) of at least >1 mmHg at 4 h after the start of the maneuver. However, an increase in peripheral oxygen saturation (SpO_2) and a decrease in driving pressure (DP) at the expense of a reduction in plateau pressure (Ppl) due to an increase in static lung compliance (Cst) may be sufficient to show improvement [3].

4 Adverse Events Related to the Prone Position in IMV

The prone position in patients under IMV is not exempt from adverse effects. Absolute contraindications to placing an intubated patient in the prone position are vertebral instability (mainly at the cervical and thoracic levels) and intracranial hypertension. The most common scenario in which both cases occur is polytrauma that includes pulmonary contusions and traumatic brain or spinal cord injury, although other causes of lung damage may be involved, such as transfusion related acute lung injury (TRALI) or sepsis. It is recommended, in case of spinal injury, to fix the spine surgically and then start the prone position. In case of suspected intracranial hypertension, it is recommended to measure intracranial pressure (ICP) invasively and not to pronate if it is >20 mmHg. If the ICP is <20 mmHg, a prone position test can be performed, but if it rises above the safety margin (>20–22 mmHg), it is recommended not to use it. Some considerations to contraindicate this posture may include severe burns to anterior regions (face, neck, chest, abdomen, or genitalia), tracheal surgery, or shock with high vasopressor or inotropic requirements. It is recommended to carry out a checklist prior to the pronation maneuver [10] (see Table 1). During or after the maneuver, some adverse events may occur, such as transient desaturation, mobilization of secretions and airway obstruction, removal of invasive devices (e.g., venous catheters, endopleural tube, orotracheal extubation), vomiting, edema in contact areas, ischemic neuropathy (commonly in

Table 1 Checklist for prone positioning (Bruni et al.)

Before the procedure
Check endotracheal tube position and fixation
Check endotracheal cuff pressure (20–30 cmH_2O)
Prepare for emergency reintubation (resuscitation bag, laryngoscope, tube, suctioning system)
Check arterial and venous catheter fixation
Lengthen lines for vascular access
Check ECMO cannulas
Check other catheters, drainage bags, or tubes whenever possible
Prepare and check patient's monitoring
Check sedation and neuromuscular blockade (if intubated)
Explain to the patient the maneuver (if awake)
Assure preoxygenation
During the run
Align arms to the body with palms up
One operator positioned at the head (coordinator)
Two operators positioned per side
Gain patient's collaboration (if awake)
After the maneuver
Check endotracheal tube (displacement, obstruction)
Check vital parameters
Check or reconnect the vascular lines (kinking)
Check patient's position (arm and head)
Protect pressure areas with dedicated materials and air mattress
Restart (and monitor) enteral nutrition

thebrachial plexus), and pressure ulcers. Pregnancy is not a contraindication for performing the prone position and should be considered in all obstetric patients with ARDS whose hypoxemia puts the life of the maternal-fetal binomial at risk [11]. Taking into account that acute respiratory failure was the first cause of death in pregnant patients during the COVID-19 pandemic, the personnel in charge must consider the associated complications and monitor frequently [12].

5 When to Return to the Supine Position?

Patients can be pronated and supinated daily if conditions allow, but the survival benefit is seen when >16 continuous strokes per day are achieved. This entails a workload for healthcare personnel, which is why it has been proposed to maintain the prone position continuously since the COVID-19 pandemic, to avoid daily turns [13]. In any case, it has been recommended to consider keeping patients in supine if a $PaO_2/FiO_2 > 150$ mmHg is maintained for more than 4 h after being supinated. A patient who again presents a considerable decrease in oxygenation could again be a candidate to be pronated; however, the benefit in this scenario is not well established [3].

6 Conclusion

The prone position is a safe and low-cost strategy that, if applied early in intubated patients under IMV with ARDS, is associated with increased oxygenation, improved ventilatory mechanics, and decreased mortality.

References

1. Gattinoni L, Carlesso E, Taccone P, Polli F, Guerin C, Mancebo J. Prone positioning improves survival in severe ARDS: a pathophysiologic review and individual patient meta-analysis. Minerva Anestesiol. 2010;76(6):448–54.
2. Johnson NJ, Luks AM, Glenny RW. Gas exchange in the prone posture. Respir Care. 2017;62(8):1097–110. https://doi.org/10.4187/respcare.05512.
3. Guérin C, Reignier J, Richard JC, et al. Prone positioning in severe acute respiratory distress syndrome. N Engl J Med. 2013;368(23):2159–68. https://doi.org/10.1056/NEJMoa1214103.
4. Papazian L, Aubron C, Brochard L, et al. Formal guidelines: management of acute respiratory distress syndrome. Ann Intensive Care. 2019;9(1):69. Published 2019 Jun 13. https://doi.org/10.1186/s13613-019-0540-9.
5. Mathews KS, Soh H, Shaefi S, et al. Prone positioning and survival in mechanically ventilated patients with coronavirus disease 2019-related respiratory failure. Crit Care Med. 2021;49(7):1026–37. https://doi.org/10.1097/CCM.0000000000004938.
6. Prone position for acute respiratory distrés síndrome: a systematic review and metanalisis. Munshi Lavenaa.

7. Hochberg C, Psoter K, Sahetya S, et al. Comparing prone positioning use in COVID-19 versus historic acute respiratory distress syndrome. Crit Care Explor. 2022;4(5):e0695. https://doi.org/10.1097/CCE.0000000000000695.
8. Shelhamer MC, Wesson PD, Solari IL, et al. Prone positioning in moderate to severe acute respiratory distress syndrome due to COVID-19: a cohort study and analysis of physiology. J Intensive Care Med. 2021;36(2):241–52. https://doi.org/10.1177/0885066620980399.
9. Langer T, Brioni M, Guzzardella A, et al. Prone position in intubated, mechanically ventilated patients with COVID-19: a multi-centric study of more than 1000 patients. Crit Care. 2021;25(1):128. Published 2021 Apr 6. https://doi.org/10.1186/s13054-021-03552-2.
10. Bruni A, Garofalo E, Longhini F. Avoiding complications during prone position ventilation. Intensive Crit Care Nurs. 2021;66:103064. https://doi.org/10.1016/j.iccn.2021.103064.
11. Deloya-Tomas E, Mondragon-Labelle T, Lopez-Fermin J, et al. Considerations for mechanical ventilation in the critically Ill obstetric patient. Crit Care Obstet Gynecol. 2020;6(4):10.
12. González-Seguel F, Pinto-Concha JJ, Aranis N, Leppe J. Adverse events of prone positioning in mechanically ventilated adults with ARDS. Respir Care. 2021;66(12):1898–911. https://doi.org/10.4187/respcare.09194.
13. Page DB, Vijaykumar K, Russell DW, et al. Prolonged prone positioning for COVID-19-induced acute respiratory distress syndrome: a randomized pilot clinical trial. Ann Am Thorac Soc. 2022;19(4):685–7. https://doi.org/10.1513/AnnalsATS.202104-498RL.

One Ventilator, Multiple Patients

Jorge E. Sinclair Ávila, Juan Pablo Herrera Berríos, Jorge Enrique Sinclair De Frias, and Allyson Hidalgo

1 Description of the Problem

Although at the beginning of the pandemic we considered COVID as a primarily pulmonary disease, the evolution of the scientific literature has led us to consider it as a multisystemic disease. The emergence of the virus drastically changed the approach through which new management guidelines are developed. The current paradigm continues to be that of evidence-based medicine, a methodology through which multiple research elements are published in order to reach a logical conclusion based on the quality of the evidence presented, usually at international meetings. Thus, a new paradigm called real-world evidence [1] emerges.

A system is defined as a complex object whose constituent parts are related to at least some of the other components either at a conceptual or at a material level. Thus, every system is in turn made up of three fundamental elements: composition, structure, and environment.

Naturally, this ventilatory strategy seeks to mitigate the damage caused by a disproportionate supply/demand of mechanical ventilation. In the field of ethics, there are criteria that differ in the selection of patients who should receive care at the expense of limiting it to another patient, a dilemma called the problem of the lesser

J. E. Sinclair Ávila
Hospital Pacífica Salud/Johns Hopkins Medicine, Panama City, Panama

J. P. Herrera Berríos
Complejo Hospitalario Dr. Arnulfo Arias Madrid, Panama City, Panama

J. E. Sinclair De Frias (✉)
Department of Physiology, Faculty of Medicine, University of Panama, Panama City, Panama

A. Hidalgo
Arizona State University, Phoenix, AZ, USA

J. Hidalgo et al. (eds.), *Personalized Mechanical Ventilation*,
https://doi.org/10.1007/978-3-031-14138-6_13

evil. Thus, the questions to consider in a scenario where a patient needs mechanical ventilation and there are no ventilators available are the following: Should the patient be connected in parallel to another patient on a single ventilator? Does it generate less harm than not doing so? Should mechanical ventilation be limited or shared?

Invasive mechanical ventilation poses a multidimensional challenge [2] to healthcare systems globally. Ventilators are a limited resource. Thus, the decision to connect a patient to a ventilator in circumstances abstracted from the pandemic is a challenge in itself. To add to the complexity, the pandemic has undermined multiple spheres of society, making obvious the gap between the demand for health sector services and the inadequacy of resources to meet that demand.

Although there is a large body of literature on COVID, the literature on the multi-patient ventilator strategy in the context of critical situations (e.g., the current pandemic) is sparse. Several authors have studied the possibility of adapting a ventilatory system to optimize the use of this resource.

2 Literature Review

The pilot study by Neyman [3] in 2006 sets out the principles of how to modify the circuit of a conventional ventilator with simulated patients. Paladino [4] conducted an experimental study in which four sheep without pulmonary pathology were ventilated, concluding that there are important variations in terms of the minute volume administered to each member of the circuit. Moreover, the results of that study are not extrapolative to the clinical context of humans. Subsequently, Branson [5, 6] showed that tidal volume varied according to changes in lung model characteristics, specifically resistance and compliance.

Further development of this concept has uncovered the problems and limitations of this technique. The consensus of several organizations is that it is impossible to manage each patient individually, and that, although patients with similar characteristics have started mechanical ventilation, the process of recovery or clinical deterioration may differ between them, a situation that merits individualized adjustments of the ventilatory mechanics. Regarding this aspect, there are currently no individual monitoring elements; all the alarms and ventilation parameters indicated correspond to the average of the patients.

The increase of more circuits can add more errors in the management of the ventilator, and additional external monitoring is required since the ventilator monitors the average pressure and volumes and not of each one. When sharing the same ventilator, there is a high risk of cross contamination, and the effectiveness of the filters is not proven in case of multiple ventilation.

Finally, in the event of cardiac arrest in a patient, it is necessary to remove the ventilation from the other patients, taking care not to generate aerosols of the virus and put healthcare personnel at risk. Even if precautions are taken, this ventilation stoppage could alter the dynamics of the ventilatory supply to the other patients.

Finally, there are ethical issues. Although the ventilator can save the life of one patient, using it with more than one patient increases the risk of critical treatment failure in all of them. This situation imposes an enormous burden on the treating physician who must decide whether to offer a technique that can save the life of a salvageable patient or subject more patients to poor treatment and consequent death.

3 Conclusions and Recommendations

Based on the current evidence, the problematic of the use of a modified ventilator for several patients involves three fundamental aspects: physiological, technical, and patient safety aspects. Thus, the use of such a circuit represents a threat to the individualized medicine approach. In the face of this, we must remember the four fundamental principles of medicine: non-maleficence, beneficence, autonomy, and justice.

The use of this technique according to the literature reviewed does not guarantee a constant respiratory minute volume for each patient coupled to the ventilatory system. Not every patient with severe COVID-19 has the same Gattinoni phenotype, so if the use of this strategy were to be considered, patients would have to be stratified based on lung compliance characteristics. In addition, the risk of pulmonary cross infection must be considered, and in the absence of resources, it is not possible to recommend the use of this strategy in a generalized manner even in the context of the current pandemic.

It is therefore advisable to develop scientific knowledge through further studies and improvement of the health infrastructure in order to provide a practical solution applicable to different institutions, whether public or private, to optimize the use of this resource in crisis situations, without compromising the quality of care provided.

The methods for implementing multiple ventilation mentioned above require specific conditions to be met, including a highly specialized center with the availability of specialists, as well as the capacity to invest in other aspects such as space conditioning, acquisition of extra material to improve monitoring, personnel training, and availability of qualified personnel 24 h a day, 7 days a week. Furthermore, it would only be indicated when all possibilities have been exhausted, including manual bagging, and could only be used for a short period of time before switching to an individual ventilator. Ethically, it must be recognized that a shared ventilator strategy is not standard medical care practice. Although the sentiment of dealing with a crisis situation such as the COVID-19 pandemic seems laudable, the available information reveals problems and uncertainties that instead of saving the life of one patient, all patients connected to the shared ventilator are put at risk. Thus, with the technical information currently available, it is not possible to support a recommendation in favor of shared ventilator to treat COVID-19 patients.

References

1. Makady A, de Boer A, Hillege H, Klungel O, Goettsch W, on behalf of GetReal Work Package 1. What is real-world data? A review of definitions based on literature and stakeholder interviews. Value Health. 2017;20(7):858–65. https://doi.org/10.1016/j.jval.2017.03.008. Epub 2017 May 11. PMID: 28712614.
2. Chang AY, Cullen MR, Harrington RA, Barry M. The impact of novel coronavirus COVID-19 on noncommunicable disease patients and health systems: a review. J Intern Med. 2021;289(4):450–62. https://doi.org/10.1111/joim.13184. Epub 2020 Oct 27. PMID: 33020988; PMCID: PMC7675448.
3. Neyman G, Irvin CB. A single ventilator for multiple simulated patients to meet disaster surge. Acad Emerg Med. 2006;13(11):1246–9. https://doi.org/10.1197/j.aem.2006.05.009. Epub 2006 Aug 2. PMID: 16885402; PMCID: PMC7164837.
4. Paladino L, Silverberg M, Charchaflieh JG, Eason JK, Wright BJ, Palamidessi N, Arquilla B, Sinert R, Manoach S. Increasing ventilator surge capacity in disasters: ventilation of four adult-human-sized sheep on a single ventilator with a modified circuit. Resuscitation. 2008;77(1):121–6. https://doi.org/10.1016/j.resuscitation.2007.10.016. Epub 2007 Dec 31. PMID: 18164798.
5. Branson RD, Rubinson L. One ventilator, multiple patients: what the data really supports. Resuscitation. 2008;79(1):171–2; author reply 172–173.
6. Branson RD, Rubinson L. A single ventilator for multiple simulated patients to meet disaster surge. Acad Emerg Med. 2006;13(12):1352–3; author reply 1353–1354.

Ventilator-Associated Pneumonia

Erika P. Plata-Menchaca, María Luisa Martínez González, and Ricard Ferrer

1 Introduction

Critically ill patients commonly need invasive mechanical ventilation (IMV) due to acute respiratory failure secondary to different pulmonary conditions. Besides, they are vulnerable to cumulative infectious complications or colonization with the local ecology of the intensive care unit (ICU).

Ventilator-associated pneumonia (VAP) represents a condition that carries a high risk of death among mechanically ventilated patients [1]. The severity of the disease and infections caused by multidrug-resistant (MDR) organisms is associated with the worst prognosis. The latest international guidelines in Europe and America serve as tools for clinical practice in VAP [1–3]. Along with the 2016 Surviving Sepsis Campaign guidelines, the European and American VAP guidelines recommend that appropriate empirical antimicrobial therapy be administered. However, the appropriateness of empirical therapy may sometimes be a challenging and

E. P. Plata-Menchaca
Vall d'Hebron Institute of Research, Vall d'Hebron Hospital Campus, Barcelona, Spain
e-mail: erika.plata@vhir.org

M. L. M. González
Intensive Care Department, Hospital Universitario General de Catalunya, Barcelona, Spain

R. Ferrer (✉)
Vall d'Hebron Institute of Research, Vall d'Hebron Hospital Campus, Barcelona, Spain

Intensive Care Department, Hospital Universitari Vall d'Hebron, Vall d'Hebron Hospital Campus, Barcelona, Spain

Centro de Investigación Biomédica en Red de Enfermedades Respiratorias (CIBER), Madrid, Spain
e-mail: r.ferrer@vhebron.net

J. Hidalgo et al. (eds.), *Personalized Mechanical Ventilation*,
https://doi.org/10.1007/978-3-031-14138-6_14

complicated process. The inherent risk of acquiring MDR organisms due to treatment may lead to adverse outcomes and increased mortality. Advances in developing tools for the early and accurate diagnosis of VAP patients and antimicrobial stewardship will reduce the change of receiving an inadequate empirical treatment and exposure to unnecessary antibiotics.

In this chapter, we propose an approach to the diagnosis, risk factors, prognosis, prevention, and management of VAP, including empirical and targeted use of antibiotics in the context of MDR organisms. In addition, carbapenem-sparing strategies will be reviewed to improve antimicrobial stewardship strategies [4, 5]. We reviewed the best available publications on each topic and simplified the research process for critical care clinicians.

2 The Impact of Ventilator-Associated Pneumonia

VAP is a frequent complication among ICU patients and is associated with adverse outcomes and increased healthcare costs [6, 7]. The mean cost of VAP in the United States oscillates between 9986 US$ and 54,503 US$, and a median increased hospital stay of 9.6 days [8]. Attributable mortality of VAP is around 13%, depending on the population studied and disease severity [9].

VAP is a common complication in mechanically ventilated patients with severe acute respiratory syndrome coronavirus 2 (SARS-CoV-2) respiratory failure (40–65%) [10, 11] and patients with acute respiratory distress syndrome (ARDS) (30%) [12]. In the general ICU population, the risk of VAP is approximately 18% [13]. In some studies, microbiological surveillance and identification of ventilator-associated events enable better recognition of VAP among mechanically ventilated patients [14]. Improved approaches to prevention and prescription of appropriate empirical and targeted treatments determine favorable outcomes.

3 Epidemiology

Firstly, clinicians should differentiate VAP from ventilated hospital-acquired pneumonia or ICU-hospital-acquired pneumonia, as clinical implications, prognosis, and approach to treatment may vary [15, 16]. VAP is a subtype of hospital-acquired pneumonia and is defined as lung infection developing after 48 h of IMV. Ventilated hospital-acquired pneumonia is pneumonia developing after 48 h of hospital admission, and its severity warrants the need for IMV. Hospital-ICU-acquired pneumonia accounts for pneumonia developing after 48 h of ICU admission without IMV. Recently, the presence of ventilator-associated tracheobronchitis (VAT) was recognized as a possible predisposing condition for VAP, and its incidence has been reported to be similar [17]. In this chapter, ventilated hospital-acquired pneumonia, hospital-ICU acquired pneumonia, and VAT will not be discussed.

Although the incidence of VAP has globally reduced, it is overwhelming. In Europe, the incidence of VAP was 8.9 episodes/1000 days of IMV, as reported by the European Centre for Disease Prevention and Control (ECDC) [18]. In the United States, the incidence reported is between 1.2 and 8.5 cases/1000 days of IMV, depending on the data source [14, 19]. In addition, the incidence of VAP may vary according to the definition used [20]. The prevalence of VAP also varies depending on the diagnostic criteria and setting [21], due to different definitions, diagnostic resources, and type of patients admitted. The highest incidence of VAP is observed in patients with SARS-CoV-2 respiratory failure [10], ARDS [12], sepsis [22], traumatic brain injury [23], and extracorporeal membrane oxygenation (ECMO) support [24].

In the ICU, nearly half of the patients will acquire an infection. The most common healthcare-acquired infections in the ICU are respiratory infections (65%) [25, 26]. From 10 to 40% of patients on IMV for more than 48 hours will develop VAP [27]. The duration of IMV is one of the most important risk factors for VAP [28], and the attributed mortality increases with the time of onset of VAP. Early-onset VAP is associated with a mortality rate of 19.2%, and late-onset VAP of 31.4% [29]. Some authors have reported that secondary infections in the ICU occur most commonly in patients with sepsis or high acute severity scores; such infections contribute modestly to overall mortality [22].

VAP is associated with adverse outcomes in critically ill patients. The presence of this condition increases the risk of 30-day mortality by 38%. However, compared with ICU-hospital-acquired pneumonia, the risk of 30-day mortality may be lower for VAP (38% vs. 82%) [30]. VAP has been associated with increased ICU stay and duration of IMV [21]. The crude mortality rates of VAP range between 24 and 72%, with high mortality associated with *Pseudomonas aeruginosa* infection [31].

3.1 Risk Factors for VAP

Among risk factors associated with VAP, patient-related factors include inadequate hand hygiene of healthcare workers, inappropriate manipulation of respiratory support devices, acute or chronic severe disease, prolonged IMV, altered mental consciousness, malnutrition, diabetes mellitus, chronic kidney disease, smoking, chronic pulmonary diseases, and alcoholism. ICU-related factors include the presence of sepsis, ARDS, support with ECMO, burns, traumatic brain injury, prolonged sedation, abdominal or thoracic surgery, intra-abdominal hypertension, use of corticosteroids or other immunosuppressive drugs, and overuse or misuse of antimicrobials [1, 12, 23, 27, 28]. Recently, hyperoxemia has been identified as an important risk factor for VAP [32]. Risk factors for VAP may also increase the risk for infections due to MDR organisms and determine prognosis.

4 Etiology

Different characteristics predispose individuals to certain pathogens; individual risk factors and disease severity are determinants. In most cases, the predominant pathogens include *P. aeruginosa*, *S. aureus*, *Acinetobacter spp.*, *Klebsiella spp.*, and *Enterobacteriaceae spp.* [13]. In a study of tertiary care hospitals in China, Huang et al. described a high incidence of MDR pathogens, such as carbapenem-resistant *Acinetobacter baumannii* (44%), carbapenem-resistant *Klebsiella pneumoniae* (44%), carbapenem-resistant *P. aeruginosa* (59.5%), methicillin-resistant *S. aureus* (MRSA) (60%), and *S. maltophilia* 3.8%. In contrast, the incidence of drug-resistant pathogens as the cause of VAP is different from these data in Spain (MRSA: 12.2%; carbapenem-resistant *A. baumannii*: 75%; carbapenem-resistant *P. aeruginosa*: 36.4%; carbapenem-resistant *K. pneumoniae* (CPK): 5.88%) [33]. Knowledge of the local ecology is a determinant of the risk of colonization of the airway and developing VAP [34].

5 Risk Factors for Multidrug-Resistant Organisms

There are significant differences in the local prevalence of MDR organisms [35], and local antibiotic resistance is strongly affected by local antibiotic prescription policies. Each institution should analyze their local epidemiological data and not rely on national or regional data. In Spain, the 2019 ENVIN-HELICS report quantified the antibiotic resistance of the most important microorganisms. The report described all data related to the expected resistance rates in the different ICUs [33].

Different risk factors have been described for VAP due to MDR organisms (Fig. 1) [2]. Some of them include local ecology with a high prevalence of MDR

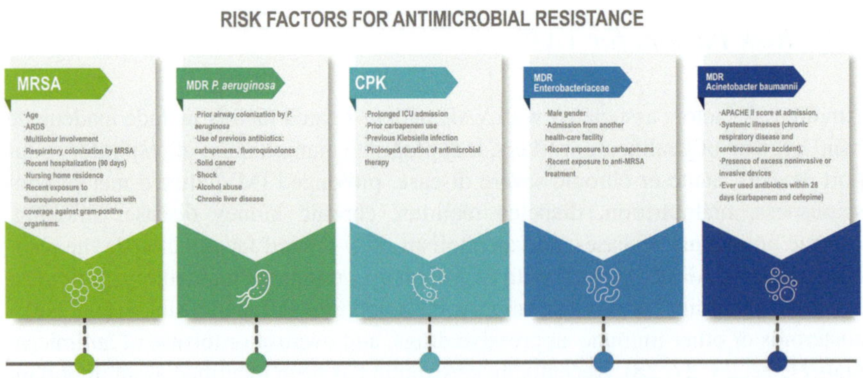

Fig. 1 Risk factors for antimicrobial resistance. [5, 36–47]. MRSA denotes methicillin-resistant *S. aureus*. *MDR* multidrug-resistant, *CPK* carbapenemase-producing *Klebsiella spp.*, *ARDS* acute respiratory distress syndrome

organisms, presence of septic shock, recent hospitalization or current hospitalization for >5 days, known colonization by MDR organisms, and previous use of broad-spectrum antibiotics. However, reliable discrimination of infection due to certain MDR organisms by only assessing individual risk factors is challenging. Microbiological surveillance and local epidemiology settle their relevance for that purpose, as well [34]. The MDR organisms most commonly involved in VAP are MDR *Pseudomonas aeruginosa*, methicillin-resistant *Staphylococcus aureus* (MRSA), extended-spectrum beta-lactamase-producing enterobacteria (ESBL-E), *Acinetobacter baumannii,* and carbapenemase-producing *Enterobacteriaceae* (CPE).

Once a patient is known to be colonized by an MDR organism, empiric antimicrobial treatment should target such a pathogen only if previously described as a potential cause of the suspected infection. The location of colonization is important.

6 Clinical and Microbiological Diagnosis

VAP is pneumonia occurring after 48 h of endotracheal intubation. Pneumonia is defined in the 2005 guidelines as a new lung infiltrate, and clinical evidence shows that it is of an infectious origin (e.g., the new onset of fever, purulent sputum, leukocytosis), with decline in oxygenation [27].

According to the US Centers for Disease Control and Prevention (CDC) metrics, VAP is an infection-related ventilator-associated complication, which includes the following [48]:

- New or progressive infiltrate, consolidation, or cavitation
- Fever (>38 °C or >100.4 °F) **OR** leukocytosis (≥12,000 WBC/μL) or leukopenia (<4000 WBC/μL)
- A positive culture for a pathogenic organism in an adequate sputum or bronchoalveolar lavage sample with observed ≥25 neutrophils/low-power field **AND**
- Decreasing oxygenation after at least two calendar days of clinical stability (≥2 days of stable or decreasing daily minimum PEEP followed by a rise in daily minimum PEEP of ≥2.5 cmH_2O, sustained for ≥2 days, or ≥2 days of stable or decreasing daily minimum FiO_2 followed by an increase in daily minimum FiO_2 of ≥0.15 points, sustained for ≥2 days).

However, clinical guidelines did not consider the CDC criteria for diagnosis at bedside, as the aim of the measurement of these events was to improve surveillance and quality improvement [1]. Thus, the 2005 guidelines' definition was not amended in the 2016 US guidelines as they are clinically useful.

Obtaining cultures before initiation of therapy is a priority in all cases, aimed at targeting treatments once a pathogen is isolated. The use of quantitative cultures and invasive sampling is a matter of controversy, and different approaches are implemented in the United States and Europe. The US guidelines advocate for the use of noninvasive samples and semiquantitative cultures [1]. The European guidelines recommend the use of invasive quantitative samples prior to the prescription of any antibiotic treatment [2]. This recommendation is intended to improve the accuracy of the results and reduce antibiotic exposure in stable patients with VAP. However, clinicians should consider possible deleterious effects of invasive techniques (e.g., bronchoscopy) on gas exchange in unstable patients with septic shock or ARDS [29]. At least one meta-analysis and a randomized controlled trial have compared qualitative and quantitative samples to diagnose VAP. Such studies found no differences in mortality or other important clinical outcomes [49, 50]. Qualitative diagnostic approaches (endotracheal aspirates) increase the chance of positivity of cultures [51]. However, overidentification of pathogens carries a risk of overtreatment if other clinical criteria are not considered.

Microbiologically confirmed VAP involves a microorganism isolated from respiratory or blood samples in a patient with a suspicion of pneumonia. Microbiological isolations should be considered as a definite etiology of VAP under clinical judgment.

7 Rapid Diagnostic Tests for Early Targeting of Treatments

The use of next-generation rapid and noninvasive diagnostic tests is promising and will optimize diagnostic approaches and empiric antibiotic treatment. Rapid diagnostic tests include the analysis of the exhalome, chromogenic tests, and multiplex polymerase chain reaction (MPCR) tests. When using bronchoalveolar lavage samples [sensitivity of 89.2% and specificity of 97.1%] and endotracheal aspirates [sensitivity of 71.8% and specificity of 96.6% (range, 95.4–97.5%)], MPCR assays are useful for the detection of microbiological agents [52, 53]. The BioFire FilmArray Blood Culture (BCID) panel has a sensitivity of 78.6%, a specificity of 98.1%, a positive predictive value of 78.6%, and a negative predictive value of 96.6% in respiratory samples for the 1-h identification of causative agents of VAP [54].

8 The Importance of Delivering an Appropriate Empirical Antibiotic Treatment

Antibiotics have become highly valuable and limited resources, and the choice of the right treatment should have a consistent and structured theoretical and practical basis. Clinicians should make their decisions based on the best available evidence. The removal of unnecessary treatments, de-escalation strategies, and awareness of potential side effects and drug interactions are our goals as critical care physicians [55, 56]. However, data from the National Surveillance Program of ICU-Acquired Infection in Europe Link for Infection Control through Surveillance (ENVIN-HELICS) [33] revealed that the likelihood of receiving inadequate empirical treatment for *P. aeruginosa* as the cause of VAP is around 30%, even in patients receiving combination treatment. Antimicrobial stewardship programs are antimicrobial optimization programs to minimize the effects associated with the use of antimicrobials, such as the emergence of resistance, and promote the use of cost-effective treatments [56, 57]. As of today, the ideal antibiotic has good in vitro activity, suitable efficacy in clinical trials, excellent safety profile, and low potential for the emergence of drug-resistant strains during treatment.

9 How Do I Choose the Best Empirical and Targeted Treatment for My Patient?

There are three main steps to choose an appropriate empirical treatment in VAP: establishing the severity of infection and knowing your local ecology, your patient's previous colonization, and pharmacodynamic/pharmacokinetic issues. According to the best available evidence [58–66], we propose a clinical algorithm for the empirical and targeted VAP treatment, considering local ecology, acute severity of the disease, time of diagnosis, previous colonization, resistance, available drugs, and known efficacy of antibiotics (Fig. 2). Also, the existence of risk factors for MDR organisms and comorbidities are factors to be considered when evaluating treatment options for empirical treatment [4, 5, 67–69].

Sepsis involves the presence of organ dysfunction due to infection [70]. Thus, early appropriate broad-spectrum empirical antibiotic treatment for critically ill patients with VAP and sepsis should be unquestioned [71]. Empirical therapy should cover MDR organisms previously known to be colonizing the patient or known to be prevalent in the unit. Rapid antimicrobial de-escalation will reduce the risk of emerging resistance due to the prescription of multiple antibiotics. The use of CarbaSCORE was recently proposed to identify critically ill patients in whom carbapenems would be suitable as empirical treatment [72]. However, the main limitation of the score is that it considers the presence of bacteremia or known previous colonization by MDR organisms. In sepsis, additional diagnostic procedures for that purpose may delay the initiation of treatment. Incorporating new fast microbiological techniques into clinical scores may aid clinical decisions. Other antimicrobials, such as ceftobiprole or tigecycline, are not recommended [62, 63]. There is a warning from the FDA against the use of tigecycline for the treatment of serious infections. Tigecycline is currently not approved for VAP treatment [73].

New-generation drugs have been clinically validated for the treatment of MDR organisms, such as MDR *P. aeruginosa* and ESBL-E. Some drugs are useful for improving carbapenem-sparing policies [64, 66]. Ceftolozane/tazobactam (CFT-TAZ), ceftazidime/avibactam (CAZ/AVI), and cefiderocol have broadened the treatment options for patients with VAP due to MDR organisms. Both antibiotics have good in vitro activity and low-resistance profiles [4, 5].

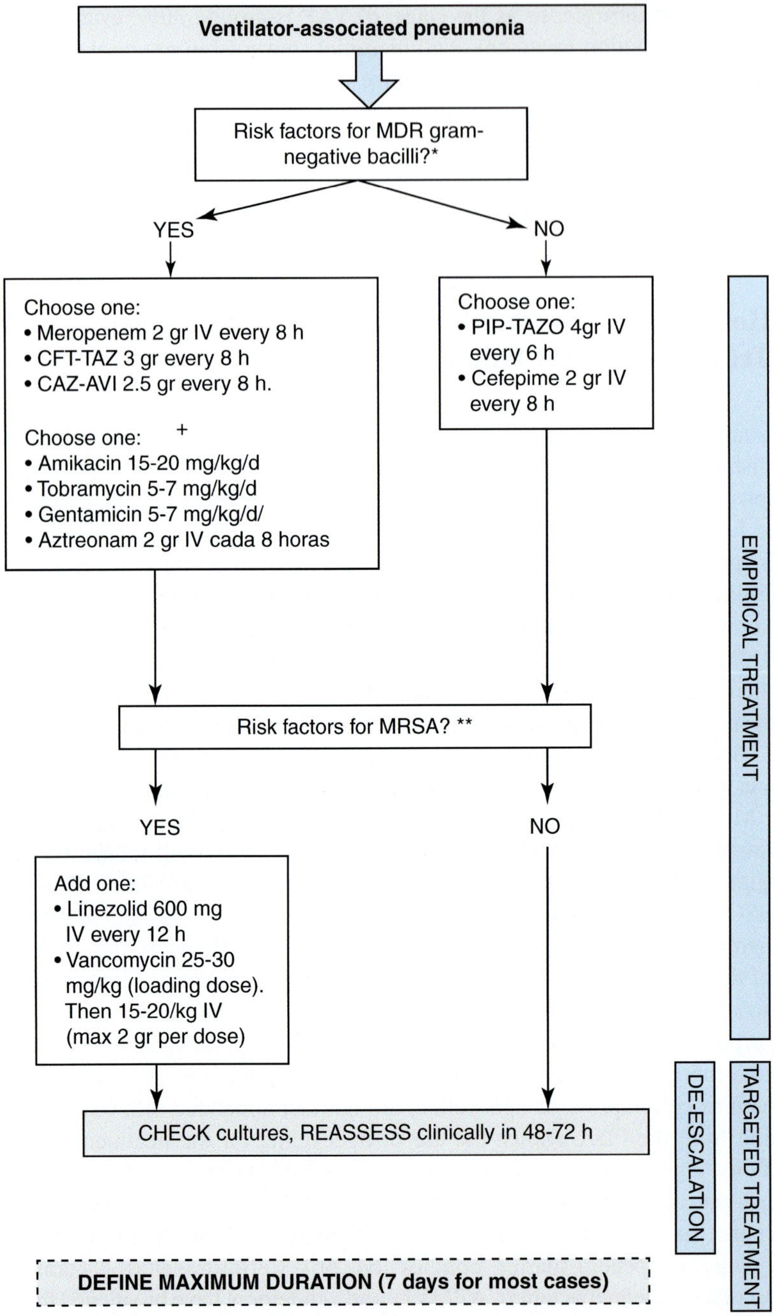

Fig. 2 Management algorithm for ventilator-associated pneumonia [58–66]. *Risk factors for MDR gram-negative bacilli: See Fig. 1. **Risk factors for MRSA: See Fig. 1. *MDR* denotes multidrug-resistant, *CFT-TAZ* ceftolozane-tazobactam, *CAZ-AVI* ceftazidime-avibactam, *PIP-TAZO* piperacillin-tazobactam, *MSRA* methicillin-resistant *S. aureus*

9.1 Suitable Antibiotics with Coverage Against Gram-Negative Organisms

Piperacillin-tazobactam. This agent is a beta-lactam/beta-lactamase inhibitor with coverage against gram-positive organisms, gram-negative organisms (including *P. aeruginosa*), and anaerobes. In patients with a low risk for MDR gram-negative bacilli (e.g., ESBL-E, MDR *P. aeruginosa*, MDR Acinetobacter spp.), this is considered an appropriate treatment for early-onset VAP, unless local ecology in the unit is unfavorable.

Meropenem. This agent is a broad-spectrum carbapenem antibiotic with excellent activity against many pathogens, including ESBL-E and *P. aeruginosa*. In patients at high risk for MDR gram-negative bacilli, it is a good option. The recommended standard dose for VAP is 2 g every 8 h [74]. Prolonged infusions of meropenem are associated with a higher clinical improvement rate and lower mortality. Thus, prolonged infusions of meropenem are recommended for patients with severe infections, such as VAP, or suspected infections due to MDR pathogens [75].

Ceftolozane/tazobactam (CFT/TAZ). This agent has the best potential to treat *P. aeruginosa* infections, presents the greatest in vitro activity against this pathogen, and has a lower resistance profile than other anti-pseudomonal agents [76]. Some in vitro studies have reported that 96% of strains are susceptible (minimum inhibitory concentration [MIC] of ≤4 μg/mL) to this agent. Thus, various experts recommend CFT/TAZ to treat *P. aeruginosa* infections [4, 67, 68]. The ASPECT-NP trial, which included 726 patients, demonstrated the non-inferiority of CFT/TAZ when compared with meropenem 1 g every 8 h. Mortality at 28 days was 24.2% vs. 37%, even in patients with initial antibiotic treatment failure (28-day mortality of 22.6% vs. 45%) [66]. The main limitation of the ASPECT-NP trial is that CFT/TAZ was compared against suboptimal doses of meropenem. The standard dose of meropenem for VAP is 2 g every 8 h [74]. The recommended dose for VAP is 3 g by intravenous infusion within 3 h every 8 h.

Ceftazidime/avibactam (CAZ/AVI). This drug is a third-generation cephalosporin with activity against serine-carbapenemase-producing *P. aeruginosa*, class A, C, and D (OXA-48) beta-lactamases. CAZ/AVI does not have activity against metallo-β-lactamases [64, 77]. Current recommendations consider the use of CAZ/AVI for the treatment of infections caused by CPK-like carbapenemase-producing *Enterobacteriaceae* [69]. There are no head-to-head comparisons between CFT/TAZ and CAZ/AVI for the treatment of MDR organisms.

Cefiderocol. This antibiotic was recently approved by the FDA to treat urinary tract infections. The CREDIBLE-CR trial found that the clinical and microbiological efficacy of cefiderocol was similar to the best available treatments in patients with infections caused by carbapenem-resistant gram-negative bacteria, including hospital-acquired pneumonia and VAP [78].

Adjunctive aerosolized antibiotics. The use of adjuvant aerosolized antibiotics for VAP is controversial, as the best available evidence does not support their use.

Two recent randomized controlled trials of VAP patients with suspected MDR gram-negative infection, the IASIS and the INHALE trials, did not achieve their primary endpoints [79, 80]. In some individual cases of VAP due to MDR *A. baumannii*, the use of aerosolized colistin may be an option as rescue therapy when other systemic treatments fail [81].

Systemic colistin is a noneffective drug for VAP. In a recent observational study, Pogue et al. compared the safety and efficacy of CFT/TAZ vs. polymyxins or aminoglycosides. CFT/TAZ was independently associated with clinical cure (adjusted odds ratio [aOR], 2.63; 95% confidence interval [CI], 1.31–5.30) [82]. The MAGIC-BULLET trial was unable to demonstrate the non-inferiority of colistin compared to meropenem, both in combination with levofloxacin [65]. Besides, intravenous colistin is not recommended, as both studies reported excessive nephrotoxicity.

9.2 Suitable Antibiotics with Coverage Against MRSA

Linezolid is an antibiotic with coverage against MRSA and can be added to empirical combined regimens for the treatment of *P. aeruginosa*. It is indicated for patients admitted in units with a prevalence of MRSA of >10–20% or for patients with known previous colonization by MRSA. Some studies show superior efficacy of linezolid than **vancomycin**, better lung tissue penetration, and lower incidence of nephrotoxicity [83, 84]. Drug-level measurements are not necessary when linezolid is used. For these reasons, we consider linezolid preferable, although clinical guidelines recommend either linezolid or vancomycin to treat MRSA infections [1]. Daptomycin should *not* be used to treat VAP, as this drug has almost no lung tissue penetrability, and it is inactivated by surfactant. For more information regarding treatment options for MRSA infections, consult the Infectious Diseases Society of America guidelines [85].

Of note, when methicillin-susceptible *S. aureus* (MSSA) is isolated, targeted treatment is indicated. Thus, treatment with linezolid or vancomycin *must* be de-escalated to cloxacillin 2 g IV every 4 h or cefazolin 2 g IV every 8 h. Continuing therapy with coverage against MRSA in patients with MSSA infections should be discouraged as it is associated with detrimental outcomes [86, 87].

Current guidelines recommend that all hospitals regularly generate and disseminate a local antibiogram. Local epidemiology registry should advise empiric treatment regimens of pathogens associated with VAP and their antimicrobial susceptibilities [1]. *Knowledge of local epidemiology and microbiological surveillance is crucial for improving clinical approaches to empirical treatment for VAP.* These data are essential for disease control and enhance antimicrobial stewardship.

10 How Do I Support my Decision to Extend, Withhold, or De-Escalate Treatment?

The indiscriminate use of antibiotic combinations can induce the emergence of highly resistant strains. For this reason, the search for the causative microorganism in respiratory samples for de-escalation represents a crucial element of comprehensive management and antimicrobial stewardship in VAP. The reassessment of an individual's clinical status at 48–72 h of initiation of treatment may reflect its adequacy. Procalcitonin-guided treatment can be useful to guide duration or prolong it in several circumstances, such as inappropriate antibiotic treatments, infections due to MDR or extensively drug-resistant (XDR) microorganisms, or when second-line antibiotics are used [2]. Some experts recommend the use of procalcitonin values in combination with relevant clinical parameters (e.g., Clinical Pulmonary Infection Score [CPIS], PaO_2/FiO_2, Sequential Organ Failure Assessment [SOFA] score) for shortening antimicrobial treatment [88].

A **7-day** course of antimicrobial therapy is widely recommended by the American and European guidelines, as prolonged courses of antibiotics promote the emergence of resistance. However, the optimal duration of therapy for MDR organisms has not been clearly defined. The Impact of the Duration of Antibiotics on Clinical Events in Patients with *Pseudomonas Aeruginosa* Ventilator-Associated Pneumonia (iDIAPASON) trial is aimed at demonstrating that a short duration (8 days) versus long duration (15 days) therapy strategy for the treatment of VAP due to *P. aeruginosa* is safe and not associated with an increased mortality or recurrence rate [89]. Clinicians should advocate for antibiotic de-escalation and reducing antibiotic exposure as part of high-quality antimicrobial stewardship (AS). AS programs have been created to support physicians' decisions and to ensure appropriate antimicrobial treatments. Each institution should create specialized teams addressed to organize AS programs, according to their available staff and available resources.

11 Prognosis

One of the most critical determinants of successful outcomes in VAP patients is having received a suitable empirical antibiotic [90]. Inappropriate treatment significantly increases the risk of death among patients with severe infections [91, 92]. Of note, receiving an inadequate antibiotic therapy is a potentially modifiable prognostic factor, which can be attenuated by implementing antimicrobial stewardship policies that consider the local ecology of the ICU.

Other patient-related and disease-related factors have been associated with adverse outcomes, as well. Comorbidities, performance status, older age, malignancy, acute severity of disease (septic shock or ARDS), lymphopenia, and infection due to an MDR organism are outstanding [93–95]. To correctly assess these factors, predictive analyses should be focused on patients who received suitable empirical treatment. Also, the natural course of disease influences outcomes. The absence of improved oxygenation during antibiotic treatment is the single most important factor determining mortality (OR 2.18 [1.24–3.84] $p = 0.007$) in VAP [96]. The persistence of fever/hypothermia in association with purulent respiratory secretions, multilobar infiltrates >50% of the lung area, and presence of septic shock or multi-organ failure have been recognized to impact patient outcomes. Clinical scales and biomarker-guided strategies may aid in the follow-up of VAP patients [88, 97].

12 Prevention of VAP: The "Pneumonia Zero" Program

Different strategies have been developed to improve the quality of care of mechanically ventilated patients and VAP prevention [29]. The Pneumonia Zero project was created as a nationwide multimodal intervention based on implementing evidence-based bundle measures. This program has been successful in reducing by 50% the incidence of VAP in Spanish ICUs [98]. Primary measures include training healthcare professionals on the appropriate manipulation of the airway (aspiration of bronchial secretions), planning on safety for patients, and hand hygiene. Other important measures are buccal hygiene with chlorhexidine (0,12% 0,2%), endotracheal tube cuff pressure over 20 cmH_2O, head elevation (30–45 °C), preferential use of noninvasive ventilation when possible, expiratory valve sets, and avoidance of routine changes of tubes, humidifiers, and breathing circuit sets. Additional measures include the continuous subglottic secretion aspiration and selective digestive decontamination. The most crucial aspect of VAP prevention is the development of institutional policies and protocols for training healthcare professionals on preventive interventions, such as the "Pneumonia Zero" project. Initiatives should be focused on improving communication between professionals, learning from errors during the management of mechanically ventilated patients, and continuous evaluation of practices learned in the program [99].

13 Conclusions

Ventilator-associated pneumonia is an ICU-related infection with significant consequences for the patient and the healthcare system. Appropriate empirical treatment and early de-escalation should be implemented to increase the chance of survival. Moreover, identifying risk factors for MDR organisms, local policies to improve antimicrobial stewardship, and knowledge of local ecology and previous colonization are of outstanding importance. Healthcare workers should be trained to implement recommended preventive measures, such as adequate hand hygiene and respiratory device management. The use of rapid diagnostic tests for pathogen identification enables the early targeting of antibiotic treatment to reduce exposure to unnecessary broad-spectrum antibiotics.

References

1. Kalil AC, Metersky ML, Klompas M, Muscedere J, Sweeney DA, Palmer LB, et al. Management of adults with hospital-acquired and ventilator-associated pneumonia: 2016 clinical practice guidelines by the Infectious Diseases Society of America and the American Thoracic Society. Clin Infect Dis. 2016;63(5):e61–e111. https://doi.org/10.1093/cid/ciw353.
2. Torres A, Niederman MS, Chastre J, Ewig S, Fernandez-Vandellos P, Hanberger H, et al. International ERS/ESICM/ESCMID/ALAT guidelines for the management of hospital-acquired pneumonia and ventilator-associated pneumonia: guidelines for the management of hospital-acquired pneumonia (HAP)/ventilator-associated pneumonia (VAP) of the European Respiratory Society (ERS), European Society of Intensive Care Medicine (ESICM), European Society of Clinical Microbiology and Infectious Diseases (ESCMID) and Asociacion Latinoamericana del Torax (ALAT). Eur Respir J. 2017;50(3):1700582. https://doi.org/10.1183/13993003.00582-2017.
3. Levy MM, Evans LE, Rhodes A. The surviving sepsis campaign bundle: 2018 update. Intensive Care Med. 2018;44(6):925–8. https://doi.org/10.1007/s00134-018-5085-0.
4. Montravers P, Bassetti M. The ideal patient profile for new beta-lactam/beta-lactamase inhibitors. Curr Opin Infect Dis. 2018;31(6):587–93. https://doi.org/10.1097/qco.0000000000000490.
5. Bassetti M, Righi E, Vena A, Graziano E, Russo A, Peghin M. Risk stratification and treatment of ICU-acquired pneumonia caused by multidrug- resistant/extensively drug-resistant/pandrug-resistant bacteria. Curr Opin Crit Care. 2018;24(5):385–93. https://doi.org/10.1097/mcc.0000000000000534.
6. Warren DK, Shukla SJ, Olsen MA, Kollef MH, Hollenbeak CS, Cox MJ, et al. Outcome and attributable cost of ventilator-associated pneumonia among intensive care unit patients in a suburban medical center. Crit Care Med. 2003;31(5):1312–7. https://doi.org/10.1097/01.Ccm.0000063087.93157.06.
7. Esperatti M, Ferrer M, Theessen A, Liapikou A, Valencia M, Saucedo LM, et al. Nosocomial pneumonia in the intensive care unit acquired by mechanically ventilated versus nonventilated patients. Am J Respir Crit Care Med. 2010;182(12):1533–9. https://doi.org/10.1164/rccm.201001-0094OC.
8. Muscedere JG, Day A, Heyland DK. Mortality, attributable mortality, and clinical events as end points for clinical trials of ventilator-associated pneumonia and hospital-acquired pneumonia. Clin Infect Dis. 2010;51(Suppl 1):S120–5. https://doi.org/10.1086/653060.
9. Melsen WG, Rovers MM, Groenwold RH, Bergmans DC, Camus C, Bauer TT, et al. Attributable mortality of ventilator-associated pneumonia: a meta-analysis of individual patient data from randomised prevention studies. Lancet Infect Dis. 2013;13(8):665–71. https://doi.org/10.1016/s1473-3099(13)70081-1.
10. Dudoignon E, Caméléna F, Deniau B, Habay A, Coutrot M, Ressaire Q, et al. Bacterial pneumonia in COVID-19 critically ill patients: a case series. Clin Infect Dis. 2020;72:905. https://doi.org/10.1093/cid/ciaa762.
11. Chang SH, Jiang J, Kon ZN, Williams DM, Geraci T, Smith DE, et al. Safety and efficacy of bronchoscopy in critically ill patients with coronavirus disease 2019. Chest. 2020;159:870. https://doi.org/10.1016/j.chest.2020.09.263.

12. Forel JM, Voillet F, Pulina D, Gacouin A, Perrin G, Barrau K, et al. Ventilator-associated pneumonia and ICU mortality in severe ARDS patients ventilated according to a lung-protective strategy. Crit Care. 2012;16(2):R65. https://doi.org/10.1186/cc11312.
13. Koulenti D, Tsigou E, Rello J. Nosocomial pneumonia in 27 ICUs in Europe: perspectives from the EU-VAP/CAP study. Eur J Clin Microbiol Infect Dis. 2017;36(11):1999–2006. https://doi.org/10.1007/s10096-016-2703-z.
14. Magill SS, Li Q, Gross C, Dudeck M, Allen-Bridson K, Edwards JR. Incidence and characteristics of ventilator-associated events reported to the National Healthcare Safety Network in 2014. Crit Care Med. 2016;44(12):2154–62. https://doi.org/10.1097/ccm.0000000000001871.
15. Saied W, Martin-Loeches I, Timsit JF. What is new in non-ventilated ICU-acquired pneumonia? Intensive Care Med. 2020;46(3):488–91. https://doi.org/10.1007/s00134-019-05859-9.
16. Zaragoza R, Vidal-Cortés P, Aguilar G, Borges M, Diaz E, Ferrer R, et al. Update of the treatment of nosocomial pneumonia in the ICU. Crit Care. 2020;24(1):383. https://doi.org/10.1186/s13054-020-03091-2.
17. Martin-Loeches I, Povoa P, Rodríguez A, Curcio D, Suarez D, Mira JP, et al. Incidence and prognosis of ventilator-associated tracheobronchitis (TAVeM): a multicentre, prospective, observational study. Lancet Respir Med. 2015;3(11):859–68. https://doi.org/10.1016/s2213-2600(15)00326-4.
18. Healthcare-associated infections in intensive care units—Annual Epidemiological Report for 2016. European Centre for Disease Prevention and Control. https://www.ecdc.europa.eu/en/publications-data/healthcare-associated-infections-intensive-care-units-annual-epidemiological-0. Accessed 10 Nov 2020.
19. Skrupky LP, McConnell K, Dallas J, Kollef MH. A comparison of ventilator-associated pneumonia rates as identified according to the National Healthcare Safety Network and American College of Chest Physicians criteria. Crit Care Med. 2012;40(1):281–4. https://doi.org/10.1097/CCM.0b013e31822d7913.
20. Martin-Loeches I, Povoa P, Nseir S. A way towards ventilator-associated lower respiratory tract infection research. Intensive Care Med. 2020;46(7):1504–5. https://doi.org/10.1007/s00134-020-06101-7.
21. Papazian L, Klompas M, Luyt CE. Ventilator-associated pneumonia in adults: a narrative review. Intensive Care Med. 2020;46(5):888–906. https://doi.org/10.1007/s00134-020-05980-0.
22. van Vught LA, Klein Klouwenberg PM, Spitoni C, Scicluna BP, Wiewel MA, Horn J, et al. Incidence, risk factors, and attributable mortality of secondary infections in the intensive care unit after admission for sepsis. JAMA. 2016;315(14):1469–79. https://doi.org/10.1001/jama.2016.2691.
23. Li Y, Liu C, Xiao W, Song T, Wang S. Incidence, risk factors, and outcomes of ventilator-associated pneumonia in traumatic brain injury: a meta-analysis. Neurocrit Care. 2020;32(1):272–85. https://doi.org/10.1007/s12028-019-00773-w.
24. Bouglé A, Bombled C, Margetis D, Lebreton G, Vidal C, Coroir M, et al. Ventilator-associated pneumonia in patients assisted by veno-arterial extracorporeal membrane oxygenation support: epidemiology and risk factors of treatment failure. PLoS One. 2018;13(4):e0194976. https://doi.org/10.1371/journal.pone.0194976.
25. Fernando SM, Tran A, Cheng W, Klompas M, Kyeremanteng K, Mehta S, et al. Diagnosis of ventilator-associated pneumonia in critically ill adult patients-a systematic review and meta-analysis. Intensive Care Med. 2020;46(6):1170–9. https://doi.org/10.1007/s00134-020-06036-z.
26. Vincent JL, Rello J, Marshall J, Silva E, Anzueto A, Martin CD, et al. International study of the prevalence and outcomes of infection in intensive care units. JAMA. 2009;302(21):2323–9. https://doi.org/10.1001/jama.2009.1754.
27. Guidelines for the management of adults with hospital-acquired, ventilator-associated, and healthcare-associated pneumonia. Am J Respir Crit Care Med. 2005;171(4):388–416. https://doi.org/10.1164/rccm.200405-644ST.
28. Wu D, Wu C, Zhang S, Zhong Y. Risk factors of ventilator-associated pneumonia in critically III patients. Front Pharmacol. 2019;10:482. https://doi.org/10.3389/fphar.2019.00482.

29. Martin-Loeches I, Rodriguez AH, Torres A. New guidelines for hospital-acquired pneumonia/ventilator-associated pneumonia: USA vs. Europe. Curr Opin Crit Care. 2018;24(5):347–52. https://doi.org/10.1097/mcc.0000000000000535.
30. Ibn Saied W, Mourvillier B, Cohen Y, Ruckly S, Reignier J, Marcotte G, et al. A comparison of the mortality risk associated with ventilator-acquired bacterial pneumonia and non-ventilator ICU-acquired bacterial pneumonia. Crit Care Med. 2019;47(3):345–52. https://doi.org/10.1097/ccm.0000000000003553.
31. Micek ST, Wunderink RG, Kollef MH, Chen C, Rello J, Chastre J, et al. An international multicenter retrospective study of Pseudomonas aeruginosa nosocomial pneumonia: impact of multidrug resistance. Crit Care. 2015;19(1):219. https://doi.org/10.1186/s13054-015-0926-5.
32. Jaffal K, Six S, Zerimech F, Nseir S. Relationship between hyperoxemia and ventilator associated pneumonia. Ann Transl Med. 2017;5(22):453. https://doi.org/10.21037/atm.2017.10.15.
33. ENVIN–HELICS [Internet]. [cited 2020 Nov 3]. http://hws.vhebron.net/envin-helics/https://hws.vhebron.net/envin-helics/Help/Informe%20ENVIN-UCI%202019.pdf.
34. Bonten MJ, Weinstein RA. The role of colonization in the pathogenesis of nosocomial infections. Infect Control Hosp Epidemiol. 1996;17(3):193–200. https://doi.org/10.1086/647274.
35. Beardsley JR, Williamson JC, Johnson JW, Ohl CA, Karchmer TB, Bowton DL. Using local microbiologic data to develop institution-specific guidelines for the treatment of hospital-acquired pneumonia. Chest. 2006;130(3):787–93. https://doi.org/10.1378/chest.130.3.787.
36. Torre-Cisneros J, Natera C, Mesa F, Trikic M, Rodríguez-Baño J. Clinical predictors of methicillin-resistant Staphylococcus aureus in nosocomial and healthcare-associated pneumonia: a multicenter, matched case-control study. Eur J Clin Microbiol Infect Dis. 2018;37(1):51–6. https://doi.org/10.1007/s10096-017-3100-y.
37. Torre-Cisneros J, Tejero García R, Natera Kindelán C, Font Ugalde P, de Luna FFA, Castón Osorio JJ et al. [Risk factors of nosocomial pneumonia caused by methicillin-resistant Staphylococcus aureus]. Med Clin (Barc). 2012;138(3):99–106. https://doi.org/10.1016/j.medcli.2011.05.028.
38. Metersky ML, Frei CR, Mortensen EM. Predictors of pseudomonas and methicillin-resistant Staphylococcus aureus in hospitalized patients with healthcare-associated pneumonia. Respirology. 2016;21(1):157–63. https://doi.org/10.1111/resp.12651.
39. Buhl M, Peter S, Willmann M. Prevalence and risk factors associated with colonization and infection of extensively drug-resistant Pseudomonas aeruginosa: a systematic review. Expert Rev Anti-Infect Ther. 2015;13(9):1159–70. https://doi.org/10.1586/14787210.2015.1064310.
40. Fernández-Barat L, Ferrer M, De Rosa F, Gabarrús A, Esperatti M, Terraneo S, et al. Intensive care unit-acquired pneumonia due to Pseudomonas aeruginosa with and without multidrug resistance. J Infect. 2017;74(2):142–52. https://doi.org/10.1016/j.jinf.2016.11.008.
41. Rojo V, Vázquez P, Reyes S, Puente Fuertes L, Cervero M. [Risk factors and clinical evolution of carbapenemase-producing Klebsiella pneumoniae infections in a university hospital in Spain. Case-control study]. Rev Esp Quimioter. 2018;31(5):427–434.
42. Wang Z, Qin RR, Huang L, Sun LY. Risk factors for Carbapenem-resistant Klebsiella pneumoniae infection and mortality of Klebsiella pneumoniae infection. Chin Med J. 2018;131(1):56–62. https://doi.org/10.4103/0366-6999.221267.
43. Gao B, Li X, Yang F, Chen W, Zhao Y, Bai G, et al. Molecular epidemiology and risk factors of ventilator-associated pneumonia infection caused by Carbapenem-resistant Enterobacteriaceae. Front Pharmacol. 2019;10:262. https://doi.org/10.3389/fphar.2019.00262.
44. Sbrana F, Malacarne P, Bassetti M, Tascini C, Vegnuti L, Della Siega P, et al. Risk factors for ventilator associated pneumonia due to carbapenemase-producing Klebsiella pneumoniae in mechanically ventilated patients with tracheal and rectal colonization. Minerva Anestesiol. 2016;82(6):635–40.
45. Peralta G, Sánchez MB, Garrido JC, De Benito I, Cano ME, Martínez-Martínez L, et al. Impact of antibiotic resistance and of adequate empirical antibiotic treatment in the prognosis of patients with Escherichia coli bacteraemia. J Antimicrob Chemother. 2007;60(4):855–63. https://doi.org/10.1093/jac/dkm279.

46. Aydemir H, Tuz HI, Piskin N, Celebi G, Kulah C, Kokturk F. Risk factors and clinical responses of pneumonia patients with colistin-resistant Acinetobacter baumannii-calcoaceticus. World J Clin Cases. 2019;7(10):1111–21. https://doi.org/10.12998/wjcc.v7.i10.1111.
47. Zheng YL, Wan YF, Zhou LY, Ye ML, Liu S, Xu CQ, et al. Risk factors and mortality of patients with nosocomial carbapenem-resistant Acinetobacter baumannii pneumonia. Am J Infect Control. 2013;41(7):e59–63. https://doi.org/10.1016/j.ajic.2013.01.006.
48. Hayashi Y, Morisawa K, Klompas M, Jones M, Bandeshe H, Boots R, et al. Toward improved surveillance: the impact of ventilator-associated complications on length of stay and antibiotic use in patients in intensive care units. Clin Infect Dis. 2013;56(4):471–7. https://doi.org/10.1093/cid/cis926.
49. Berton DC, Kalil AC, Teixeira PJ. Quantitative versus qualitative cultures of respiratory secretions for clinical outcomes in patients with ventilator-associated pneumonia. Cochrane Database Syst Rev. 2014;(10):CD006482. https://doi.org/10.1002/14651858.CD006482.pub4.
50. Canadian Critical Care Trials Group. A randomized trial of diagnostic techniques for ventilator-associated pneumonia. N Engl J Med. 2006;355(25):2619–30. https://doi.org/10.1056/NEJMoa052904.
51. Solé Violán J, Fernández JA, Benítez AB, Cardeñosa Cendrero JA, Rodríguez de Castro F. Impact of quantitative invasive diagnostic techniques in the management and outcome of mechanically ventilated patients with suspected pneumonia. Crit Care Med. 2000;28(8):2737–41. https://doi.org/10.1097/00003246-200008000-00009.
52. Millot G, Voisin B, Loiez C, Wallet F, Nseir S. The next generation of rapid point-of-care testing identification tools for ventilator-associated pneumonia. Ann Transl Med. 2017;5(22):451. https://doi.org/10.21037/atm.2017.11.05.
53. Clavel M, Barraud O, Moucadel V, Meynier F, Karam E, Ploy MC, et al. Molecular quantification of bacteria from respiratory samples in patients with suspected ventilator-associated pneumonia. Clin Microbiol Infect. 2016;22(9):812.e1–7. https://doi.org/10.1016/j.cmi.2016.06.013.
54. Pulido MR, Moreno-Martínez P, González-Galán V, Fernández Cuenca F, Pascual Á, Garnacho-Montero J, et al. Application of BioFire FilmArray blood culture identification panel for rapid identification of the causative agents of ventilator-associated pneumonia. Clin Microbiol Infect. 2018;24(11):1213.e1–4. https://doi.org/10.1016/j.cmi.2018.06.001.
55. Tabah A, Bassetti M, Kollef MH, Zahar JR, Paiva JA, Timsit JF, et al. Antimicrobial de-escalation in critically ill patients: a position statement from a task force of the European Society of Intensive Care Medicine (ESICM) and European Society of Clinical Microbiology and Infectious Diseases (ESCMID) Critically Ill Patients Study Group (ESGCIP). Intensive Care Med. 2020;46(2):245–65. https://doi.org/10.1007/s00134-019-05866-w.
56. Ruiz J, Ramirez P, Gordon M, Villarreal E, Frasquet J, Poveda-Andres JL, et al. Antimicrobial stewardship programme in critical care medicine: a prospective interventional study. Med Intensiva. 2018;42(5):266–73. https://doi.org/10.1016/j.medin.2017.07.002.
57. De Waele JJ, Schouten J, Beovic B, Tabah A, Leone M. Antimicrobial de-escalation as part of antimicrobial stewardship in intensive care: no simple answers to simple questions—a viewpoint of experts. Intensive Care Med. 2020;46(2):236–44. https://doi.org/10.1007/s00134-019-05871-z.
58. Freire AT, Melnyk V, Kim MJ, Datsenko O, Dzyublik O, Glumcher F, et al. Comparison of tigecycline with imipenem/cilastatin for the treatment of hospital-acquired pneumonia. Diagn Microbiol Infect Dis. 2010;68(2):140–51. https://doi.org/10.1016/j.diagmicrobio.2010.05.012.
59. Rubinstein E, Lalani T, Corey GR, Kanafani ZA, Nannini EC, Rocha MG, et al. Telavancin versus vancomycin for hospital-acquired pneumonia due to gram-positive pathogens. Clin Infect Dis. 2011;52(1):31–40. https://doi.org/10.1093/cid/ciq031.
60. Kollef MH, Chastre J, Clavel M, Restrepo MI, Michiels B, Kaniga K, et al. A randomized trial of 7-day doripenem versus 10-day imipenem-cilastatin for ventilator-associated pneumonia. Crit Care. 2012;16(6):R218. https://doi.org/10.1186/cc11862.
61. Wunderink RG, Niederman MS, Kollef MH, Shorr AF, Kunkel MJ, Baruch A, et al. Linezolid in methicillin-resistant Staphylococcus aureus nosocomial pneumonia: a randomized, controlled study. Clin Infect Dis. 2012;54(5):621–9. https://doi.org/10.1093/cid/cir895.

62. Ramirez J, Dartois N, Gandjini H, Yan JL, Korth-Bradley J, McGovern PC. Randomized phase 2 trial to evaluate the clinical efficacy of two high-dosage tigecycline regimens versus imipenem-cilastatin for treatment of hospital-acquired pneumonia. Antimicrob Agents Chemother. 2013;57(4):1756–62. https://doi.org/10.1128/aac.01232-12.
63. Awad SS, Rodriguez AH, Chuang YC, Marjanek Z, Pareigis AJ, Reis G, et al. A phase 3 randomized double-blind comparison of ceftobiprole medocaril versus ceftazidime plus linezolid for the treatment of hospital-acquired pneumonia. Clin Infect Dis. 2014;59(1):51–61. https://doi.org/10.1093/cid/ciu219.
64. Torres A, Zhong N, Pachl J, Timsit JF, Kollef M, Chen Z, et al. Ceftazidime-avibactam versus meropenem in nosocomial pneumonia, including ventilator-associated pneumonia (REPROVE): a randomised, double-blind, phase 3 non-inferiority trial. Lancet Infect Dis. 2018;18(3):285–95. https://doi.org/10.1016/s1473-3099(17)30747-8.
65. Cisneros JM, Rosso-Fernández CM, Roca-Oporto C, De Pascale G, Jiménez-Jorge S, Fernández-Hinojosa E, et al. Colistin versus meropenem in the empirical treatment of ventilator-associated pneumonia (Magic Bullet study): an investigator-driven, open-label, randomized, noninferiority controlled trial. Crit Care. 2019;23(1):383. https://doi.org/10.1186/s13054-019-2627-y.
66. Kollef MH, Nováček M, Kivistik Ü, Réa-Neto Á, Shime N, Martin-Loeches I, et al. Ceftolozane-tazobactam versus meropenem for treatment of nosocomial pneumonia (ASPECT-NP): a randomised, controlled, double-blind, phase 3, non-inferiority trial. Lancet Infect Dis. 2019;19(12):1299–311. https://doi.org/10.1016/s1473-3099(19)30403-7.
67. Bassetti M, Vena A, Russo A, Croxatto A, Calandra T, Guery B. Rational approach in the management of Pseudomonas aeruginosa infections. Curr Opin Infect Dis. 2018;31(6):578–86. https://doi.org/10.1097/qco.0000000000000505.
68. Mensa J, Barberán J, Soriano A, Llinares P, Marco F, Cantón R, et al. Antibiotic selection in the treatment of acute invasive infections by Pseudomonas aeruginosa: guidelines by the Spanish Society of Chemotherapy. Rev Esp Quimioter. 2018;31(1):78–100.
69. Bassetti M, Righi E, Carnelutti A, Graziano E, Russo A. Multidrug-resistant Klebsiella pneumoniae: challenges for treatment, prevention and infection control. Expert Rev Anti-Infect Ther. 2018;16(10):749–61. https://doi.org/10.1080/14787210.2018.1522249.
70. Singer M, Deutschman CS, Seymour CW, Shankar-Hari M, Annane D, Bauer M, et al. The third international consensus definitions for sepsis and septic shock (Sepsis-3). JAMA. 2016;315(8):801–10. https://doi.org/10.1001/jama.2016.0287.
71. Rhodes A, Evans LE, Alhazzani W, Levy MM, Antonelli M, Ferrer R, et al. Surviving sepsis campaign: international guidelines for management of sepsis and septic shock: 2016. Intensive Care Med. 2017;43(3):304–77. https://doi.org/10.1007/s00134-017-4683-6.
72. Teysseyre L, Ferdynus C, Miltgen G, Lair T, Aujoulat T, Lugagne N, et al. Derivation and validation of a simple score to predict the presence of bacteria requiring carbapenem treatment in ICU-acquired bloodstream infection and pneumonia: CarbaSCORE. Antimicrob Resist Infect Control. 2019;8:78. https://doi.org/10.1186/s13756-019-0529-z.
73. FDA Drug Safety Communication. Increased risk of death with Tygacil (tigecycline) compared to other antibiotics used to treat similar infections. https://www.fda.gov/drugs/drug-safety-and-availability/fda-drug-safety-communication-increased-risk-death-tygacil-tigecycline-compared-other-antibiotics. Accessed 10 Nov 2020.
74. Monajati M, Ala S, Aliyali M, Ghasemian R, Heidari F, Ahanjan M, et al. Clinical effectiveness of high dose versus standard dose of meropenem in ventilator-associated pneumonia caused by multidrug-resistant bacteria: a randomized single-blind clinical trial. Infect Disord Drug Targets. 2021;21(2):274–83. https://doi.org/10.2174/1871526520666200227102013.
75. Yu Z, Pang X, Wu X, Shan C, Jiang S. Clinical outcomes of prolonged infusion (extended infusion or continuous infusion) versus intermittent bolus of meropenem in severe infection: a meta-analysis. PLoS One. 2018;13(7):e0201667. https://doi.org/10.1371/journal.pone.0201667.

76. Goodlet KJ, Nicolau DP, Nailor MD. In vitro comparison of Ceftolozane-Tazobactam to traditional Beta-lactams and Ceftolozane-Tazobactam as an alternative to combination antimicrobial therapy for Pseudomonas aeruginosa. Antimicrob Agents Chemother. 2017;61(12):e01350–17. https://doi.org/10.1128/aac.01350-17.
77. Alraddadi BM, Saeedi M, Qutub M, Alshukairi A, Hassanien A, Wali G. Efficacy of ceftazidime-avibactam in the treatment of infections due to Carbapenem-resistant Enterobacteriaceae. BMC Infect Dis. 2019;19(1):772. https://doi.org/10.1186/s12879-019-4409-1.
78. Bassetti M, Echols R, Matsunaga Y, Ariyasu M, Doi Y, Ferrer R, et al. Efficacy and safety of cefiderocol or best available therapy for the treatment of serious infections caused by carbapenem-resistant gram-negative bacteria (CREDIBLE-CR): a randomised, open-label, multicentre, pathogen-focused, descriptive, phase 3 trial. Lancet Infect Dis. 2021;21:226–40. https://doi.org/10.1016/s1473-3099(20)30796-9.
79. Kollef MH, Ricard JD, Roux D, Francois B, Ischaki E, Rozgonyi Z, et al. A randomized trial of the amikacin Fosfomycin inhalation system for the adjunctive therapy of gram-negative ventilator-associated pneumonia: IASIS trial. Chest. 2017;151(6):1239–46. https://doi.org/10.1016/j.chest.2016.11.026.
80. Niederman MS, Alder J, Bassetti M, Boateng F, Cao B, Corkery K, et al. Inhaled amikacin adjunctive to intravenous standard-of-care antibiotics in mechanically ventilated patients with gram-negative pneumonia (INHALE): a double-blind, randomised, placebo-controlled, phase 3, superiority trial. Lancet Infect Dis. 2020;20(3):330–40. https://doi.org/10.1016/s1473-3099(19)30574-2.
81. Niederman MS. Adjunctive nebulized antibiotics: what is their place in ICU infections? Front Med (Lausanne). 2019;6:99. https://doi.org/10.3389/fmed.2019.00099.
82. Pogue JM, Kaye KS, Veve MP, Patel TS, Gerlach AT, Davis SL, et al. Ceftolozane/Tazobactam vs Polymyxin or aminoglycoside-based regimens for the treatment of drug-resistant Pseudomonas aeruginosa. Clin Infect Dis. 2020;71(2):304–10. https://doi.org/10.1093/cid/ciz816.
83. An MM, Shen H, Zhang JD, Xu GT, Jiang YY. Linezolid versus vancomycin for methicillin-resistant Staphylococcus aureus infection: a meta-analysis of randomised controlled trials. Int J Antimicrob Agents. 2013;41(5):426–33. https://doi.org/10.1016/j.ijantimicag.2012.12.012.
84. Stein GE, Wells EM. The importance of tissue penetration in achieving successful antimicrobial treatment of nosocomial pneumonia and complicated skin and soft-tissue infections caused by methicillin-resistant Staphylococcus aureus: vancomycin and linezolid. Curr Med Res Opin. 2010;26(3):571–88. https://doi.org/10.1185/03007990903512057.
85. Liu C, Bayer A, Cosgrove SE, Daum RS, Fridkin SK, Gorwitz RJ, et al. Clinical practice guidelines by the Infectious Diseases Society of America for the treatment of methicillin-resistant Staphylococcus aureus infections in adults and children. Clin Infect Dis. 2011;52(3):e18–55. https://doi.org/10.1093/cid/ciq146.
86. Wong D, Wong T, Romney M, Leung V. Comparative effectiveness of beta-lactam versus vancomycin empiric therapy in patients with methicillin-susceptible Staphylococcus aureus (MSSA) bacteremia. Ann Clin Microbiol Antimicrob. 2016;15:27. https://doi.org/10.1186/s12941-016-0143-3.
87. McDanel JS, Perencevich EN, Diekema DJ, Herwaldt LA, Smith TC, Chrischilles EA, et al. Comparative effectiveness of beta-lactams versus vancomycin for treatment of methicillin-susceptible Staphylococcus aureus bloodstream infections among 122 hospitals. Clin Infect Dis. 2015;61(3):361–7. https://doi.org/10.1093/cid/civ308.
88. Torres A, Artigas A, Ferrer R. Biomarkers in the ICU: less is more? No. Intensive Care Med. 2021;47:97. https://doi.org/10.1007/s00134-020-06271-4.
89. Bouglé A, Foucrier A, Dupont H, Montravers P, Ouattara A, Kalfon P, et al. Impact of the duration of antibiotics on clinical events in patients with Pseudomonas aeruginosa ventilator-associated pneumonia: study protocol for a randomized controlled study. Trials. 2017;18(1):37. https://doi.org/10.1186/s13063-017-1780-3.

90. Dupont H, Mentec H, Sollet JP, Bleichner G. Impact of appropriateness of initial antibiotic therapy on the outcome of ventilator-associated pneumonia. Intensive Care Med. 2001;27(2):355–62. https://doi.org/10.1007/s001340000640.
91. Zilberberg MD, Shorr AF, Micek ST, Vazquez-Guillamet C, Kollef MH. Multi-drug resistance, inappropriate initial antibiotic therapy and mortality in gram-negative severe sepsis and septic shock: a retrospective cohort study. Crit Care. 2014;18(6):596. https://doi.org/10.1186/s13054-014-0596-8.
92. Kollef MH. Treatment of ventilator-associated pneumonia: get it right from the start. Crit Care Med. 2003;31(3):969–70. https://doi.org/10.1097/01.Ccm.0000055381.70829.94.
93. Ranzani OT, Ferrer M, Esperatti M, Giunta V, Bassi GL, Carvalho CR, et al. Association between systemic corticosteroids and outcomes of intensive care unit-acquired pneumonia. Crit Care Med. 2012;40(9):2552–61. https://doi.org/10.1097/CCM.0b013e318259203d.
94. Ranzani OT, Prina E, Torres A. Nosocomial pneumonia in the intensive care unit: how should treatment failure be predicted? Rev Bras Ter Intensiva. 2014;26(3):208–11. https://doi.org/10.5935/0103-507x.20140032.
95. Ceccato A, Panagiotarakou M, Ranzani OT, Martin-Fernandez M, Almansa-Mora R, Gabarrus A, et al. Lymphocytopenia as a predictor of mortality in patients with ICU-acquired pneumonia. J Clin Med. 2019;8(6) https://doi.org/10.3390/jcm8060843.
96. Esperatti M, Ferrer M, Giunta V, Ranzani OT, Saucedo LM, Li Bassi G, et al. Validation of predictors of adverse outcomes in hospital-acquired pneumonia in the ICU. Crit Care Med. 2013;41(9):2151–61. https://doi.org/10.1097/CCM.0b013e31828a674a.
97. Póvoa P, Martin-Loeches I, Ramirez P, Bos LD, Esperatti M, Silvestre J, et al. Biomarkers kinetics in the assessment of ventilator-associated pneumonia response to antibiotics—results from the BioVAP study. J Crit Care. 2017;41:91–7. https://doi.org/10.1016/j.jcrc.2017.05.007.
98. Álvarez-Lerma F, Palomar-Martínez M, Sánchez-García M, Martínez-Alonso M, Álvarez-Rodríguez J, Lorente L, et al. Prevention of ventilator-associated pneumonia: the multimodal approach of the Spanish ICU "Pneumonia Zero" program. Crit Care Med. 2018;46(2):181–8. https://doi.org/10.1097/ccm.0000000000002736.
99. Pujante-Palazón I, Rodríguez-Mondéjar JJ, Armero-Barranco D, Sáez-Paredes P. [Prevention of ventilator-associated pneumonia: a comparison of level of knowledge in three critical care units]. Enferm Intensiva. 2016;27(3):120–8. https://doi.org/10.1016/j.enfi.2015.10.001.

Mechanical Ventilation in Pregnant Woman

Carlos Montufar

1 Introduction

Respiratory failure remains one of the leading causes of maternal mortality; in addition, it is an important cause of admission to an intensive care unit [1, 2].

Respiratory failure can present in a hypoxemic form (type 1), characterized by a $PaO_2 < 60$ mmHg, with normal or decreased $PaCO_2$ levels, or a hypercapnic form (type 2) characterized by a $PaCO_2 > 50$ mmHg. Type 1 is by far the most common.

Dilutional anemia of pregnancy produces a decrease in arterial oxygen content. Thus, in pregnant women, oxygen delivery becomes dependent on cardiac output [3]. As gestation progresses, oxygen consumption increases throughout pregnancy, and consequently cardiac output must increase in such a way that oxygen delivery is higher than oxygen consumed [4–6].

The use of analgesics and sedatives is important for good ventilation. But international guidelines recommend maintaining light levels of sedation in the ICU with the use of established tools, such as the Richmond Agitation and Sedation Scale [7].

2 Physiological Changes

The pregnant patient suffers from important anatomical changes in her airway, which can facilitate a greater proportion of complications of the respiratory system [8]. In addition, these changes increase the degree of complexity to ventilate a

C. Montufar (✉)
Gynecology, Critical Care Obstetrics Unit, Critical Care Obstetrics, Complejo Hospitalario, Caja de Seguro Social, Panama City, Panama

Department of Obstetrics, Critical Care Obstetric Unit, Complejo Hospitalario, Caja de Seguro Social, Panamá City, Panamá

J. Hidalgo et al. (eds.), *Personalized Mechanical Ventilation*,
https://doi.org/10.1007/978-3-031-14138-6_15

pregnant patient and even prevent successful endotracheal intubation. These changes include edema and hyperemia of the upper airways. Capillary engorgement of the mucosa throughout the respiratory tract causes swelling of the nasal and oral pharynx, larynx, and trachea [9, 10].

Minute ventilation increases by up to 40 to 50% at term, with an increase in tidal volume (hyperpnea) rather than respiratory rate being responsible [11]. This results in a respiratory alkalosis, with the normal $PaCO_2$ in pregnancy sitting between 28 and 32 mmHg, with a compensatory metabolic acidosis resulting in a bicarbonate level of 18–21 mEq/L [12].

An elevated diaphragm due to the enlarging uterus (up to 5 cm) decreases compliance of the ventilatory system (reduction of chest wall compliance). There are physiological changes of pregnancy of great importance, which modify the ventilatory dynamics of the pregnant woman with a strong impact on the mother's gas exchange, and repercussions of the supply of O_2 and elimination of CO_2 in the fetus. In addition, these changes precipitate the development of respiratory failure in the pregnant patient earlier and require prompt decisions regarding the availability of an advanced airway (intubation).

In addition, there are hormone-mediated changes, mainly progesterone, which can facilitate respiratory failure. These changes include reduced tonus of the lower esophagus sphincter, increased respiratory drive with greater tidal volume leading to increased minute ventilation due to elevated levels of progesterone, and decreased functional residual capacity (FRC) [8, 13, 14].

The degree of complexity for the management of the airway becomes greater when it comes to morbidly obese patients [15]. Hood et al. showed that difficult intubation was encountered more frequently in morbidly obese parturient (>130 kg) [16].

The incidence of failed intubation is approximately eight times higher in the obstetric population compared to non-obstetric patients [17], and the incidence of fatal failed intubation is 13 times higher in the obstetric population [18].

Pregnancy has a major effect on lung volumes. It is associated with a 30–50% increase in tidal volume (TV), which occurs at the expense of the functional residual capacity (FRC). This transformation of the residual volume into tidal volume improves the supply of oxygen to the fetus [13]. This "transformation" of the residual lung volume into tidal volume makes the pregnant woman very susceptible to hypoxemia. Progesterone-induced stimulation is one of the factors in achieving this phenomenon.

Acute respiratory failure with need of ventilator support is infrequent in pregnant patients in developed countries, although the percentage is higher in low- and middle-income countries [14, 19]. Fewer than 2% of women in the peripartum period need treatment in the intensive care unit [14, 19].

Endotracheal intubation in pregnancy is technically difficult. The incidence of failed intubation among the pregnant population is estimated to be up to eight times that of the nonpregnant population [20].

There are key determinants to achieve correct fetal oxygenation, which must be taken into account when giving ventilatory support to a pregnant patient, such as uterine blood flow, maternal arterial oxygen content, concentration of maternal hemoglobin, and hemoglobin–oxygen dissociation curve of mother and the fetus [21].

The combination of the physiological and anatomical changes of pregnancy, including high baseline oxygen consumption, airway edema, breast enlargement, and reduced FRC, makes managing the maternal airway challenging.

Dyspnea of pregnancy refers to a commonly encountered condition in pregnancy. When a pregnant woman complains of dyspnea, distinguishing between underlying disease and normal pregnancy-related dyspnea can be a difficult diagnostic problem.

3 Causes

Shortness of breath is a common complaint in pregnancy, with most of the pregnant women experiencing some form of it during the gestation period. Dyspnea of pregnancy refers to a commonly encountered condition in pregnancy in which women describe a sense of "air hunger." When a pregnant woman complains of dyspnea, distinguishing between underlying disease and normal pregnancy-related dyspnea can be a difficult diagnostic problem.

Among the most frequent causes of respiratory distress in pregnant women, we have bacterial pneumonia, asthmatic crisis, pulmonary edema (e.g., preeclampsia), bronchial aspiration pneumonia, pulmonary embolism, amniotic fluid embolism, acute respiratory distress syndrome (e.g., sepsis), trauma, transfusions, and cardiac pulmonary edema.

Pneumonia remains a major cause of non-obstetric complications in pregnant women, and even a cause of death [22, 23].

Among the agents that most frequently generate pneumonia are *Streptococcus pneumoniae*, *Haemophilus influenzae*, and atypical pathogens like *Mycoplasma pneumoniae*, *Legionella pneumophila*, *Chlamydia pneumoniae*, varicella, and influenza A [24].

Potential indications for ICU admissions, according to the American Thoracic Society/Infectious Diseases Society of America, include but are not limited to the need for mechanical ventilation, septic shock requiring vasopressors, respiratory rate of >30 breaths per minute, and PaO_2/FiO_2 ratio [25].

It is estimated that approximately 8% of pregnant women have asthma [26]. Severe exacerbations of asthma can cause preterm deliveries, low-birth-weight fetuses, and neonatal death [27].

Pulmonary embolism is one of the main causes of maternal death, being the first in high-income countries, with a 5–6 times greater risk of it occurring in a pregnant woman, when compared to the non-obstetric population [28].

Pulmonary edema in pregnant women can be caused by a cardiovascular condition, by fluid misuse or in a mixed way as in preeclampsia.

The risk of aspiration rises in pregnancy due to increase of abdominal pressure, relaxation of the lower esophagus sphincter, and delayed gastric emptying. Aspiration can lead to acute bronchospasm, airway obstruction, and finally, in most cases, chemical pneumonitis (Mendelson syndrome) or an aspiration pneumonia.

Amniotic fluid embolism (AFE) is a rare, but catastrophic event in the intrapartum or early postpartum period, which produces cardiogenic shock, acute pulmonary hypertension, left ventricular failure, severe respiratory failure, and anaphylactic reactions [29].

Dramatic physiological changes in the pregnant patient (decrease in residual functional capacity and decrease in serum bicarbonate) cause her to have a low tolerance to hypoxemic and acidotic states, and this, in turn, produces a great susceptibility of these states to the fetus. This forces us to modify the oxygenation goals to be achieved when we treat an obstetric patient with ventilatory failure, having to achieve a minimum pO_2 of 70 mmHg and an O_2 saturation of 95%.

4 Oxygenation and Ventilation Goal in Pregnancy

Indications for intubation and mechanical ventilation in pregnancy remain the same as those of nonpregnant patients, which include progressive or unremitting hypoxia, apnea, upper airway obstruction, respiratory acidosis, maternal fatigue, altered mental status, and hemodynamic instability [30].

The ARDSNet trial of 2000 showed that both high volumes and high plateau pressures increase mortality. Pregnant patients were not included in this trial; however, in the absence of any evidence to the contrary, tidal volumes should be set to ≤6 ml/kg ideal body weight and plateau airway pressures should not exceed 30 cmH2O (the lower the better) in pregnant patients also [31].

With lung-protective ventilation, low tidal volumes and low minute ventilation can lead to hypercapnia. This hypercapnia produced, called "permissive hypercapnia," serves as a protective measure in cases of ARDS, in non-obstetric patients. Hypercapnia has a relevance in the possibility of the fetus to eliminate CO_2, which is carried out through a mother/fetus CO_2 gradient.

There is some evidence that permissive hypercarbia in neonates (45–55 mmHg) is well tolerated, although there have been no well-conducted randomized controlled trials in this population.

The choice of an initial ventilatory rate, tidal volume, oxygen percentage, and need for positive end-expiratory pressure (PEEP) should be balanced against the potential inducement of barotrauma from an unequal distribution of compliant alveoli or from bronchoconstriction.

The usual pressure limits of the common recommendation may not be fully applicable in pregnant patients because of the increased chest wall compliance and the higher abdominal pressure of the uterus [31]. Therefore, a higher peak inspiratory pressure and positive end-expiratory pressure (PEEP) should be set in pregnant patients.

Apart from barotrauma, volutrauma, and atelectrauma, another complication of mechanical ventilation is ventilator-associated pneumonia.

As explained previously, hypoxia and acidosis are poorly tolerated by mother and fetus. The oxygenation goal in all kinds of respiratory failure should be a maternal SpO_2 of 95% or a PaO_2 of 70 mm Hg or higher [32].

The ventilatory support has the objective of supporting the patient in severe respiratory distress, with the goal of helping the fatigued muscles in charge of ventilatory mechanics to rest, while maintaining an adequate gas exchange.

There is no strong evidence to make a difference in the way a pregnant patient is given ventilatory support. Some interventions can be established that are better adapted to the gestation condition.

A reasonable starting point for mechanical ventilation may use the following settings: assisted controlled mode, respiratory rate 10–14 breaths/min, tidal volume 5–8 mL/kg, minute ventilation less than 115 mL/kg, extrinsic PEEP only as needed to improve oxygenation, FiO_2 beginning at 100%, and weaning as tolerated to <50% while maintaining an oxygen saturation of greater than 94%.

From the Amato et al. study, it was demonstrated that using low levels of tidal volume (<6 ml/kg), versus the use of conventional tidal volume (12 ml/kg), generated a lower mortality at 28 days (38% vs. 71%) and a lower incidence of barotrauma [33]. The Acute Respiratory Distress Syndrome Network Study (ARDSNet) found the same results, using the same strategy of applying a tidal volume of 6 ml/kg [31]. This maneuver remains valid for pregnant patients.

In third-trimester pregnancies, the uterus compresses the aortocaval system, which compromises venous return. Mechanical ventilation delivers oxygen at positive pressure, which increases intrathoracic pressure and worsens venous return. Placing the patient in the left lateral decubitus position or tilting her to the left by placing a wedge under the right hip might be helpful strategies.

The usual pressure limits of the common recommendation may not be fully applicable in pregnant patients because of the increased chest wall compliance and the higher abdominal pressure of the uterus. Therefore, a higher peak inspiratory pressure and positive end-expiratory pressure (PEEP) should be set in pregnant patients [34].

The application of PEEP during mechanical ventilation in the management of ARDS is important as PEEP increases functional residual capacity. Although there are no studies aimed at determining adequate PEEP levels for a pregnant patient, we can assume that the use of higher levels of PEEP could improve residual functional capacity, which is decreased in pregnant women.

Difficulty accessing an airway in a pregnant woman becomes even more increased when the patient is morbidly obese. Obesity confers them a risk of developing diabetes, chronic arterial hypertension, and preeclampsia more frequently [16, 35]. In addition, they are at increased risk of developing postpartum hemorrhage [36]. To add, patients with morbid obesity have more anatomical difficulties, chronic cardiopulmonary dysfunctions, greater perioperative morbidity and mortality, and greater surgical technical challenges [15].

Current evidence establishes that non-deep sedation offers better clinical results and should be our way of approaching our patients.

Regarding the use of sedatives, we know that propofol crosses the placenta and will have a sedative effect depending on the dose. It does not have important fetal effects nor is it dangerous if used as an anesthesia inducer, but it will have a greater fetal depressant effect if it is used for a long time.

Long-acting benzodiazepines (diazepam) should be avoided in pregnant patients as they have a cumulative effect on the fetus. The negative effect is less with midazolam. All benzodiazepines can cause fetal malformations [37].

Fentanyl is not recommended for use in pregnant patients, as it is associated with respiratory depression in the newborn and neurological disorders.

Dexmedetomidine is a good alternative for sedation in pregnant patients due to its rapid clearance [38, 39].

Although pregnancy is often an exclusion criterion for trials of prone positioning, prone positioning has been used successfully in pregnancy according to published case reports [40–42]. There is no contraindication for prone positioning during pregnancy, although fetal monitoring during positioning would seem reasonable.

Regardless of these suggestions, the important thing is to achieve with the different ventilatory maneuvers a maternal $PaO_2 \geq 70$ mmHg and a $SaO_2 \geq 95\%$, without compromising maternal hemodynamics or uteroplacental perfusion.

5 Noninvasive Positive-Pressure Ventilation (NIPPV)

In recent years, full-awake, not-sedated patients have become more and more important to improve outcome in the ICU. This has led to increased use of noninvasive ventilation (NIV) to avoid intubation and use of sedation drugs and to reduce the incidence of delirium.

NIV refers to positive-pressure ventilation delivered to the patient without the need for endotracheal intubation. Some have considered that an increased risk of aspiration due to lower resting gastroesophageal sphincter tone and suboptimal ventilation due to pregnancy-associated airway edema can occur [43].

With respect to parturient with ARDS, several case reports describe the use of noninvasive ventilation as a means of ventilatory support [44, 45].

In our experience, we have not had cases of bronchial aspiration, and it was effective for ventilatory support in pregnant patients with mild and moderate ARDS [46]. The ideal candidate should meet at least the following criteria: adequate respiratory drive, ability to control one's own airway, ability to tolerate tight-fitting mask, hemodynamic stability, and not be at high risk for aspiration.

6 Fetus

In addition to providing maternal support and avoiding death, our goals of approach must be achieving to maintain the fetal-placenta compartment in acid-base balance and a good fetal oxygenation.

There are very important determinants necessary to guarantee the delivery of oxygen to the fetus and to avoid hypoxemic aggression: uterine blood flow, maternal arterial oxygen content, concentration of maternal hemoglobin, and hemoglobin–oxygen dissociation curve of mother and the fetus [21].

Animal studies showed that a maternal O_2 saturation of 88–95% resulted in the fetal saturation of 55–70% [47].

Maternal hypoxic states result in reduced placental flow because of vasoconstriction of the uterine and placental vessels, causing a decrease in oxygen transfer to the fetus [48].

Animal studies showed that a maternal O_2 saturation of 95–88% resulted in a fetal saturation of 70–55% [47].

In pregnancy, oxygen saturation should be maintained slightly higher (>95%) to prevent hypoxia to the fetus.

To guarantee good uterine perfusion, it is advisable to avoid states of both maternal hypocapnia ($pCO_2 < 30$ mmHg) and hypercapnia ($pCO_2 > 60$ mmHg) [49, 50].

In cases such as abruption, severe preeclampsia, or eclampsia, the termination of pregnancy will be carried out at any gestational age as soon as the stabilization of the patient is achieved. In the case of cardiac arrest, the cesarean section will be performed within 4 min of the event.

In other cases, the termination of pregnancy will be carried out depending on the risks to the fetus of prematurity with the risks of continued exposure to a "hostile" uterine environment, direct risks to the mother of limiting treatment modalities because of her pregnancy, and risks of delivery, given the maternal stability or the lack of it.

Studies that have specifically examined whether delivery has improved maternal outcome, however, have not supported this hypothesis and, in fact, may support avoiding delivery for non-obstetric indications. In their retrospective case series, Tomlison et al. reported the outcomes of ten women who required intubation for respiratory failure and who delivered while on ventilatory support. Although these women experienced a 28% decrease in the fraction of inspired oxygen required, overall respiratory function was not improved [51].

Fetal heart rate decelerations, loss of variability, and sudden onset of uterine contractions can be early signs of maternal hypovolemia or deteriorating maternal status, and therefore continuous fetal heart rate monitoring of the viable fetus may be useful in monitoring not only fetal status, but maternal status as well.

Nutritional support should begin as soon as possible, preferably within 24–48 h, as the higher metabolic needs of pregnancy lead very quickly to a "starvation" state.

Early recognition of an episode of respiratory distress is important, and thus achieve adequate and timely ventilatory support. It is necessary to know the different changes inherent to pregnancy, both anatomical and physiological. They can either be misinterpreted as disease or mask a compromised status.

References

1. Kaunitz AM, Hughes JM, Grimes DA, et al. Causes of maternal mortality in the United States. Obstet Gynecol. 1985;65:605–12.
2. United States Public Health Service. Progress toward achieving the 1990 objectives for pregnancy and infant health. MMWR. 1988;37:405.
3. Barron W, Lindheimer M. Medical disorders during pregnancy. 1st ed. St. Louis: Mosby – Year Book; 1991. p. 234.
4. Pernoll ML, Metcalf J, Schlenker TL, et al. Oxygen consumption at rest and during exercise in pregnancy. Respir Physiol. 1975;25:285–93.
5. Gemzell CA, Robbe H, Strom G, et al. Observations on circulatory changes and muscular work in normal labor. Acta Obstet Gynecol Scand. 1957;36:75–93.
6. Ueland K, Hansen JM. Maternal cardiovascular hemodynamics. II. Posture and uterine contractions. Am J Obstet Gynecol. 1969;103:1–7.
7. Barr J, Fraser GL, Puntillo K, et al. Clinical practice guidelines for the management of pain, agitation, and delirium in adult patients in the intensive care unit. Crit Care Med. 2013;41:263–306.
8. Torgersen KL, Curran CA. A systematic approach to the physiologic adaptations of pregnancy. Crit Care Nurs Q. 2006;29(1):2–19.
9. Jouppila R, Jouppila P, Hollmen A. Laryngeal oedema as an obstetric anaesthesia complication: case reports. Acta Anaesthesiol Scand. 1980;24(2):97–8.
10. Kuczkowski KM, Reisner LS, Benumof JL. Airway problems and new solutions for the obstetric patient. J Clin Anesth. 2003;15(7):552–63.
11. Elkus R, Popovich J Jr. Respiratory physiology in pregnancy. Clin Chest Med. 1992;13(4):555–65.
12. Ickx BE. Fluid and blood transfusion management in obstetrics. Eur J Anaesthesiol. 2010;27(12):1031–5.
13. Tan EK, Tan EL. Alterations in physiology and anatomy during pregnancy. Best Pract Res Clin Obstet Gynaecol. 2013;27(6):791–802.
14. Weinberger SE, Weiss ST, Cohen WR, et al. Pregnancy and the lung. Am Rev Respir Dis. 1980;121(3):559–81.
15. Saravanakumar K, Rao SG, Cooper GM. The challenges of obesity and obstetric anaesthesia. Curr Opin Obstet Gynecol. 2006;18(6):631–5.
16. Hood DD, Dewan DM. Anesthetic and obstetric outcome in morbidly obese parturients. Anesthesiology. 1993;79(6):1210–8.
17. Lyons G, Failed intubation. Six years' experience in a teaching maternity unit. Anaesthesia. 1985;40(8):759–62.
18. Glassenberg R. General anesthesia and maternal mortality. Semin Perinatol. 1991;15(5):386–96.
19. Pollock W, Rose L, Dennis CL. Pregnant and postpartum admissions to the intensive care unit: a systematic review. Intensive Care Med. 2010;36(9):1465–74.
20. Quinn AC, Milne D, Columb M, et al. Failed tracheal intubation in obstetric anaesthesia: 2 yr national case-control study in the UK. Br J Anaesth. 2013;110(1):74–80.
21. Lapinsky SE. Cardiopulmonary complications of pregnancy. Crit Care Med. 2005;33(7):1616–22.
22. Rigby FB, Pastorek JG. Pneumonia during pregnancy. Clin Obstet Gynecol. 1996;39(1):107–19.
23. Goodnight WH, Soper DE. Pneumonia in pregnancy. Crit Care Med. 2005;33(10 Suppl):S390–7.
24. Sheffield JS, Cunningham FG. Community-acquired pneumonia in pregnancy. Obstet Gynecol. 2009;114(4):915–22.
25. Mandell LA, Wunderink RG, Anzueto A, et al. Infectious Diseases Society of America/American Thoracic Society consensus guidelines on the management of community-acquired pneumonia in adults. Clin Infect Dis. 2007;44(Suppl. 2):S27–72.
26. Kwon HL, Triche EW, Belanger K, et al. The epidemiology of asthma during pregnancy: prevalence, diagnosis, and symptoms. Immunol Allergy Clin N Am. 2006;26(1):29–62.

27. Tamási L, Horváth I, Bohács A, et al. Asthma in pregnancy–immunological changes and clinical management. Respir Med. 2011;105(2):159–64.
28. Brown HL, Hiett AK. Deep vein thrombosis and pulmonary embolism in pregnancy: diagnosis, complications, and management. Clin Obstet Gynecol. 2010;53(2):345–59.
29. McDonnell NJ, Percival V, Paech MJ. Amniotic fluid embolism: a leading cause of maternal death yet still a medical conundrum. Int J Obstet Anesth. 2013;22(4):329–36.
30. Maselli DJ, Adams SG, Peters JI, et al. Management of asthma during pregnancy. Ther Adv Respir Dis. 2013;7(2):87–100.
31. The Acute Respiratory Distress Syndrome Network. Ventilation with lower tidal volumes as compared with traditional tidal volumes for acute lung injury and the acute respiratory distress syndrome. N Engl J Med. 2000;342:1301–8.
32. Powrie R, Camann W, editors. De Swiet's medical disorders in obstetric practice. 5th ed. Oxford: Blackwell Publishing Limited; 2010.
33. Amato MBP, Barbas CSV, Medeiros DM, et al. Effect of a protective-ventilation strategy on mortality in the acute respiratory distress syndrome. N Engl J Med. 1998;338:347–54.
34. Campbell LA, Klocke RA. Implications for the pregnant patient. Am J Respir Crit Care Med. 2001;163(5):1051–4.
35. Kaiser PS, Kirby RS. Obesity as a risk factor for cesarean in a low-risk population. Obstet Gynecol. 2001;97(1):39–43.
36. Pathi A, Esen U, Hildreth A. A comparison of complications of pregnancy and delivery in morbidly obese and non-obese women. J Obstet Gynaecol. 2006;26(6):527–30.
37. McElhatton PR. The effects of benzodiazepine use during pregnancy and lactation. Reprod Toxicol. 1994;8(6):461–75.
38. Ala-Kokko TI, Pienimäki P, Lampela E, et al. Transfer of clonidine and dexmedetomidine across the isolated perfused human placenta. Acta Anaesthesiol Scand. 1997;41(2):313–9.
39. Tariq M, Cerny V, Elfaki I, et al. Effects of subchronic versus acute in utero exposure to dexmedetomidine on foetal developments in rats. Basic Clin Pharmacol Toxicol. 2008;103(2):180–5.
40. Samanta S, Samanta S, Wig J, Baronia AK. How safe is the prone position in acute respiratory distress syndrome at late pregnancy? Am J Emerg Med. 2014;32:687.e1–3.
41. Kenn S, Weber-Carstens S, Weizsaecker K, Bercker S. Prone positioning for ARDS following blunt chest trauma in late pregnancy. Int J Obstet Anesth. 2009;18:268–71.
42. Sun Q, Qiu H, Huang M, Yang Y. Lower mortality of COVID19 by early recognition and intervention: experience from Jiangsu Province. Ann Intensive Care. 2020;10:33.
43. Allred CC, Matias Esquinas A, Caronia J, et al. Successful use of noninvasive ventilation in pregnancy. Eur Respir Rev. 2014;23(131):142–4.
44. Frassanito L, Draisci G, Pinto R, et al. Successful application of helmet non-invasive ventilation in a parturient with acute respiratory distress syndrome. Minerva Anestesiol. 2011;77:1121–3.
45. Djibre M, Berkane N, Salengro A, et al. Noninvasive management of acute respiratory distress syndrome related to influenza a (H1N1) virus pneumonia in a pregnant woman. Intensive Care Med. 2010;36:373–4.
46. Montufar-Rueda C, Ditisheim A, Gei AF, Pinilla R, Dinh E, Velez J, Castillo b, Farias L. Noninvasive positive pressure ventilation (NIPPV) in the pregnant patient: a case series. Open J Obstet Gynecol. 2020;10:1563–72.
47. Meschia G. Fetal oxygenation and maternal ventilation. Clin Chest Med. 2011;32(1):15–9, vii
48. Hampl V, Jakoubek V. Regulation of fetoplacental vascular bed by hypoxia. Physiol Res. 2009;58(Suppl 2):S87–93.
49. Peng AT, Blancato LS, Motoyama EK. Effect of maternal hypocapnia v. eucapnia on the foetus during caesarean section. Br J Anaesth. 1972;44(11):1173–8.
50. Ivankovic AD, Elam JO, Huffman J. Effect of maternal hypercarbia on the newborn infant. Am J Obstet Gynecol. 1970;107(6):939–46.
51. Tomlison M, Cauthers T, Whitty J. Does delivery improve maternal condition in the respiratory-compromised gravida? Obstet Gynecol. 1998;91:108–11.

Weaning and Liberation from Mechanical Ventilation

Pedro Arriaga

When to start and how to liberate critically ill patients on mechanical ventilation in the ICU are very important processes. How to carry out the practice of weaning and liberation of patients from mechanical ventilation has a tremendous impact on the morbi-mortality of patients in the ICU [1]. We should start evaluating the readiness for liberation as soon as possible, using clinical criteria and physiological tests based on protocols. Once this is done, we can reduce the degree of support from the ventilator (weaning) followed by extubation (liberation).

Different institutions and organizations around the world have developed a variety of methods for weaning and liberation. The use of daily awakening trials (DAT) and spontaneous breathing trials (SBT) has been globally accepted. These methods can be manual or computer generated, but there is not enough evidence that one is superior to the other. Manual methods are the most common ones and the ones with more experience, but they are also more time consuming.

The use of a protocolized weaning process has been widely supported in clinical trials as compared to the ones using only clinical judgment [2–6].

Prerequisites for liberation of patients from mechanical ventilation are the following:

1. The underlying condition for intubation has been corrected.
2. The patient is hemodynamically stable.
3. The patient must be able to maintain satisfactory gas exchange using minimal settings.
4. The neurological status of the patient is good enough to protect the airway (the presence of cough and gag reflex; the amount of secretions) [5, 7–9].

P. Arriaga (✉)
Division of Critical Care, Karl Heusner Memorial Hospital, Belize City, Belize

J. Hidalgo et al. (eds.), *Personalized Mechanical Ventilation*,
https://doi.org/10.1007/978-3-031-14138-6_16

1 Weaning Parameters

A series of parameters to evaluate the readiness of a patient on when and how to start the weaning process are the following:

1. The patient oxygenation status (PaO_2, P/F ratio, PaO_2/PAO_2 ratio, A-a DO_2 gradient).
2. The performance of the respiratory muscles in a particular patient (respiratory rate, tidal volume, levels of $PaCO_2$, minute ventilation, Pimax, forced vital capacity, maximum voluntary ventilation, ultrasonographic evaluation of the diaphragm).
3. The work of breathing of the patient (dynamic and static compliance).
4. The central respiratory drive of the patient (P0.1, mean inspiratory flow) [8–10].

2 Weaning Predictors

These are physiological tests that help us to predict the readiness of our patients to tolerate the weaning process and to initiate spontaneous breathing trials.

2.1 Rapid Shallow Breathing Index (RSBI) Test.

In 1991, Yang and Tobin described this index as the ratio of respiratory rate (RR) to tidal volume (VT) with a threshold value of >105 breaths/min/L as predicted of liberation failure, while a value <105 breaths/min/L was linked to a successful liberation.

The RSBI has a moderate sensitivity and poor specificity for predicting extubation (liberation) success. The conditions that can affect the results of the RSBI are sepsis, fever, supine position, anxiety, restrictive lung disease, female gender, diameter of the endotracheal tube that we are using in our patients, and suctioning [8–10].

2.2 Cuff Leak Test

The presence of an endotracheal tube has been linked to the development of laryngeal edema, especially when the patient has been on mechanical ventilation for several days (and/or manipulation of the airway during intubation). This increases the incidence of post-extubation stridor that potentially is a risk factor for re-intubation. The cuff leak test is used to assess the risk for potential stridor in patients post-extubation [11, 12].

To perform the test:

1. Patients must be properly suctioned with the cuff.
2. The inspiratory and expiratory tidal volumes with the cuff must be recorded.
3. The cuff has to be deflated.
4. The expiratory tidal volume over the next six breathing cycles must be recorded, and an average of the three lowest values should be taken.
5. The difference between the inspiratory tidal volume (before the cuff was deflated) and the averaged expiratory tidal volume will be the cuff leak volume [11, 12].

The suggested cutoff value is >110 ml or 10% of the tidal volume for a patient to have risk of post-extubation stridor [11, 12].

This test has good specificity but moderate sensitivity for the possibility of post-extubation stridor. According to the latest guidelines from the American Thoracic Society, a cuff leak test is important for:

1. Patients that have had a traumatic intubation.
2. Patients intubated for longer than 6 days.
3. Patients that were using large endotracheal tubes.
4. Female patients.

The guidelines suggest that the use of systemic steroids should be considered at least 4 h before extubation for patients who failed a cuff leak test but passed a SBT and are ready for liberation [11, 12].

3 Daily Awakening Trials (DATs)

A DAT is a time interval when sedatives are held in order to evaluate the degree of response of the patient and need for continuity of using such medications. The use of DATs and SBTs is the foundation to decide when to liberate our patients from mechanical ventilation. Teamwork, proper communication, and use of protocols are critical in order to perform valid DATs and SBTs [12, 13].

A safety screen must be performed in order to determine if the patient is a candidate for a DAT.

This safety screen must take into consideration:

1. The underlying conditions and the indication for intubation.
2. The mode of ventilation and the ventilator parameters that are being used on the patient.
3. Associated conditions like the previous neurological status.
4. The use of medications and alcohol.
5. The metabolic state of the patient.
6. The level of agitation.

Daily eligibility should be performed on each patient. Once the patient passes this safety screen, a DAT should be performed. If the patient fails the DAT, the level of sedation, type of sedatives, and doses have to be reconsidered (reduction to half of the previous dose). Once the patient passes a DAT, a SBT must be performed [12, 13].

4 Spontaneous Breathing Trial (SBT)

A SBT consists of a time interval when mechanical ventilation is held or used with minimal settings (PEEP 5 and PSV 5), which helps us to decide if the patient can breathe without or with minimal assistance and to consider liberation from mechanical ventilation. When we compare patients who have been evaluated using SBTs to patients who have been weaned according to the discretion of the treating physician, BTS-based protocols reduce the duration of mechanical ventilation [14–16].

During an SBT, the patient is placed on continuous positive airway pressure (CPAP) of 5 cm, a low level of pressure support ventilation (5 cm), and a $FiO_2 < 50\%$ (minimal settings). Typically, the time period of the trial should be between 30 min and 2 h. The time of the trial must depend on the indication and duration of the mechanical ventilation or how the patient performed on previous SBTs [15–17].

4.1 Eligibility Criteria for SBT

Improved or solved respiratory failure.

Patient is able to breathe spontaneously.

$FiO_2 < 50\%$, $PaO_2/FiO_2 > 150$, PEEP 8 cm, H_2O $SPO_2 > 88\%$.

No agitation.

Respiratory rate <35 breaths/min, minute volume < 5 L/min.

Hemodynamically stable (none or minimal vasopressor use, mean arterial blood pressure >60 mm Hg, no arrhythmia).

No agitation, stable intracranial pressure in neurological patients.

Hemoglobin level >7 g/L [7, 13, 18, 19].

4.2 Criteria for a Failed SBT

1. Respiratory rate >35 breaths/min for 5 min or <6 breaths/min (use of accessory muscles/paradoxical breathing patterns).
2. Peripheral saturation <90% (we must consider the oxygenation status and the comorbidities that patients have before intubation).
3. Heart rate >140 beats/min or increase 25% above baseline or <60 beats/min.
4. New-onset dysrhythmias.

5. Systolic blood pressure >180 mm Hg or <90 mm Hg.
6. Changes in mental status (agitations, delirium, somnolence).
7. Diaphoresis.

Once the patient fulfills the criteria for a successful SBT (30% of patients that never satisfy the previous criteria may be weaned), has appropriate cough, has a gag reflex present, handles secretions well, and has a positive cuff leak test, he or she should be extubated (liberated) as soon as possible [20, 21].

5 Conclusion

Weaning and liberation are important processes in mechanically ventilated patients. Based on evidence, these processes can be effectively performed when a protocolized method is used. A successful weaning and liberation process needs teamwork with excellent communication.

References

1. Baker AM, et al. Effect on the duration of mechanical ventilation of identifying patient capable of breathing spontaneously. NEJM. 1996;335(25):1864.
2. Kolleff MH, et al. A randomized controlled trial of protocol-directed versus physician directed weaning from mechanical ventilation. Crit Care Med. 1997;25(4):567–74.
3. Blackwood B, et al. Protocolized versus non protocolized weaning for reducing the duration of mechanical ventilation in critically ill adult patients Cochrane database. Syst Rev. 2014;2014(11):CD006904.
4. Brochard L, et al. Comparison of three methods of gradual withdrawal from ventilatory support during weaning from mechanical ventilation. AM J Respir Crit Care Med. 1994;150(4):896.
5. Baker E. The prognostic significance of passing a daily screen of weaning parameters. Intensive Care Med. 1999;25(6):581.
6. Nurns KE, et al. Wean earlier and automatically with new technology (the WEAN study). A multicenter, pilot randomized control trial. Am J Respir Crit Care Med. 2013;187(11):1203.
7. Girard TD, et al. An official American Thoracic Society/American College of Chest Physicians clinical practice guideline: liberation from mechanical ventilation in critically ill adults: rehabilitation protocols, ventilator liberation protocols and cuff leak test. Am J Respir Crit Care Med. 2017;195 (1:120–33.
8. Yang KL, Tobin MJ. A prospective study of indexes predicting the outcome of trials of weaning from mechanical ventilation. N Engl J Med. 1991;324:1445–50.
9. Karthika M, et al. Rapid shallow breathing index. Anna Thoracidc Med. 2016;11(3):167–76.
10. Trivedi V, et al. The usefulness of the rapid shallow breathing index in predicting successful extubation: a systemic review and meta-analysis. Chest. 2022;161(1):97–111.
11. Kuriyama A. Performance of the cuff leak test in adults in predicting post extubation airway complications - a systemic review and metanalysis. Crit Care. 2020;24(1):640.
12. Girard TD, et al. An official American Thoracic Society/American College of Chest Physicians clinical practice guideline: liberation from mechanical ventilation in critically ill adults: rehabilitation protocols, ventilator liberation protocols and cuff leak test. Am J Respir Crit Care Med. 2017;195:120–33.

13. Girard TD, et al. Efficacy and safety of a paired sedation and ventilation weaning protocol for mechanically ventilated patients in intensive care(awakening and breathing controlled trial) a randomized controlled trial. Lancet. 2008;371:126–34.
14. Esteban A, et al. A comparison of four methods of weaning patients from mechanical ventilation Spanish lung failure collaborative. NEJM. 1995;332:345.
15. Blackwood B, et al. Protocolized versus non-protocolized weaning for reducing of duration of mechanical ventilation in critically ill adult patients. Cochrane Database Sys Rev. 2014;2014:CD006904.
16. Ely EW, et al. Effect on the duration of mechanical ventilation of identifying patients capable of breathing spontaneously. NEJM. 1996;335(25):1864.
17. Brochard L, et al. Inspiratory pressure support compensates for the additional work of breathing caused by the endotracheal tube. Anesthesiology. 1991;75:739–45.
18. MacIntyre NR, et al. Evidence base guidelines for weaning and discontinuing ventilator support: a collective task force facilitated by the American College of Chest Physicians; the American Association for Respiratory Care: and the American college of Critical Care Medicine. Chest. 2001;120:375S–95S.
19. Collective Task force American College Chest Physicians/American Association for respiratory Care/American College of Critical Care Medicine. Evidence based guidelines for weaning and discontinuing ventilator support. Respir Care. 2002;47(1):69–90.
20. Herbert PC, et al. DO blood transfusions improve outcomes related to mechanical ventilation? Chest. 2001;1119(6):1850.
21. Ely EW, et al. The prognostic significance of passing a daily screen of weaning parameters. Intensive Care Med. 1999;25(6):581.

Mechanical Ventilation in Septic Shock

Adel Mohamed Yasin Alsisi, Jorge Hidalgo, Jorge E. Sinclair De Frías, and Allyson Hidalgo

1 Introduction

Mechanical ventilation, over the years, has been one of the cornerstone strategies in critical care and one of the most utilized life support measures used in a critically ill patient. Mechanical ventilation and critical care units are historically linked. In the last decade, we have seen important progress in the strategies offering mechanical ventilation to support the respiratory system, having into consideration physiological and gas exchange as well as the histology and biomolecular aspects of the lung tissue and more friendly use of mechanical ventilators. A lot of effort has been put into well-defined mechanical ventilator support strategies [1].

Shock is a state characterized for a tissue hypoxia and also dysregulated oxygen delivery that can lead to multi-organ failure. Most frequently, shock is caused by sepsis and it is common to see this patient admitted in the intensive care unit (ICU) because of the need for close hemodynamic monitoring (see Table 1).

The patients with sepsis are always a clinical challenge [2]. Sepsis is a major syndromic cause of intensive care unit admission, and sepsis is associated with high

A. M. Y. Alsisi
ICU Department, Prime Healthcare Group, Dubai, UAE

Critical Care Department, Cairo University, Cairo, Egypt

Prime Hospital, Dubai, UAE

J. Hidalgo (✉)
Critical Care Division, Belize Healthcare Partners, Belize, Belize

J. E. Sinclair De Frías
Faculty of Medicine, University of Panama, Panama City, Panama

A. Hidalgo
Biochemistry, Arizona State University, Phoenix, AZ, USA

J. Hidalgo et al. (eds.), *Personalized Mechanical Ventilation*,
https://doi.org/10.1007/978-3-031-14138-6_17

Table 1 Shock

Shock is most frequently caused by sepsis and is a common reason for ICU admission Needs close hemodynamic monitoring. Clinical manifestation: – Systemic arterial: SBP < 90 mmHg or mean arterial pressure (MAP) 70 mmHg – Tissue hypoperfusion: Cool and clammy skin versus warmed and flushed, low urine output 0.5 ml/kg/h, and altered mental status – Metabolic acidosis: Serum lactate level > 2 mmol/L and anion gap
Causes and pathophysiology: Septic shock is a form of distributive shock and is the most common etiology of shock seen in the ICU. However, other etiologies should be considered as follows: – Distributive shock: (vasodilation) sepsis and anaphylaxis; by echocardiography, normal cardiac chambers and preserved contractility – Hypovolemic shock: (loss of plasma or blood volume) hemorrhage, internal fluid losses (third spacing), external fluid losses(GI losses); by echocardiography, small cardiac and we can see normal or high contractility – Obstructive shock: (obstruction, pericardial tamponade) pulmonary embolism, cardiac tamponade, or tension pneumothorax. By echocardiography, we can see pericardial effusion, small right and left ventricle, and dilated inferior vena cava, in pulmonary embolism of pneumothorax: Dilated right ventricle, small left ventricle – Cardiogenic shock: (ventricular failure) acute myocardial infarction, end-stage cardiomyopathy, advanced valvular heart disease, myocarditis, cardiac arrhythmias, pump failure, or dysfunction. By echocardiography, large ventricles and poor contractility
Identifying the etiology of shock is crucial for adequate treatment, and each of the categories of shock listed above requires a specific management strategy.

morbidity and mortality [3]. The progression of an organ failure requiring support is expected in the septic patient; the path of recovery is slow, with a profound impact on quality of life even months after the onset of sepsis [3]. Sepsis can affect any organ, and the lungs are usually an important concern [4]. In order to reduce the possibility of lung injury, a proper sepsis care should therefore consider ventilatory support to achieve our goals.

1.1 Sepsis-Associated Lung Injury

The clinical relevance of sepsis-related lung injury is very important and, regardless of its source, sepsis (including pneumonia, which is one of the most common causes of ARDS) can induce lung inflammation through several mechanisms that are independent of mechanical ventilation, including [1, 2, 4]:

Inflammatory mediators as

- Cytokines.
- Collagen and fibronectin deposits.
- Apoptosis of the alveolar cells (mediated by Fas/Fas-L).
- Peroxynitrite production and also depending on the causative agent [5].

During sepsis-associated lung injury, the different inflammatory mediators vary as the condition evolves. Inflammatory response to the underlying injury leads to damage to the epithelial barriers and causes an accumulation of protein-rich edema fluid in the alveoli. Physiologically, the alveolar damage results in a ventilatory-perfusion mismatch (V/Q mismatch) with an increased shunting (alveoli unable to exchange oxygen) and an increase in dead space (microvascular injury leading to lack of perfusion). On the other hand, neutrophil activation in the lung increased throughout the progression of lung injury [6]. Some studies report that harmful ventilatory strategies show important systemic effects and also impact mortality, and also we notice an increase in the susceptibility of the lung to ventilator injury [7, 8].

2 Mechanical Ventilation Consideration

After we address the severity of the lung damage, the next step we need to work on is the supportive care that limits ventilator-induced lung injury (see Tables 2 and 3).

2.1 *Low Tidal Volume*

An important improvement in survival rates and reduction of mechanical ventilator-related injuries like barotrauma have been seen with the use of lung-protective and pressure-limited ventilatory strategies, and the recommendations are to use a low tidal volume of 5–8 ml/Kg, employ a longer inspiratory time, and not exceed a transpulmonary pressure of 30 cm water. Permissive hypercapnia may occur with lesser tidal volumes, but it is tolerated [1, 9].

We need to set the mechanical ventilation goals as follows (see Table 4):

- Improving gas exchange.
- Reducing work of breathing.
- Avoiding oxygen toxicity.

Table 2 Causes of ventilator-induced lung injury

Volutrauma (barotrauma)	Atelectrauma	Biotrauma
Delivering too much volume/pressure leads to overdistention to the alveoli. Because the compliance of the ARDS lungs is heterogeneous, the same airway pressure may cause under-distention of a more affected lung region with low compliance and overdistention of a less affected region	Allowing alveoli to collapse completely during each breath cycle with too little airway pressure leads to shear stress and denaturation of surfactants	The physical forces and trauma of ventilation lead to release of mediators that sustain inflammation and translocation of proinflammatory products and bacteria through already permeable barriers, causing systemic damage

Table 3 Lung injury caused by forces generated by ventilation at low and high lung volumes

Ventilation at low lung volume: Atelectotrauma Lung inhomogeneity	**Ventilation at high volumes:** Hyperinflation, air leaks Overdistention		
Structural consequences: Epithelial-mesenchymal transformation, surfactant dysfunction, fibroproliferation, sloughing of bronchial epithelium, hyaline membranes, pulmonary edema, increased alveolar-capillary permeability			
Biologic alterations: – Increased concentration of – Hydroxyproline, transforming growth factor b – Interleukin-8 **Release of mediators:** – Tumor necrosis factor a (TNFa), B-catenin – Interleukin-6 (IL-6), interleukin-1B (IL-1B) Recruitment of – Pulmonary alveolar macrophages (PAMs) – Neutrophils – Activation of epithelium and endothelium	**Physiological abnormalities:** – Physiological dead space – Compliance – PaO_2 – $PaCO_2$		
Systemic effects: **Translocation of**			
Lipopolysaccharides (LPS)	Multiple mechanism	Multiorgan	Death
Bacteria	Apoptosis dysfunction		
Various mediators			

- Minimizing high airway pressures.
- Avoiding further lung damage.
- Allowing the injured lung to heal.

We also need to have in consideration that low tidal volume side effects are increased CO_2 levels (hypercapnia) [10]. The actual agreement says that we can tolerate hypercapnia as long as the pH levels are more than 7.20, and also hypercapnia is associated with a reduction on sepsis-induced inflammation; however, the immunosuppressive effects may cause a reduction in bacterial clearance and deleterious effects in lung injury [11, 12]. ARDS is a dynamic condition, and the goals need to be set based on that.

2.2 PEEP

We must apply some degree of PEEP in ARDS patients [2]. Nevertheless, the precise definition of how much PEEP is required and the best method to calculate it is not standardized. Commonly we set predefined PEEP values, based on the FIO_2 and our oxygenation goals; The ARDS-net PEEP table calculation is another valuable tool. And another option involves setting PEEP at the maximum possible value until plateau reaches 30 cm H_2O [13], with proper titration using pulmonary mechanics

Table 4 Mechanical Ventilation goals

<table>
<tr><td>Ventilator settings</td><td>Tidal volume</td><td colspan="9">Oxygen titration and PEEP</td></tr>
<tr><td>Calculated predicted body weight (PBW) for males or females</td><td>Goals of plateau pressure
pPlat < 30 cm H_2O</td><td colspan="9">Set oxygenation goals: paO_2 55–80 mmHg or SpO_2 88–95%</td></tr>
<tr><td rowspan="3">Initial mode as volume assist control: Initial tidal volume to 6 ml/kg PBW</td><td rowspan="3">Check inspiratory plateau pressure with 0.5 s inspiratory pause at least every 4 h and after each change in PEEP or tidal volume</td><td colspan="9">Use FIO_2/PEEP combination to achieve oxygen goals:</td></tr>
<tr><td>FIO_2</td><td>0.3</td><td>0.4</td><td>0.5</td><td>0.6</td><td>0.7</td><td>0.8.</td><td>0.9</td><td>1.0</td></tr>
<tr><td>PEEP</td><td>5</td><td>5–8</td><td>8–10</td><td>10</td><td>10–14</td><td>14</td><td>14–18</td><td>18–24</td></tr>
<tr><td>Initial ventilation rate < 35 breaths/min with the idea to match baseline minute ventilation</td><td>pPlat >30 cm H_2O, tidal volume in 1 ml/kg PBW to 5 or if necessary to 4 ml/kg PBW
pPlat 25 cm H_2O and tidal volume < 6 ml/kg, tidal volume by 1 ml/kg PBW until pPlat >25 cm H_2O or tidal volume = 6 ml/kg
In case auto-PEEP or severe dyspnea occurs, tidal volume may be increased to 7 or 8 ml/kg PBW if pPlat remains 30 cm H_2O</td><td colspan="9">PEEP should be applied starting with the minimum value for a given FIO_2</td></tr>
<tr><td colspan="2">Volume cycled</td><td colspan="9">Pressure controlled</td></tr>
<tr><td>Advantages</td><td>Guaranteed tidal volume and VE, and most of the time the familiarity of the clinician</td><td colspan="2">Advantages</td><td colspan="7">Airway pressures controlled and better patient tolerance</td></tr>
<tr><td>Disadvantages</td><td>Airway pressure not controlled and patient tolerance is worse</td><td colspan="2">Disadvantages</td><td colspan="7">VT and VE not guaranteed and less clinician familiarity</td></tr>
</table>

and imaging techniques [10, 11]. Probably, a reduced ARDS mortality is seen when we apply high numbers of PEEP [12]. One approach we can use is to set the PEEP according to the high values of the ALVEOLI trial PEEP table [14, 15]. One of the special considerations we need to have in mind is in those patients with right ventricle failure, commonly seen in ARDS patients, and this is an important marker of poor prognosis. In this situation, an increase in PEEP values may worsen the hemodynamic status of the patient.

2.3 *Lung-Protective Ventilation in Sepsis Without Lung Injury*

The use of lung-protective strategies outside acute lung injury is not clear. A recent meta-analysis suggested that low tidal volume ventilation could be associated with clinical benefits; the majority of the publication is more in surgical patients [1, 16].

Low tidal volumes may reduce the progression to lung injury even in non-ARDS patients [14]. This is based on the concept that patients with sepsis are more prone to ventilatory-induced lung injury. Due to that, it is advisable to initiate lung-protective ventilatory strategies as soon as possible with the septic patients [17].

2.4 *Open the Lung and Maneuvers of Recruitment*

The systematic increase in the airway pressure addressed to open the closed alveolar units is called maneuver recruitment. Since the closing pressure is lower than the opening pressure, units will remain open at lower airway pressures once opened. This will result in an increase in residual lung capacity and, therefore, may theoretically decrease dynamic lung strain. Nevertheless, there is no consensus regarding how and when a recruitment maneuver should be performed. A recent systematic review suggested that recruitment maneuvers were associated with mortality improvement, but it was underpowered [17–19]. Therefore, recruitment maneuvers are an interesting second-tier therapy for hypoxemia in ARDS (see Table 5).

The use of PEEP may reduce or prevent ventilator-induced lung injury. Sufficient PEEP to recruit atelectatic alveolar units and increase lung volumes so that respiration happens on the most compliant part of the pressure-volume curve is recommended. On a regular clinical day, this can be achieved by measuring plateau pressures and calculating lung compliance at different levels of PEEP.

Table 5 Mechanical ventilation consideration, based on lung-protective strategies

Tidal volume	The current standard of care for MV in ARDS includes lung-protective ventilation targeting a low tidal volume Low tidal volume: 4–6 ml/kg (predictive body weight). Each patient will present with their own individual challenges. Requires evaluation of end-expiratory lung volume (EELV) and inspiratory capacity (IC), artificial intelligence, and closed-loop systems that can contribute to better monitoring
PEEP	PEEP represents an essential component in ARDS management. PEEP allows alveolar recruitment to potentially open collapsed or edematous and inhomogeneously distributed areas of the ARDS "baby lung." important to set our oxygenation goals (PaO_2: 55-80 mmHg, or SPO_2: 88–92%) and we need to titrate the PEEP: Mild ARDS: Low peep <12 cm H_2O; in moderate-to-severe ARDS: High PEEP >12–15 cm H_2O
Plateau pressure	Plateau pressure: <27 cm H_2O. We need to maintain low driving pressure < 13 cm H_2O. The driving pressure helps to individualize tidal volume and PEEP levels
Flow rate	IFR = comfort: 60–80 L × min; with this variable, we control how quickly the air goes in
Rate	Rate = ventilation: Initially, we set it at 18 and we made adjustments based on the ventilatory needs
Transpulmonary pressure	PL represents the distending force of the lung determined by the equation PAW—PP L (where PAW is airway pressure and PP L is the pleural pressure), and it is estimated by esophageal pressure (PE S). In ARDS, both lung and chest wall elastance (ECW) is often impaired. It is critical to have a good physiological interpretation
Mechanical power	Mechanical power (MP) is the product of mechanical energy and respiratory rate, also defined as the amount of energy per unit of time
Driving pressure	Driving pressure (ΔP) represents the ratio between VT and CRS or the airway plateau pressure minus PEEP (PP LAT – PEEP)
Alveolar recruitment	We need to identify the patients that can benefit from a recruitment maneuver
Oxygenation	Is one of the most common targets in setting ventilation as well as gas exchange; also we need to consider other key variables as dead space, ventilatory ratio, and oxygen transport
Personalized medicine	The use of phenotypes can be used for stratification, but the translation to clinical practice requires more research

3 Final Points

Septic shock is a common cause of lung injury and increases lung susceptibility to VILI. However, the particularities of the management of sepsis-induced pulmonary lesions are still not yet well defined. The recommendation is to use a lung-protective mechanical ventilation approach for all patients with sepsis. We need to approach each patient individually based on lung physiology and morphology, etiology, lung imaging, and identification of the phenotypes; this can benefit the management of these patients in the future.

References

1. Pelosi P, Ball L, et al. Personalized mechanical ventilation in acute respiratory distress syndrome. Crit Care. 2021;25:250. https://doi.org/10.1186/s13054-021-03686-3.
2. Esteban A, Anzueto A, Frutos F, Alía I, Brochard L, Stewart TE, Benito S, Epstein SK, Apezteguía C, Nightingale P, Arroliga AC, Nightingale P, et al. Characteristics and outcomes in adult patients receiving mechanical ventilation. JAMA. 2002;287(3):345–55.
3. Evans L, Rhodes A, Annane D. Surviving Sepsis Campaign: international guidelines for management of severe sepsis and septic shock. Crit Care Med. 2021;49(11):e1063–143.
4. Angus DC, van der Poll T. Severe sepsis and septic shock. N Engl J Med. 2013;369(9):840–51.
5. Sevransky JE, Levy MM, Marini JJ. Mechanical ventilation in sepsis-induced acute lung injury/ acute respiratory distress syndrome: an evidence-based review. Crit Care Med. 2004;32(11 Suppl):S548–53.
6. Rubenfeld GD, Caldwell E, Peabody E, Weaver J, Martin DP, Neff M, Stern EJ, Hudson LD. Incidence and outcomes of acute lung injury. N Engl J Med. 2005;353(16):1685–93.
7. Villar J, Blanco J, Añón JM, Santos-Bouza A, Blanch L, Ambrós A, Gandía F, Carriedo D, Mosteiro F, Basaldúa S, et al. The ALIEN study: incidence and outcome of acute respiratory distress syndrome in the era of lung protective ventilation. Intensive Care Med. 2011;37(12):1932–41.
8. Kojicic M, Li G, Hanson AC, Lee KM, Thakur L, Vedre J, Ahmed A, Baddour LM, Ryu JH, Gajic O. Risk factors for the development of acute lung injury in patients with infectious pneumonia. Crit Care. 2012;16(2):R46.
9. Dos Santos CC, Slutsky AS. Invited review: mechanisms of ventilator-induced lung injury: a perspective. J Appl Physiol. 2000;89(4):1645–55.
10. Abraham E, Singer M. Mechanisms of sepsis-induced organ dysfunction. Crit Care Med. 2007;35(10):2408–16.
11. Waikar SS, Liu KD, Chertow GM. Diagnosis, epidemiology and outcomes of acute kidney injury. Clin J Am Soc Nephrol. 2008;3(3):844–61.
12. Protti A, Andreis DT, Monti M, Santini A, Sparacino CC, Langer T, Votta E, Gatti S, Lombardi L, Leopardi O, et al. Lung stress and strain during mechanical ventilation: any difference between statics and dynamics? Crit Care Med. 2013;41(4):1046–55.
13. Slutsky AS, Ranieri VM. Ventilator-induced lung injury. N Engl J Med. 2013;369(22):2126–36.
14. Wellman TJ, Winkler T, Costa EL, Musch G, Harris RS, Zheng H, Venegas JG, Vidal Melo MF. Effect of local tidal lung strain on inflammation in normal and lipopolysaccharide-exposed sheep. Crit Care Med. 2014;42(7):e491–500.
15. Martınez-Caro L, Nin N, Sánchez-Rodríguez C, Ferruelo A, El Assar M, de Paula M, Fernández-Segoviano P, Esteban A, Lorente JA. Inhibition of nitro- oxidative stress attenuates pulmonary and systemic injury induced by high – tidal volume mechanical ventilation. Shock. 2015;44(1):36–43.
16. Rojas M, Woods CR, Mora AL, Xu J, Brigham KL. Endotoxin-induced lung injury in mice: structural, functional, and biochemical responses. Am J Physiol Lung Cell Mol Physiol. 2005;288(2):L333–41.
17. Kitamura Y, Hashimoto S, Mizuta N, Kobayashi A, Kooguchi K, Fujiwara I, Nakajima H. Fas/ FasL-dependent apoptosis of alveolar cells after lipopolysaccharide-induced lung injury in mice. Am J Respir Crit Care Med. 2001;163(3):762–9.
18. Sousse LE, Jonkam CC, Traber DL, Hawkins HK, Rehberg SW, Traber LD, Herndon DN, Enkhbaatar P. Pseudomonas aeruginosa is associated with increased lung cytokines and asymmetric dimethylarginine compared with methicillin-resistant Staphylococcus aureus. Shock. 2011;36(5):466–70.
19. Lange M, Szabo C, Traber DL, Horvath E, Hamahata A, Nakano Y, Traber LD, Cox RA, Schmalstieg FC, Herndon DN, et al. Time profile of oxidative stress and neutrophil activation in ovine acute lung injury and sepsis. Shock. 2012;37(5):468–72.

Monitoring of Mechanical Ventilation

Khaled Ismail and Dipak Lodhe

1 Introduction

Mechanical ventilation is an essential part of treatment for patients undergoing general anesthesia or experiencing respiratory failure requiring intensive care. The use of mechanical ventilation carries a risk and does have complications that could compromise the care of those patients who might have more serious health issues. The use of mechanical ventilation monitoring is required to identify early signs of clinical worsening and to minimize the risk of iatrogenic harm. The use of plethysmography and capnography became a standard and mandatory part of monitoring during mechanical ventilation both under anesthesia and in intensive care. They ensure that adequate oxygenation and ventilation are provided. Measurement of airway pressures like plateau pressure, peak airway pressure, transpulmonary pressure, and pressure-volume loop is performed to ensure that adequate PEEP is applied and protect the patients against barotrauma. The monitoring and frequent adjustment of airway cuff pressures are performed to minimize the risk of airway injury and ventilator-associated pneumonia. We will discuss monitoring during mechanical ventilation with a focus on the accuracy, ease of use, and effectiveness in preventing harm for each of these monitoring modalities. Finally, we need to be able to assess the goal of ventilation for a particular patient (safety, comfort, or liberation) and then match the available technology to the patient's needs. This, of course, involves selecting the most appropriate mode of ventilation. But perhaps the more challenging problem is to select the optimum settings.

K. Ismail (✉)
Critical Medicine, Cleveland Clinic, Abu Dhabi, UAE

D. Lodhe
Anesthesia and Intensive Care Medicine, SSMC, Abu Dhabi, UAE

J. Hidalgo et al. (eds.), *Personalized Mechanical Ventilation*,
https://doi.org/10.1007/978-3-031-14138-6_18

Different ventilation strategies have been suggested in the past in patients with acute respiratory distress syndrome (ARDS) . Airway pressure monitoring alone is inadequate to assure optimal ventilatory support in ARDS patients. The assessment of transpulmonary pressure (P_{TP}) can help clinicians to tailor mechanical ventilation to the individual patient needs. Transpulmonary pressure monitoring, defined as airway pressure (P_{aw}) minus intrathoracic pressure (ITP), provides essential information about chest wall mechanics and its effects on the respiratory system and lung mechanics.

2 Gas Exchange

2.1 *Pulse Oximetry and Transcutaneous Carbon Dioxide Monitoring* (Fig. 1)

Pulse oximetry (SpO_2) is a standard monitoring device in intensive care units (ICUs), currently used to guide therapeutic interventions.

Pulse oximetry is widely used in anesthesiology and intensive care and, in intensive care unit (ICU) patients, has a bias of less than 1% and a good-to-moderate precision [1]; accuracy decreases in hypoxemia (oxygen saturation as measured by pulse oximetry, or SpO_2, of less than 90%). Among the intrinsic limitations of pulse oximetry are that it is insensitive to changes in arterial partial pressure of oxygen (PaO_2) at high PaO_2 levels and cannot distinguish between normal hemoglobin and methemoglobin or carboxyhemoglobin. Nail polish may affect the measurement by about 2% (not really clinically relevant) [2], and pulse oximetry can slightly underestimate arterial oxygen saturation (SaO_2) in patients with darkly pigmented skin

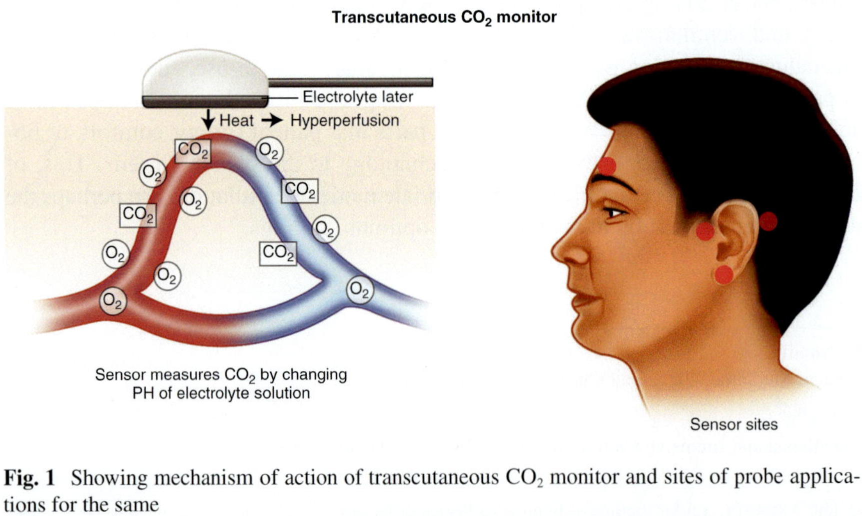

Fig. 1 Showing mechanism of action of transcutaneous CO_2 monitor and sites of probe applications for the same

[3]. Altered skin perfusion and carboxy-hemoglobin can also lead to inaccurate pulse oximetry readings. The type of probe can make a difference, and accuracy is usually better for finger than for earlobe probes [4]. False alarms are common, usually because of motion artifacts, particularly in the pediatric population.

Pulse oximetry readings should be used to provide an early warning sign, decreasing the need for blood gas measurements. In a randomized controlled trial in more than 20,000 surgical patients [5], pulse oximetry was not associated with decreased postoperative complications or mortality, but 80% of the anesthesiologists felt more secure when a pulse oximeter was used!

Transcutaneous partial pressure of carbon dioxide (PCO_2) monitors has also been developed with probes generally placed on the earlobe. Precision of transcutaneous PCO_2 measurements has improved as technology has advanced, and devices have become smaller but still need regular recalibration [6]. Their place in the respiratory monitoring of ICU patients has not yet been defined.

3 Volumetric Capnography and Dead Space Calculation

The expiratory capnogram provides qualitative information on the waveform patterns associated with mechanical ventilation and quantitative estimation of expired CO_2. Capnography tracings show three phases (Fig. 1) [7]: phase I contains gas from the apparatus and anatomic dead space (airway), phase II represents increasing CO_2 concentration resulting from progressive emptying of alveoli, and phase III represents alveolar gas. Phase III is often referred to as the plateau, and its appearance is relatively flat or has a small positive slope; the highest point is the end-tidal PCO_2 ($PetCO_2$). The almost rectangular shape of the expired capnogram depends on the homogeneity of the gas distribution and alveolar ventilation. Lung heterogeneity creates regional differences in CO_2 concentration, and gas from high V/Q regions first appears in the upper airway during exhalation. This sequential emptying contributes to the rise of the alveolar plateau; the greater the V/Q heterogeneity, the steeper the expired CO_2 slope. Accordingly, the slope of the alveolar plateau has been shown to correlate with the severity of airflow obstruction [8] (Fig. 2).

Physiologic dead space (Vd_{phys}) can be easily calculated from the Enghoff modification of the Bohr equation by using arterial partial pressure of carbon dioxide ($PaCO_2$) with the assumption that $PaCO_2$ is similar to alveolar PCO_2:

$$Vd_{phys}/V_T = (PaCO_2 - P_ECO_2)/PaCO_2, Vd_{phys} / V_T = \left(PaCO_2 - P_ECO_2\right) / PaCO_2,$$

where V_T is the tidal volume and P_ECO_2 is the partial pressure of CO_2 in mixed expired gas and is equal to the mean expired CO_2 fraction multiplied by the difference between the atmospheric pressure and the water vapor pressure. Vd_{phys} is increased in acute respiratory distress syndrome (ARDS), and a high dead space fraction represents an impaired ability to excrete CO_2 because of any kind of V/Q

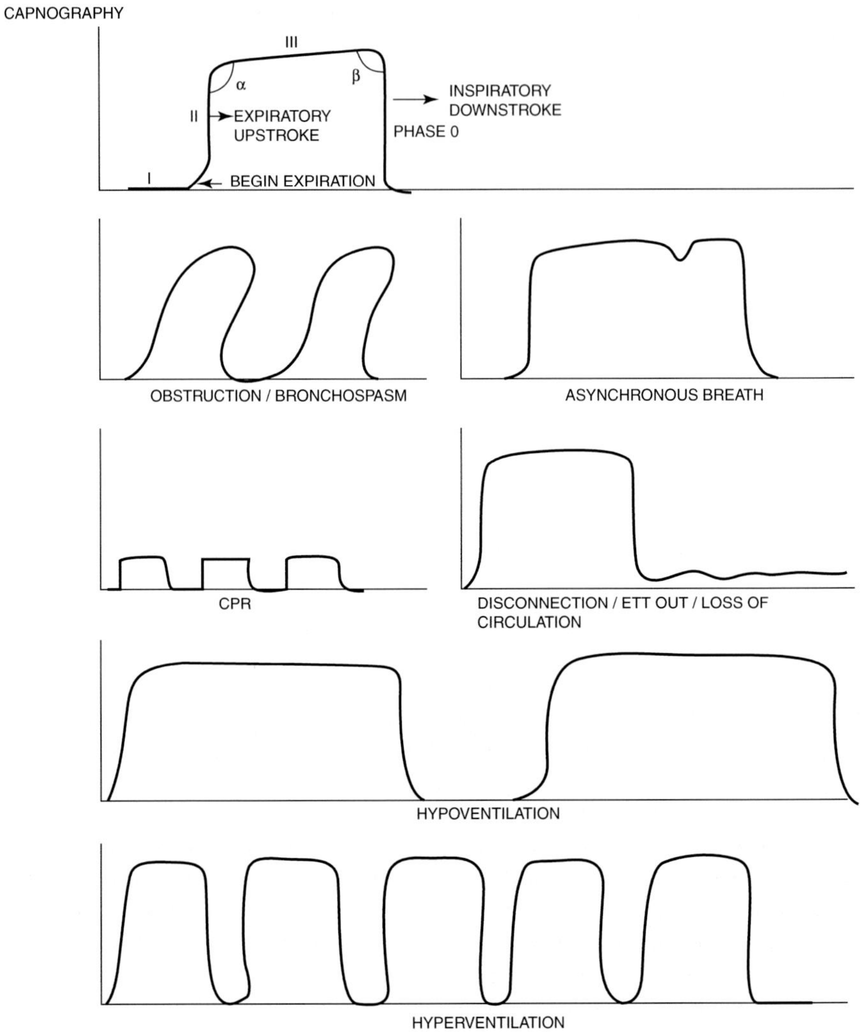

Fig. 2 Showing parts of capnograph and various patterns

mismatch. Several authors [9, 10] have demonstrated that increased Vd_{phys} values are independently associated with an increased risk of death in these patients.

Since Vd_{phys}/V_T measures the fraction of each tidal breath that is wasted on alveolar dead space (Vd_{alv}) and airway dead space(Vd_{aw}), the Vd_{aw} must be subtracted from Vd_{phys}/V_T to obtain the Vd_{alv}/V_T [11]. By using the $PetCO_2$ instead of P_ECO_2 in the equation, the Vd_{alv} can be calculated. Equating the alveolar PCO_2 to the arterial $PaCO_2$ is, however, valid only in healthy subjects. In patients with high right-to-left shunt, $PaCO_2$ is higher than alveolar PCO_2 because of the shunted blood with high $PvCO_2$ (partial pressure of carbon dioxide in mixed venous blood). Without correction [12], it must be remembered that a high dead space also includes the shunt effect.

$PaCO_2$ can be grossly estimated by $PetCO_2$. Monitoring $PetCO_2$ can also help to track $PaCO_2$ when changes in $PaCO_2$ are to be avoided (especially in critically ill, neurological patients with normal lungs). The gradient between $PaCO_2$ and $PetCO_2$ widens in ARDS and correlates across the different levels of Vd_{phys} [13]. The difference between $PaCO_2$ and $PetCO_2$ is reduced busing the maximal values of $PetCO_2$ over time [14].

In patients with sudden pulmonary vascular occlusion due to pulmonary embolism, the resultant V/Q mismatch produces an increase in Vd_{alv}. When volumetric capnography is used as a bedside technique, the association of a normal D-dimer assay result plus a normal Vd_{alv} is a highly sensitive screening test to rule out the diagnosis of pulmonary embolism [15]. Volumetric capnography has also been shown to be an excellent tool for monitoring thrombolytic efficacy in patients with pulmonary embolism [16].

When the application of positive end-expiratory pressure (PEEP) results in global lung recruitment, physiologic and alveolar dead space decrease [17]; the reverse is true when PEEP application results in lung overdistension [18]. Therefore, volumetric capnography may also be helpful to identify overdistension or better alveolar gas diffusion [19].

In summary, volumetric capnography has important potential for monitoring the difficult-to-ventilate patient. Volumetric capnography needs sophisticated equipment, and this has limited its widespread use.

3.1 Blood Gases

The PaO_2/inspired fraction of oxygen (PaO_2/FiO_2) ratio is still the most frequently used variable for evaluating the severity of lung failure and is included in the current definition of acute lung injury/ARDS [20]. The PaO_2/FiO_2 ratio is often a curvilinear (U-shaped) relationship, being at its lowest for moderate ranges of FiO_2, depending on the shunt level, the hemoglobin value, and the arteriovenous difference in O_2 content [21–23]. For a given PaO_2/FiO_2 ratio, the higher the FiO_2, the poorer the prognosis [24]. In patients with ARDS, the PaO_2/FiO_2 ratio is dependent on the PEEP level and can be a surrogate, though imperfect, marker of recruitment [25]. Hemodynamic status (via the mixed venous oxygen tension, or PvO_2) and intracardiac shunt (patent foramen ovale) also influence the PaO_2/FiO_2 ratio [26]. Despite its limitations, this ratio remains the most commonly used means of assessing the severity of lung disease. The oxygen index ([mean airway pressure × FiO_2 × 100]/PaO_2) accounts better for the influence of ventilator pressures on oxygenation value [27].

$PaCO_2$-related variables are tightly correlated to outcome [28] and to lung structural changes [29] sometimes better than oxygen-related variables (such as shunt fraction) [30, 31].

4 Alveolar-Arterial Oxygen Partial Pressure ($P_{(A\text{-}a)}\ O_2$)

Difference between alveolar oxygen partial pressure and arterial oxygen partial pressure is known as the alveolar-arterial oxygen difference ($P_{(A\text{-}a)}\ O_2$). The alveolar-arterial oxygen difference of oxygen gives us the opportunity to evaluate pulmonary gas exchange:

$$\text{Formula}: P_{(A-a)}O_2 = PAO_2 - PaO_2$$

Normal reference range: 8 mmHg (1.07 kPa), ranging 5–10 mmHg, in healthy young adults less than 30 years of age. It may increase to 24 mmHg (3.20 kPa) by the age of 60–80 years. Increase in age causes $P_{(A\text{-}a)}\ O_2$ to rise in a linear manner [32].

Clinical significance: $P_{(A\text{-}a)}\ O_2$ helps the clinician to judge whether the function of gas exchange in the lung is normal or not. Factors that affect $P_{(A\text{-}a)}\ O_2$ are anatomical shunt, imbalance of ventilation and perfusion ratio, and diffusion disorder of alveolar-capillary barrier [33].

Therefore, the changes in positive end-expiratory pressure, intrapulmonary blood flow rate, prolonged inspiratory time, and oxygen concentration can result in the change of $P_{(A\text{-}a)}\ O_2$. The higher the difference of $P_{(A\text{-}a)}\ O_2$ is, the greater the difference of oxygen content between arterial blood and alveoli will be, which suggests the impaired diffusion function of the lung. Ventilatory dysfunction often results in the rise of $P_{(A\text{-}a)}\ O_2$ difference, such as chronic obstructive pulmonary disease. In the denouement, the oxygen partial pressure difference of the alveolar artery comprehensively reflects the function of the ventilation and diffusion in the lung [34–37] (Fig. 3).

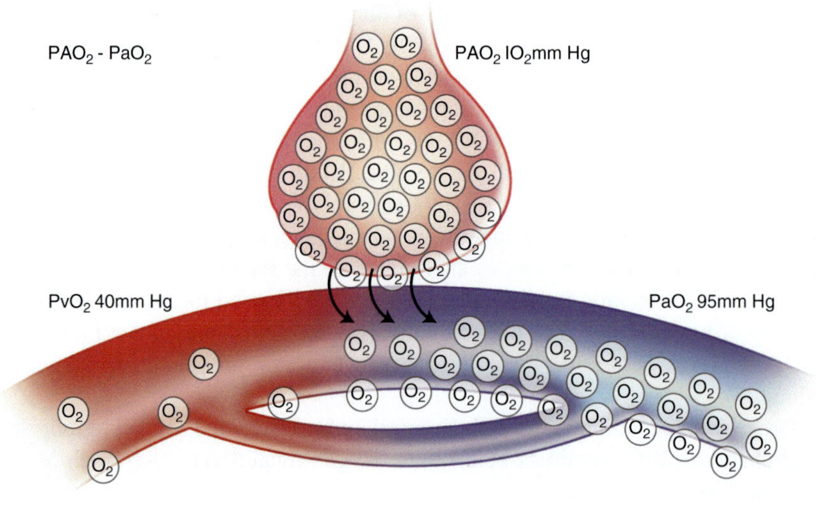

Fig. 3 $PAO_2 - PaO_2$

5 Arterial Oxygen Content (CaO_2)

The oxygen in arterial blood is in the form of physical solution and chemical binding.

Reference value: 8.55–9.45 mmol/L

Clinical significance: CaO_2 denotes the oxygen content of red blood cells and plasma. The decrease of arterial oxygen content (CaO_2) may be due to the reduction in hemoglobin, the decrease of blood oxygen saturation, or the decrease of PO_2. The normal content of oxygen in arterial blood cannot rule out tissue hypoxia.

6 Respiratory Mechanics

6.1 Compliance and Resistance (Figs. 4 and 5)

Monitoring airway pressures can provide important information. In flow (volume)-controlled mode, peak airway pressure is determined by both resistance and compliance—a high peak pressure with a much lower plateau pressure indicates a high resistance related either to the patient (bronchospasm) or to the equipment (small-diameter endotracheal tube [ETT] or narrow or obstructed tubing). Plateau pressure measurement requires a pause at end insufflation of at least 200 to 500 ms with a quasi-steady pressure. Longer pauses may be required to precisely estimate lung homogeneities or pendelluft phenomena, but their clinical role is unclear. Patients must be relaxed during this measurement.

Compliance is easily calculated as the ratio between V_T and plateau pressure minus PEEP (Fig. 2). Elastance is the reverse of compliance (how much pressure we need for a given volume). A low compliance-high elastance reflects mainly a small aerated lung available for ventilation. High plateau pressure may be related to either low compliance or high end-expiratory pressure (flow limitation or dynamic hyperinflation). Peak airway pressure is very sensitive to changes in respiratory mechanics; performing end-inspiratory and end-expiratory pauses may allow the exact cause of a high peak airway pressure to be determined. Compliance is not easily assessed on pressure-predetermined modes, especially when the expiratory phase starts before flow stops. In such cases, an end-inspiratory occlusion test should be performed to assess plateau pressure, even in time-cycled pressure-limited modes.

Measurements of respiratory mechanics are simple to perform and provide useful and relevant information for severity assessment and ventilator management. They are really reliable only in passive conditions of ventilation, in which plateau pressure monitoring is essential for adequate ventilatory management.

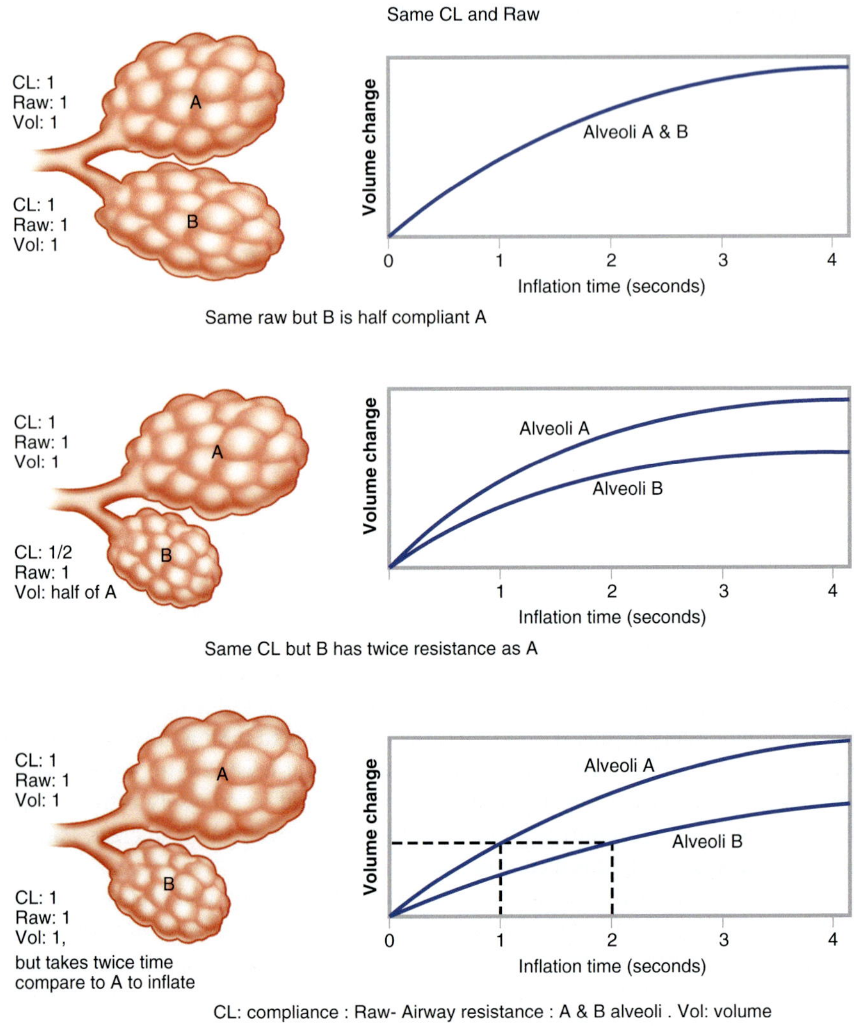

Fig. 4 Relation between compliance, resistance, and volume

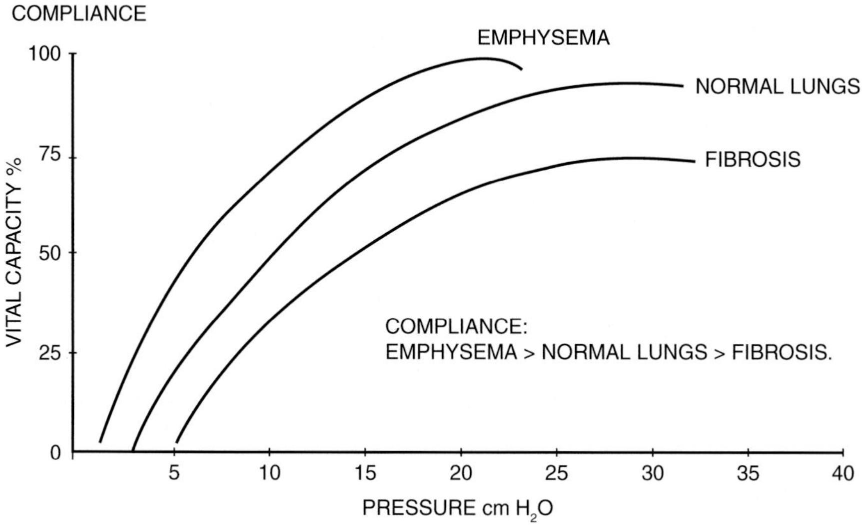

Fig. 5 Compliance in different lung conditions

7 Pressure-Volume Curves

The study of lung mechanics is particularly helpful in patients with ARDS. Study of pressure-volume (P-V) curves requires insufflations at very low flow to avoid the influence of the resistive components [38–40]. The accent has often been placed on the identification of the lower (LIP) [41] and upper (UIP) [42] inflection points on the P-V curve, but this approach has limitations. First, identifying the LIP or UIP is sometimes difficult. Second, recruitment takes place throughout the P-V curve [43, 44], and recruitment and overdistension can occur at the same time. Third, application of an optimal PEEP level should, ideally, be assessed from the expiratory rather than the inspiratory limb of this relationship.

Interpretation of P-V curves is difficult in the presence of altered chest compliance [45]. Chest wall compliance may be decreased in cases of increased abdominal pressure, thoracic trauma, large pleural effusions, obesity, and so on. Measuring esophageal pressure (surrogate of pleural pressure) allows pressure dissipated through the chest wall to be differentiated from pressure distending the lungs (transpulmonary pressure). In medical patients, the chest wall has little to modest impact on respiratory pressures [45]; whether this is different in patients with abdominal surgery or obesity needs further study. Nevertheless, the concept remains that ventilating down to too low a pressure may result in the so-called atelectrauma (opening and closing the alveoli repeatedly), and inflating the lungs too much when most of the recruitment has already occurred may result in overdistension.

The difference between the inspiratory and expiratory parts of the P-V curve is related, in part, to hysteresis [46], which reflects whether PEEP should be increased or not. If the two limbs of the curve are superimposed, increasing PEEP will not help; if there is a large difference in volume between inspiratory and expiratory portions, PEEP may help (Fig. 3). Quantification of recruitment requires multiple P-V curves [47], and, although P-V curves are now more frequently available on commercial ventilators, the lack of an estimate of recruitment still limits clinical usefulness. The P-V curve technique has thus been used mainly as a research tool.

During constant flow insufflations, a stress index (Fig. 2*)* can be calculated from the shape of the airway pressure-versus-time curve (which is essentially the opposite of the P-V curve since during constant flow time equals volume) [48]. If there is downward concavity, compliance improves over time (stress index of less than 1), reflecting tidal recruitment of collapsed alveoli; if the curve is straight (stress index of 1), compliance is constant, reflecting ventilation of the normal lung; and if there is upward concavity (stress index of greater than 1), it means that compliance is decreasing over time during insufflations, reflecting overinflation. A stress index of less than 1 may suggest a need to increase PEEP; a stress index of greater than 1 may suggest a need to reduce V_T [49]. The same limitations described for the P-V curve (that is, recruitment and overdistension) apply to this kind of analysis. The clinical place and reliability of the stress index are still debated [50] (Fig. 6).

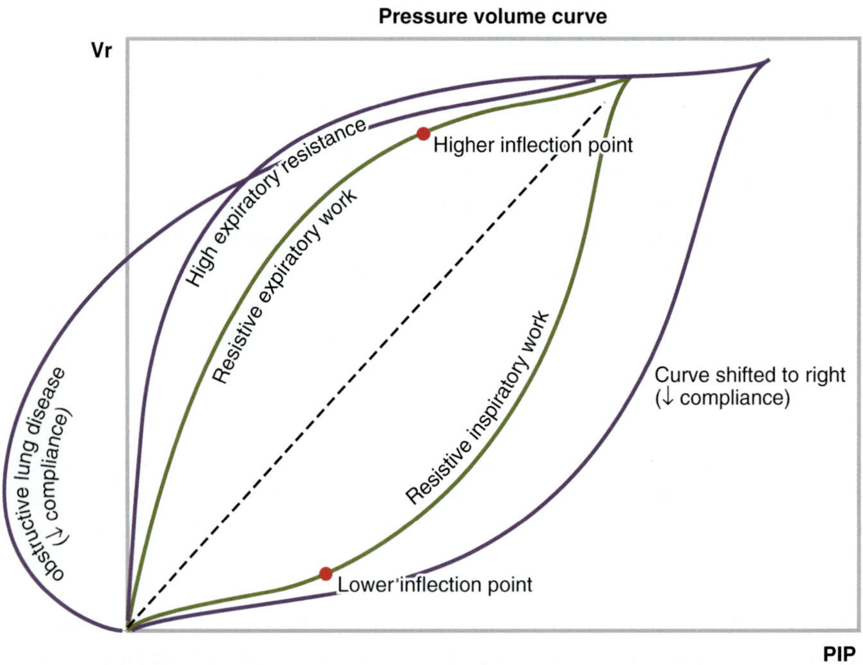

Fig. 6 Pressure-volume curve in various lung conditions. *PIP* peak inspiratory pressure, *VT* tidal volume

8 Diaphragmatic Function

Mechanical ventilation has been associated with ventilator-induced diaphragmatic dysfunction [51]. Diaphragmatic function can be altered early and is related to the duration of mechanical ventilation [52]. The transdiaphragmatic pressure difference (gastric minus esophageal pressure) reflects diaphragmatic function but only in patients who have spontaneous ventilatory breaths and who can cooperate. Magnetic phrenic stimulation can be used to assess diaphragmatic function [53] as a noninvasive method in sedated and non-sedated patients but remains a test of respiratory muscle function rather than a monitoring tool and is used mainly in research.

Measurements of diaphragmatic electrical activity are now possible and have been used to drive the ventilator during neurally adjusted ventilatory assist [54]. Although it does not provide absolute values, monitoring diaphragmatic electrical activity may be of potential interest to detect patient-ventilator asynchrony.

8.1 Pressure and Flow Monitoring to Assess Asynchrony

A considerable amount of information can be obtained from pressure- and flow-time curve analysis [55]. The airflow trace can reveal the presence of auto-PEEP, when flow does not return to zero at the end of expiration (Fig. 4). Desynchrony can be caused by poor or delayed ventilator triggering or cycling or both. Excessive levels of pressure support may result in ineffective triggering because they are associated with long inspiratory times and intrinsic PEEP [56], and insufficient assistance (for example, because of a short inspiratory time during assist/control ventilation) can also result in dyssynchrony. Auto-cycling, which results in excessive assistance and can be due to excessive triggering sensitivity or leaks, is difficult to detect. It may be revealed by reducing trigger sensitivity during a short series of "test" breaths. Decreasing levels of pressure support and increasing expiratory trigger are the most effective solutions for ineffective efforts, whereas applying some PEEP may help but does not always work [57].

Recognizing dyssynchrony is important because it can indicate dynamic hyperinflation and may lead to excessive ventilatory assistance [57] and induce delays in weaning from mechanical ventilation [58] and severe sleep disruption [59]. There is no automatic method to detect dyssynchrony. Because of the clinical importance of dyssynchrony, one must learn how to recognize it from traces on the ventilator (this can be relatively easy, at least for gross asynchronies) [58] (Fig. 5), and improved bedside training of curve reading is needed. Electromyography can also be of use in determining the presence of dyssynchrony but is rather complex for clinical use [60].

9 Occlusion Pressure ($P_{0.1}$)

The occlusion pressure, also referred to as $P_{0.1}$, reflects the respiratory drive to breathe and is correlated to WOB for a given patient. Measurements of $P_{0.1}$, now automatically provided on ventilators, may be useful to assess the patient's response to titration of ventilator settings (that is, flow rate, PEEP, and so on) and could be used as a surrogate of WOB to help titrate pressure support or external PEEP in cases of intrinsic PEEP [61, 62]. A $P_{0.1}$ of less than 2 cm H_2O is considered normal. This measure has been restricted largely to research. However, because the $P_{0.1}$ is now more widely available in the ICU and is an extremely simple and rapid way to estimate central respiratory drive, its potential clinical role needs to be evaluated.

10 Pressure-Time Product

The pressure-time product is the integral of the pressure performed by the respiratory muscles during inspiration or expiration and time or both. The pressure-time product is an alternative to WOB and has some theoretical and practical advantages over WOB calculations. The pressure-time product is associated with oxygen consumption by the respiratory muscles [63] and could be considered a surrogate to quantify the metabolic expense of respiratory effort. Since it is independent from the ability of the patient to generate volume, the pressure-time product is relevant in situations in which there is a disconnection between effort and volume (for example, during asynchrony) [64]. Normal values for the pressure-time product range between 60 and 150 cmH_2O/s per minute [65].

11 Driving Pressure

Definition: Amount of pressure required to push the given tidal volume into the patient's lung.

Two methods to calculate driving pressure:

A. Pplat—PEEP
B. p▲ = TV/Cstat

Logically, low VT will generate low pressures and will cause less harm to normal or diseased lungs. But the question is how low VT should be given.

11.1 Baby Lung Concept [26]

In ARDS, lungs are heterogeneously involved. We get some area of consolidation and some area of normal aeration lungs. The author of baby lung concept proposed that in adult patients with severe ARDS, the volume of aerated lung is approximately similar to the volume of a 5–6-year-old child. This in turn gives rise to the notion that ventricular associated lung injury is a regional phenomenon, i.e., whatever tidal volume is delivered under positive pressure gets preferentially delivered to normal lungs. So, if we deliver normal VT, it leads to excessive regional dynamic and static strain on the pulmonary tissue. From the discussion above, it makes sense that targeting a VT that matches physiology and physics of only aerated lung rather than ideal normal lung will be the best approach.

To achieve this goal, one has to measure functional lung size visually or physiologically and set VT as a fraction of function lung [28]. Simple trick is to assume that Cstat correlates with functional lung size. In a retrospective reanalysis of 3562 patients, it has been found that driving pressure was more strongly associated with survival than VT, Pstat, or PEEP [29]; on the basis of this reanalysis, it is proposed that if driving pressure is more than 15, it leads to drastic increase in barotrauma and mortality [29]. In another retrospective cohort of 700+ patients, an incremental increase in mortality has been reported in patients with driving pressure of more than 19 cm H_2O. It can be concluded that even a normal 6-8 ml/kg predicted body weight may be excessive if driving pressure is excessive, i.e., >15–19 cm H_2O.

To summarize, driving pressure represents the stress applied to the lung tissue. Our goal should be no or little harm to lung tissue by keeping check on driving pressure by managing a delicate balance between VT, Pplat, PEEP, and Cstat. Current body of evidences and literature supports the routine monitoring of driving pressure to ensure that we are not damaging whatever normal lung is left for us (Fig. 7).

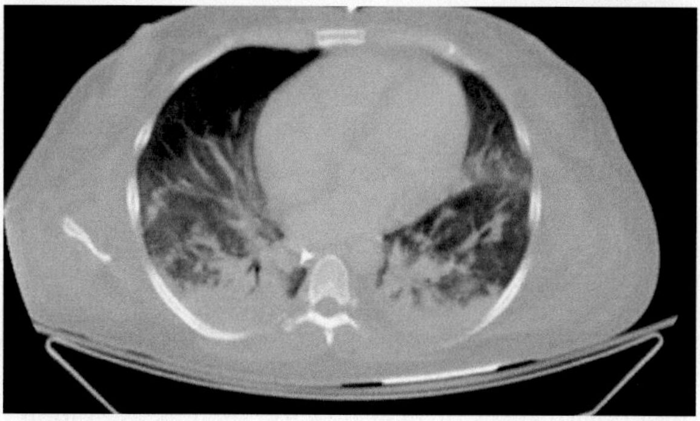

Fig. 7 (Baby lung concept) Showing that the amount of tissue taking part in gas exchange in ARDS is equivalent to baby aged 5–6 years leading to the concept of baby lungs

12 Lung Imaging

Modalities of use in the ICU for mechanically ventilated patients are chest X-ray and ultrasound.

12.1 Chest X-Ray

In addition to detecting abnormalities in lung before, during, or later in the course of mechanical ventilation, X-ray helps to assess the position of multiple catheters like nasogastric tube, central venous catheter, ET tube, and tracheostomy tube. Chest X-ray (CXR) can help detect the following abnormalities:

12.1.1 Atelectasis

A decrease in the volume of air in the lungs leading to the formation of opacity on CXR is called as atelectasis. It is the most common cause of chest X-ray opacity in ICU patients [66]. The most common areas of atelectasis in that sequence are lower left lobe, lower right lobe, and upper right lobe [67].

The X-Ray of Atelectasis Manifests as Direct X-Ray Signs and Indirect X-Ray Signs

Direct signs include reduced lung transparency and increase in the density of uniformity in the area of lung affected by atelectasis. Lobular atelectasis gives the picture in the shape of obtuse and triangular, with broad surfaces facing the costal diaphragmatic pleural surfaces and the tips pointing to the hilum of the lungs.

Indirect X-ray signs of atelectasis show hilum shadow shifting to atelectasis, and mediastinum, heart, and trachea are shifted to the affected side, especially when the whole lung shows atelectasis. However, CT is a more sensitive and accurate diagnosis of atelectasis.

12.1.2 Pneumonia

Patients in ICU have a higher incidence of pneumonia due to invasive respiratory support and complex conditions. The X-ray manifestation of pneumonia can be multi-focused or focal consolidation. Pneumonia may be difficult to distinguish from other causes of lung opacity, such as aspiration pneumonia, atelectasis, and pulmonary edema.

Pneumothorax

Pneumothorax can result from inappropriate respiratory support levels and some invasive procedures. Most of the radiographs with pneumothorax have clear pneumothorax lines, which are the boundary lines between atrophic lung tissue and gas in the pleural cavity. Mediastinal structure migration to the healthy side can be seen in a large amount of pneumothorax. Pleural effusion with pneumothorax will show gas-liquid level. Most of the ICU CXRs are performed in supine position. Such images often do not show the traditional pneumothorax, but deep sulcus may be observed [68]. As the pneumothorax increases in volume, the intrapleural air accumulates from the anteromedial region to the laterocaudal region. Deep sulcus sign is a deep and lucent costophrenic angle, which extends more inferiorly than usual. CT scan remains the gold standard for diagnosing pneumothorax.

Pleural Fluid

Pleural effusion in CXR appears as a blunt costophrenic angle. But as mentioned above, almost all CXRs in ICU are taken in supine position, and chest radiographs in the supine position are not sensitive to the diagnosis of pleural effusion and may present only as hazy opacification (Fig. 8).

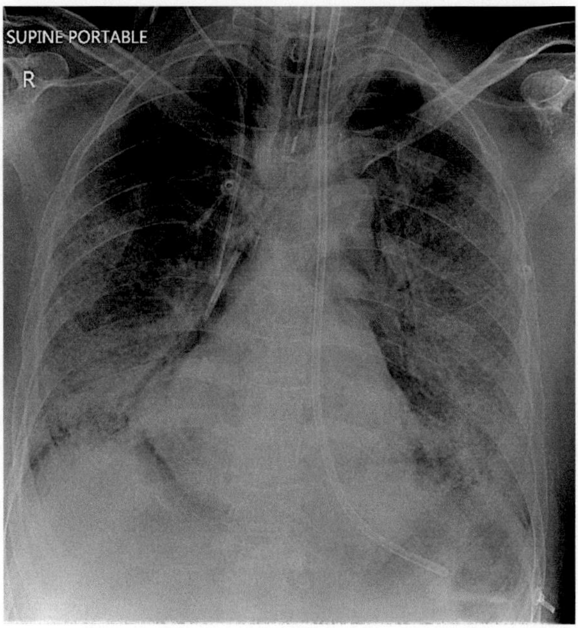

Fig. 8 Showing the importance of monitoring of CXR in the determination of positions of various invasive catheters, e.g., NG tube, ET tube, central venous catheter, and vascath for dialysis along with the effect of ventilation leading to surgical emphysema and pneumomediastinum or pneumothorax

13 Diaphragm Ultrasound

The diaphragm is a very important respiratory muscle. During spontaneous breathing, diaphragm plays an important role in generating tidal volume [69]. Many factors in ICU such as neuromuscular disease, mechanical ventilation, sepsis, and phrenic nerve injury after abdominal or cardiac surgery can lead to diaphragm dysfunction and thus increase the risk of failure to wean and prolonged mechanical ventilation [70]. Diaphragm can be examined with the help of multiple modalities like

- Electromyography.
- Transdiaphragmatic pressure.
- X-ray.
- Magnetic resonance imaging.

Most of these techniques are invasive and time consuming or involve radioactivity. Ultrasound has the advantages of being noninvasive, real time, and highly repeatable, and most importantly it is bedside. In addition to evaluating the shape of diaphragm, it also evaluates the function of diaphragm. It has been widely used in clinical diagnosis and treatment of critical care patients.

14 What Is Measured in Diaphragm Ultrasound

The thickness and the change of thickness between the left and right diaphragms are measured. Right diaphragm measurement is easier and repeatable than left [71]. It is necessary to evaluate the function of the two diaphragms separately [72].

Diaphragmatic thickness refers to the distance between the peritoneum and pleura of the diaphragms. With inhalation, the diaphragm contracts and its thickness increases. Change rate of diaphragmatic thickness = (maximum end-inspiratory diaphragmatic thickness—end-expiratory diaphragmatic thickness)/end-expiratory diaphragmatic thickness × 100% [73, 74]. In normal conditions, when the lung volume increases from functional residual volume to TLC, the average thickness of diaphragm increases by 54% (range: 42–78%) [75, 76].

For B-mode measurement, place a high-frequency probe with a frequency of 7.5 MHz or more between the anterior axillary line and the midaxillary line between the eighth and tenth intercostals, which is the junction of the diaphragm and the chest wall. The probe is kept perpendicular to the chest wall. One can see two parallel hyperechoic layers at a distance of 1.5–3 cm from the skin. The hyperechoic layer close to the skin is the pleura layer and the peritoneal layer at a distance. The area with low echo between the two hyperechoic layers is the diaphragm [77]. The thickness of diaphragm is the distance between two hyperechoic layers, i.e., pleura and peritoneum. The position of M-mode ultrasound measurement is the same as B-mode.

15 Use of Diaphragmatic Ultrasound in Mechanically Ventilated Patients

15.1 Weaning

Diaphragmatic ultrasound gives us the strength of diaphragm, as diaphragm is a very important muscle of respiration; it in turn gives an idea about the success of weaning. The results of Ferrari et al. [78] showed that the sensitivity and specificity of the change rate of diaphragmatic thickness >36% were 82% and 88%, respectively. Dinino et al. [79] reported that the sensitivity and specificity for predicting the success of weaning were 88% and 71%, respectively, when change rate of diaphragmatic thickness was more than 30%.

16 Lung Ultrasound (LUS)

Ultrasound has the advantage of being noninvasive and can be employed for the bedside assessment of the lung reliably. Ultrasound provides insights into the presence of lung pathologies like consolidation, pleural effusion, or interstitial-alveolar syndrome. LUS gives the peculiar pictures of lung like A lines, B lines, bat sign, lung sliding sign, sign of interstitial syndrome, tissue-like sign, debris sign, bronchial inflation sign, stratospheric/bar code sign, quadrilateral/sinusoidal sign, and curtain sign (Fig. 9).

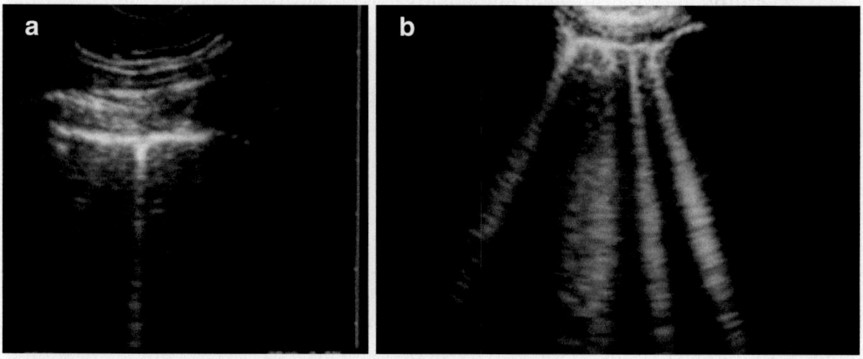

Fig. 9 Showing **a** lines (left) and **b** lines (right) in lung ultrasound

17 Ventilation Score

To calculate ventilation score, each lung is divided into three parts by anterior axillary line and posterior axillary line: anterior, lateral, and posterior. The three zones are again divided into upper and lower zones. Thus, each side of the chest wall of the patients was divided into 6 zones and 12 zones on both sides. Lung ultrasound (LUS) was performed in each area and scored according to the following criteria:

Normal pulmonary ventilation (0 points): the presence of lung sliding and horizontal A lines or no more than two B lines.

Moderate pulmonary ventilation reduction (1 point): the presence of multiple uniformly or unevenly segregated B lines.

Severe pulmonary ventilation reduction (2 points): multiple rib spaces with combined B lines.

Pulmonary consolidation (3 points): The lungs show tissue-like echoes accompanied by dynamic or static bronchial inflation signs.

According to these criteria, the total score of 12 regions ranges from 0 to 36. LUS can accurately reflect the changes of pulmonary ventilation before and after the implementation of any particular treatment measures that may affect pulmonary ventilation function, thus guiding the future decision-making. Many studies have shown that the clinical value of pulmonary ultrasound in assessing the degree of pulmonary inflation corelates well with chest CT.

18 Monitoring Lung Recruitment

Lung reaeration after recruitment maneuvers can be assessed by direct and real-time visualization [80]. The level of pulmonary collapse was found to be positively correlated with the pressure-volume curve (P-V curve). Therefore, ultrasound can guide the parameter setting of mechanical ventilation. It can also detect the possible barotrauma caused by lung recruitment.

19 Prone Position

Ultrasound can be helpful in evaluating and managing prone position ventilation therapy. Pulmonary tissue in the gravity-dependent area of ARDS patients in supine position is difficult to reopen due to the influence of gravity, abdominal pressure, and chest motion amplitude. Prone position can improve the degree of pulmonary tissue expansion in gravity-dependent areas either alone or in combination with recruitment maneuver, thus improving oxygenation and reducing mortality [81].

In the prone position of ARDS patients, ultrasound can assess the lung lesions, homogeneity, and lung recruitment in gravity-dependent areas. The degree of lung recruitment assessed by lung ultrasound after 3 h in prone position was correlated with clinical positive outcome [82]. Therefore, the effectiveness of prone position can be predicted by ultrasound, which can also help to decide the time and frequency of prone position.

20 Weaning

While weaning, ultrasound changes of pulmonary ventilation can predict the success or failure of extubation in patients who successfully passed the 1 h of spontaneous breathing test (SBT). There was no significant change in the overall pulmonary ventilation during SBT in patients who succeeded in extubation. However, in patients with post-extubation distress, pulmonary ventilation decreased during the spontaneous breathing trial [83].

21 Airway Cuff Pressure

Why we use cuff on an ETT/tracheostomy tube?

(a) Maintains Paw during mechanical ventilation.
(b) Prevents leakage of secretions into lungs.

Old ETT (e.g., red rubber) had low-volume high-pressure cuff leading to significant focal pressure injury to lungs. In a cohort study [57], they studied the extent of damage to airway in patients with tracheostomy who died, and they found the damage from the superficial erosion to extensive baring of cartilage to perforation through posterior tracheal wall.

As this potential for tracheal damage was recognized, high-volume low-pressure cuff ETT came into practice, which has become the standard in nowadays' practice. With large volume, cough pressure is distributed more evenly across the mucosa and achieves seal with much lower pressure. But it is found that newer high-volume low-pressure cuff reduces airway injury; however, it does not eliminate it [58].

In one study done as early as 1980 with the use of endoscopic photographic technique, they found that capillary blood flow to tracheal mucosa was impaired at a cuff pressure of 30 cm H_2O and capillary blood flow to tracheal rings was absent at and above cuff pressure of 50 cm H_2O [59].

In another cohort, they found that cuff pressure as low as 27 cm H_2O leads to tracheal mucosal injury ranging from moderate mucosal inflammation or edema to mucosal ulceration. They concluded that along with cuff pressure, prolonged duration of cuff pressure > 27 cm H_2O corelated well with increased risk of tracheal mucosa and cartilage injury on autopsy [60].

As mentioned in the first para of airway cuff pressure monitoring, we use cuff to maintain Paw and to stop secretion from entering inside. Cuff pressure should be just above the Paw, e.g., if Paw is <\25 cm H_2O, cuff pressure can easily be maintained below capillary perfusion pressure of 30 cm H_2O. Avoiding damage to tracheal mucosa becomes difficult if Paw is >25, in which case cuff pressure approaches near to capillary perforation pressure leading to more chances of injury.

Other issue of leakage is very difficult to tackle. It can be delayed but cannot be eliminated (97). In laboratory model, they found that cuff pressure as high as 60 cm H_2O cannot prevent aspiration of fluid around ETT. Modern high-volume low-pressure polyvinyl cuff forms longitudinal ridges/folds when inflated, leading to formation of tracks for drainage. Leakage of secretion around ETT was only prevented by greater tracheal pressure, higher than the height of fluid column above the cuff [61, 84, 85]. ETT cuff made up of different materials such as polyurethane has been tested.

It is evident from the discussion above that high cuff pressure does not eliminate leakage of fluid around ETT cuff but we do not have lower threshold of cuff pressure where leakage is significantly increased. As an example, in a model in laboratory, leakage around cuff occurred independent of CPAP or PEEP (Fig. 10).

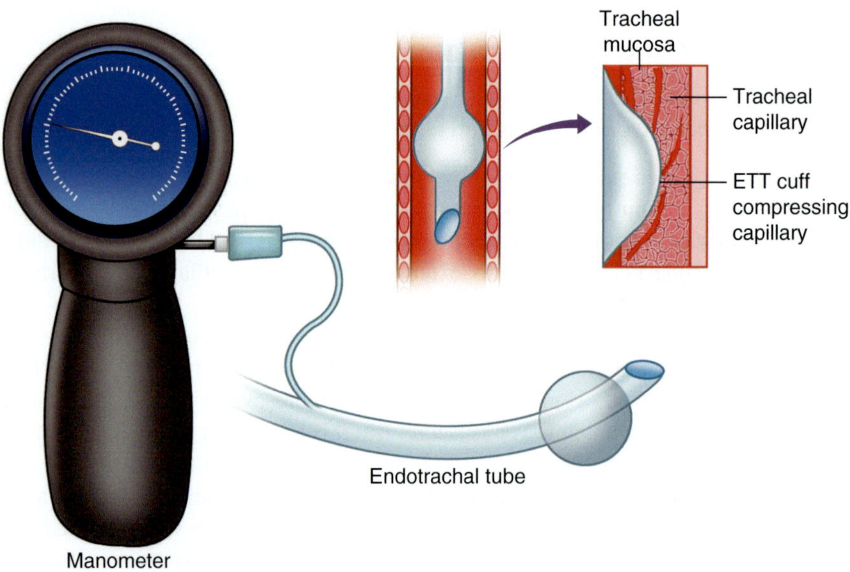

Fig. 10 Importance of ETT cuff manometry

22 In Summary

1. Cuff pressure > 30 cmH_2O impairs capillary perfusion.
2. Cuff pressure < 30 cmH_2O can easily eliminate air leak.
3. Leakage of secretion occurs independent of cuff material and high cuff pressure.
4. Leakage increases significantly when cuff pressure drops < 20 cmH_2O.

For all these reasons, it is important to monitor airway cuff pressure to decrease the risk of Paw injury and leakage of secretions. As per the current data available, an airway cuff pressure of 20–30 cmH_2O should be maintained.

23 Near-Infrared Spectroscopy

Near-infrared spectroscopy (NIRS) is a noninvasive technique used to monitor the peripheral tissue oxygenation saturation (StO_2) [86–89]. NIRS can indicate the status of tissue oxygen utilization, and it can be a valuable supplement to other physiological monitoring modalities [90]. It measures oxygen metabolism at cellular level and microvascular dysfunction, especially in conditions such as septic shock and other types of shock in which there is poor tissue perfusion.

A lower ascending slope of StO_2 is a bad prognostic factor in patients with ARDS [91]. A fall of StO_2 can be observed in patients who fail the spontaneous breathing trial.

NIRS has got some limitations. Firstly, it cannot distinguish between arterial and venous blood. Second, NIRS is affected by many factors like tissue edema, temperature, environment, age, obesity, and vascular tone due to use of vasoactive drugs [88]. In short, NIRS is a low-cost, noninvasive monitoring modality, and more research is warranted before its routine use in clinical practice.

24 Esophageal Pressure

Esophageal pressure (Pes) could be obtained by a specific catheter with a balloon placed in the lower two-thirds of the intrathoracic esophagus [92]. However, the results could also be influenced by mediastinal loading, variations of esophageal elastance, and amplitude of cardiac oscillations [93]. Even though Pes monitoring is a minimally invasive procedure and gives accurate detection of asynchronies, it is not routinely used in the clinical setting.

25 Electrical Activity of the Diaphragm

The electrical activity of the diaphragm (EAdi) indicates the patient's neural respiratory drive, which could be used to monitor the onset of neural inspiration and expiration. EAdi can be obtained easily through a nasogastric tube, which has multiple electrodes and is recorded by the software. EAdi has been used by some authors to detect patient-ventilator asynchronies, which is more accurate and sensitive than airway pressure and flow waveforms [94, 95]. However, considering its invasiveness, cost, technical challenges, and contraindications, such as severe coagulopathy, diagnosed or suspected esophageal varices, and history of esophageal or gastric surgery, EAdi is not routinely used to monitor asynchronies in the clinical practice. Some authors have demonstrated the relationship between EAdi and respiratory muscle surface electromyography (EMG), which may also be used to detect the activity of inspiratory muscles in patients who are being mechanically ventilated [96].

26 Extravascular Lung Water

Extravascular lung water (EVLW) is a quantitative measure of pulmonary edema and is correlated, in multiple patient populations, to mortality [29]. Normal values are 5–7 mL/kg (indexed to predicted body weight), and quantities above 10 mL/kg are associated with adverse clinical outcomes [97].

Indicator dilution techniques for measuring EVLW are available for bedside use in critically ill patients. The single-indicator technique is now well validated and offers the additional value of simultaneously measuring cardiovascular performance (cardiac output, fluid responsiveness, and filling volumes). Current technology uses an injection of cold saline into the right atrium and assesses transpulmonary thermodilution in the arterial system by using a femoral or brachial catheter. Limitations of the technique include requirements for good indicator mixing without loss and for constant blood flow and temperature. EVLW can be assessed only in perfused areas of the lung [98].

EVLW measurements may be used in combination with other cardiovascular and pulmonary parameters to diagnose pulmonary edema. Complementary information from indicator dilution techniques, such as cardiac filling volumes, helps to differentiate between hydrostatic/cardiogenic pulmonary edema and permeability edema [99]. Although repeated measures could be used to assess response to interventions [100], it is unclear how fast the response time is and whether this technique can be used as a tool to guide therapy.

References

1. Weiser TG, Haynes AB, Molina G, Lipsitz SR, Esquivel MM, Uribe-Leitz T, et al. Size and distribution of the global volume of surgery in 2012. Bull World Health Organ. 2016;94(3):201F–9F.
2. Wunsch H, Wagner J, Herlim M, Chong DH, Kramer AA, Halpern SD. ICU occupancy and mechanical ventilator use in the United States. Crit Care Med. 2013;41(12):2712–9.
3. Barrett MSM, Elixhauser A, Honigman LS, Pines JM. Utilization of intensive care services, 2011. Statistical Brief #185. Healthcare Cost and Utilization Project. Rockville, MD: Agency for Healthcare Research and Quality; 2014.
4. Acute Respiratory Distress Syndrome Network, Brower RG, Matthay MA, Morris A, Schoenfeld D, Thompson BT, Wheeler A. Ventilation with lower tidal volumes as compared with traditional tidal volumes for acute lung injury and the acute respiratory distress syndrome. N Engl J Med. 2000;342(18):1301–8.
5. Guerin C, Reignier J, Richard JC, Beuret P, Gacouin A, Boulain T, et al. Prone positioning in severe acute respiratory distress syndrome. N Engl J Med. 2013;368(23):2159–68.
6. Tusman G, Bohm SH, Suarez-Sipmann F. Advanced uses of pulse oximetry for monitoring mechanically ventilated patients. Anesth Analg. 2017;124(1):62–71.
7. Inman KJ, Sibbald WJ, Rutledge FS, Speechley M, Martin CM, Clark BJ. Does implementing pulse oximetry in a critical care unit result in substantial arterial blood gas savings? Chest. 1993;104(2):542–6.
8. Van de Louw A, Cracco C, Cerf C, Harf A, Duvaldestin P, Lemaire F, et al. Accuracy of pulse oximetry in the intensive care unit. Intensive Care Med. 2001;27(10):1606–13.
9. Pedersen T, Nicholson A, Hovhannisyan K, Moller AM, Smith AF, Lewis SR. Pulse oximetry for perioperative monitoring. Cochrane Database Syst Rev. 2014;3:CD002013.
10. Long term domiciliary oxygen therapy in chronic hypoxic cor pulmonale complicating chronic bronchitis and emphysema. Report of the Medical Research Council Working Party. Lancet. 1981;1(8222):681–6.
11. Continuous or nocturnal oxygen therapy in hypoxemic chronic obstructive lung disease: a clinical trial. Nocturnal Oxygen Therapy Trial Group. Ann Intern Med. 1980;93(3):391–8.
12. Mikkelsen ME, Christie JD, Lanken PN, Biester RC, Thompson BT, Bellamy SL, et al. The adult respiratory distress syndrome cognitive outcomes study: long-term neuropsychological function in survivors of acute lung injury. Am J Respir Crit Care Med. 2012;185(12):1307–15.
13. Kilgannon JH, Jones AE, Shapiro NI, Angelos MG, Milcarek B, Hunter K, et al. Association between arterial hyperoxia following resuscitation from cardiac arrest and in-hospital mortality. JAMA. 2010;303(21):2165–71.
14. Girardis M, Busani S, Damiani E, Donati A, Rinaldi L, Marudi A, et al. Effect of conservative vs conventional oxygen therapy on mortality among patients in an intensive care unit: the oxygen-ICU randomized clinical trial. JAMA. 2016;316(15):1583–9.
15. Rice TW, Wheeler AP, Bernard GR, Hayden DL, Schoenfeld DA, Ware LB. Comparison of the SpO2/FIO2 ratio and the PaO2/FIO2 ratio in patients with acute lung injury or ARDS. Chest. 2007;132(2):410–7.
16. Alian AA, Galante NJ, Stachenfeld NS, Silverman DG, Shelley KH. Impact of central hypovolemia on photoplethysmographic waveform parameters in healthy volunteers. Part 1: time domain analysis. J Clin Monit Comput. 2011;25(6):377–85.
17. Nassar BS, Schmidt GA. Capnography during critical illness. Chest. 2016;149(2):576–85.
18. Anderson CT, Breen PH. Carbon dioxide kinetics and capnography during critical care. Crit Care. 2000;4(4):207–15.
19. Lam T, Nagappa M, Wong J, Singh M, Wong D, Chung F. Continuous pulse oximetry and capnography monitoring for postoperative respiratory depression and adverse events: a systematic review and meta-analysis. Anesth Analg. 2017;125(6):2019–29.

20. Saunders R, Struys M, Pollock RF, Mestek M, Lightdale JR. Patient safety during procedural sedation using capnography monitoring: a systematic review and meta-analysis. BMJ Open. 2017;7(6):e013402.
21. Yamanaka MK, Sue DY. Comparison of arterial-end-tidal PCO2 difference and dead space/tidal volume ratio in respiratory failure. Chest. 1987;92(5):832–5.
22. Warner KJ, Cuschieri J, Garland B, Carlbom D, Baker D, Copass MK, et al. The utility of early end-tidal capnography in monitoring ventilation status after severe injury. J Trauma. 2009;66(1):26–31.
23. Russell GB, Graybeal JM. The arterial to end-tidal carbon dioxide difference in neurosurgical patients during craniotomy. Anesth Analg. 1995;81(4):806–10.
24. Verscheure S, Massion PB, Verschuren F, Damas P, Magder S. Volumetric capnography: lessons from the past and current clinical applications. Crit Care. 2016;20(1):184.
25. Rackley CR, MacIntyre NR. Low tidal volumes for everyone? Chest. 2019;156(4):783–91.
26. Gattinoni L, Pesenti A. The concept of baby lung. Intensive Care Med. 2005;31(6):776–84.
27. Gattinoni L, Pesenti A, Avalli L, Rossi F, Bombino M. Pressure-volume curve of total respiratory system in acute respiratory failure: computed tomographic scan study. Am Rev Respir Dis. 1987;136(3):730–6.
28. Gattinoni L, Tonetti T, Quintel M. Regional physiology of ARDS. Crit Care. 2017;21(Suppl 3):312.
29. Amato MB, Meade MO, Slutsky AS, Brochard L, Costa EL, Schoenfeld DA, et al. Driving pressure and survival in the acute respiratory distress syndrome. N Engl J Med. 2015;372(8):747–55.
30. Villar J, Martin-Rodriguez C, Dominguez-Berrot AM, Fernandez L, Ferrando C, Soler JA, et al. A quantile analysis of plateau and driving pressures: effects on mortality in patients with acute respiratory distress syndrome receiving lung-protective ventilation. Crit Care Med. 2017;45(5):843–50.
31. Aoyama H, Pettenuzzo T, Aoyama K, Pinto R, Englesakis M, Fan E. Association of driving pressure with mortality among ventilated patients with acute respiratory distress syndrome: a systematic review and meta-analysis. Crit Care Med. 2018;46(2):300–6.
32. Mellemgaard K. The alveolar-arterial oxygen difference: its size and components in normal man. Acta Physiol Scand. 1966;67(1):10–20.
33. Wong JJ, Loh TF, Testoni D, et al. Epidemiology of pediatric acute respiratory distress syndrome in Singapore: risk factors and predictive respiratory indices for mortality. Front Pediatr. 2014;25(2):78.
34. Floyd J, Wu L, Hay BD, et al. Evaluating the impact of pulse oximetry on childhood pneumonia mortality in resource-poor settings. Nature. 2015;528(7580):S53–9.
35. Cressoni M, Caironi P, Polli F, et al. Anatomical and functional intrapulmonary shunt in acute respiratory distress syndrome. Crit Care Med. 2008;36(3):669–75.
36. Elliott JE, Duke JW, Hawn JA, et al. Increased cardiac output, not pulmonary artery systolic pressure, increases intrapulmonary shunt in healthy humans breathing room air and 40% O2. J Physiol. 2014;592(20):4537–53.
37. Kawamura G, Kitamura T, Homma I, et al. Mechanisms underlying the improvement of arte-rial oxygenation using positive end-expiratory pressure during surgery under sevoflurane anesthesia and propofol anesthesia: a retrospective clinical study. Masui. 2013;62(6):652–9.
38. Brower RG, Lanken PN, MacIntyre N, Matthay MA, Morris A, Ancukiewicz M, et al. Higher versus lower positive end-expiratory pressures in patients with the acute respiratory distress syndrome. N Engl J Med. 2004;351(4):327–36.
39. Briel M, Meade M, Mercat A, Brower RG, Talmor D, Walter SD, et al. Higher vs lower positive end-expiratory pressure in patients with acute lung injury and acute respiratory distress syndrome: systematic review and meta-analysis. JAMA. 2010;303(9):865–73.
40. Beitler JR, Sarge T, Banner-Goodspeed VM, Gong MN, Cook D, Novack V, et al. Effect of titrating positive end-expiratory pressure (PEEP) with an esophageal pressure-guided strategy vs an empirical high PEEP-FIO2 strategy on death and days free from mechanical ventilation among patients with acute respiratory distress syndrome: a randomized clinical trial. JAMA. 2019;321(9):846–57.

41. Thille AW, Rodriguez P, Cabello B, Lellouche F, Brochard L. Patient-ventilator asynchrony during assisted mechanical ventilation. Intensive Care Med. 2006;32(10):1515–22.
42. Colombo D, Cammarota G, Alemani M, Carenzo L, Barra FL, Vaschetto R, et al. Efficacy of ventilator waveforms observation in detecting patient-ventilator asynchrony. Crit Care Med. 2011;39(11):2452–7.
43. Yoshida T, Fujino Y, Amato MB, Kavanagh BP. Fifty years of research in ARDS. Spontaneous breathing during mechanical ventilation: risks, mechanisms, and management. Am J Respir Crit Care Med. 2017;195(8):985–92.
44. Brochard L, Slutsky A, Pesenti A. Mechanical ventilation to minimize progression of lung injury in acute respiratory failure. Am J Respir Crit Care Med. 2017;195(4):438–42.
45. Brochard L. Ventilation-induced lung injury exists in spontaneously breathing patients with acute respiratory failure: yes. Intensive Care Med. 2017;43(2):250–2.
46. Lu Q, Rouby JJ. Measurement of pressure-volume curves in patients on mechanical ventilation: methods and significance. Crit Care. 2000;4(2):91–100.
47. Harris RS. Pressure-volume curves of the respiratory system. Respir Care. 2005;50(1):78–98. discussion 98–79
48. Gattinoni L, Mascheroni D, Basilico E, Foti G, Pesenti A, Avalli L. Volume/pressure curve of total respiratory system in paralysed patients: artefacts and correction factors. Intensive Care Med. 1987;13(1):19–25.
49. Matamis D, Lemaire F, Harf A, Brun-Buisson C, Ansquer JC, Atlan G. Total respiratory pressure-volume curves in the adult respiratory distress syndrome. Chest. 1984;86(1):58–66.
50. Suter PM, Fairley B, Isenberg MD. Optimum end-expiratory airway pressure in patients with acute pulmonary failure. N Engl J Med. 1975;292(6):284–9.
51. Harris RS, Hess DR, Venegas JG. An objective analysis of the pressure-volume curve in the acute respiratory distress syndrome. Am J Respir Crit Care Med. 2000; 161(2 Pt 1):432–9.
52. Chen L, Del Sorbo L, Grieco DL, Shklar O, Junhasavasdikul D, Telias I, et al. Airway closure in acute respiratory distress syndrome: an underestimated and misinterpreted phenomenon. Am J Respir Crit Care Med. 2018;197(1):132–6.
53. Jonson B, Svantesson C. Elastic pressure-volume curves: what information do they convey? Thorax. 1999;54(1):82–7.
54. Roupie E, Dambrosio M, Servillo G, Mentec H, el Atrous S, Beydon L, et al. Titration of tidal volume and induced hypercapnia in acute respiratory distress syndrome. Am J Respir Crit Care Med. 1995;152(1):121–8.
55. Demory D, Arnal JM, Wysocki M, Donati S, Granier I, Corno G, et al. Recruitability of the lung estimated by the pressure volume curve hysteresis in ARDS patients. Intensive Care Med. 2008;34(11):2019–25.
56. Mead J, Whittenberger JL, Radford EP Jr. Surface tension as a factor in pulmonary volume-pressure hysteresis. J Appl Physiol. 1957;10(2):191–6.
57. Cooper JD, Grillo HC. The evolution of tracheal injury due to ventilatory assistance through cuffed tubes: a pathologic study. Ann Surg. 1969;169(3):334–48.
58. Mathias DB, Wedley JR. The effects of cuffed endotracheal tubes on the tracheal wall. Br J Anaesth. 1974;46(11):849–52.
59. Seegobin RD, van Hasselt GL. Endotracheal cuff pressure and tracheal mucosal blood flow: endoscopic study of effects of four large volume cuffs. Br Med J (Clin Res Ed). 1984;288(6422):965–8.
60. Stauffer JL, Olson DE, Petty TL. Complications and consequences of endotracheal intubation and tracheotomy: a prospective study of 150 critically ill adult patients. Am J Med. 1981;70(1):65–76.
61. Inada T, Uesugi F, Kawachi S, Inada K. The tracheal tube with a high-volume, low-pressure cuff at various airway inflation pressures. Eur J Anaesthesiol. 1998;15(6):629–32.
62. Jain MK, Tripathi CB. Endotracheal tube cuff pressure monitoring during neurosurgery: manual vs. automatic method. J Anaesthesiol Clin Pharmacol. 2011;27(3):358–61.

63. Stewart SL, Secrest JA, Norwood BR, Zachary R. A comparison of endotracheal tube cuff pressures using estimation techniques and direct intracuff measurement. AANA J. 2003;71(6):443–7.
64. Valencia M, Ferrer M, Farre R, Navajas D, Badia JR, Nicolas JM, et al. Automatic control of tracheal tube cuff pressure in ventilated patients in semirecumbent position: a randomized trial. Crit Care Med. 2007;35(6):1543–9.
65. Babic SA, Chatburn RL. Laboratory evaluation of cuff pressure control methods. Respir Care. 2020;65(1):62–7.
66. Bentz MR, Primack SL. Intensive care unit imaging. Clin Chest Med. 2015;36(2):219–34.
67. Cadman A, Lawrance JA, Fitzsimmons L, et al. To clot or not to clot? That is the question in central venous catheters. Clin Radiol. 2004;59(9):349–55.
68. Liu SY, Tsai IT, Yang PJ. Pneumothorax and deep sulcus sign. QJM. 2016;109(9):621–2.
69. Umbrello M, Formenti P. Ultrasonographic assessment of diaphragm function in critically ill subjects. Respir Care. 2016;61(4):542–55.
70. Demoule A, Jung B, Prodanovic H, et al. Diaphragm dysfunction on admission to the intensive care unit. Prevalence, risk factors, and prognostic impact—a prospective study. Am J Respir Crit Care Med. 2013;188(2):213–9.
71. Boussuges A, Gole Y, Blanc P. Diaphragmatic motion studied by M-mode ultrasonography. Chest. 2009;135(2):391–400.
72. Mayo P, Volpicelli G, Lerolle N, et al. Ultrasonography evaluation during the weaning process: the heart, the diaphragm, the pleura and the lung. Intensive Care Med. 2016;42(7):1107–17.
73. Gottesman E, Mccool FD. Ultrasound evaluation of the paralyzed diaphragm. Am J Respir Crit Care Med. 1997;55(5):1570–4.
74. Summerhill EM, El-Sameed YA, Glidden TJ, et al. Monitoring recovery from diaphragm paralysis with ultrasound. Chest. 2008;133(3):737–43.
75. David C, Benditt JO, Scott E, et al. Diaphragm thickening during inspiration. J Appl Physiol. 1997;83(1):291–6.
76. Ueki J, De Bruin PF, Pride NB. In vivo assessment of diaphragm contraction by ultrasound in normal subjects. Thorax. 1995;50(11):1157–61.
77. Ayoub J, Cohendy R, Dauzat M, et al. Non-invasive quantification of diaphragm kinetics using m-mode sonography. Can J Anaesth. 1997;44(7):739–44.
78. Ferrari G, De Filippi G, Elia F, et al. Diaphragm ultrasound as a new index of discontinuation from mechanical ventilation. Crit Ultrasound J. 2014;6(1):8.
79. Dinino E, Gartman EJ, Sethi JM, et al. Diaphragm ultrasound as a predictor of successful extubation from mechanical ventilation. Thorax. 2014;69(5):431–5.
80. Tusman G, Acosta CM, Costantini M. Ultrasonography for the assessment of lung recruitment maneuvers. Crit Ultrasound J. 2016;8(1):8.
81. Mancebo J, Fernández R, Blanch L, et al. A multicenter trial of prolonged prone ventilation in severe acute respiratory distress syndrome. Am J Respir Crit Care Med. 2006;173(11):1233–9.
82. Wang XT, Ding X, Zhang HM, et al. Lung ultrasound can be used to predict the potential of prone positioning and assess prognosis in patients with acute respiratory distress syndrome. Crit Care. 2016;20(1):385.
83. Soummer A, Perbet S, Brisson H, et al. Ultrasound assessment of lung aeration loss during a successful weaning trial predicts postextubation distress. Crit Care Med. 2012;40(7):2064–72.
84. Young PJ, Rollinson M, Downward G, Henderson S. Leakage of fluid past the tracheal tube cuff in a benchtop model. Br J Anaesth. 1997;78(5):557–62.
85. Lucangelo U, Zin WA, Antonaglia V, Petrucci L, Viviani M, Buscema G, et al. Effect of positive expiratory pressure and type of tracheal cuff on the incidence of aspiration in mechanically ventilated patients in an intensive care unit. Crit Care Med. 2008;36(2):409–13.
86. Lipcsey M, Woinarski NC, Bellomo R. Near infrared spectroscopy (NIRS) of the thenar eminence in anesthesia and intensive care. Ann Intensive Care. 2012;2(1):11.
87. Creteur J. Muscle StO2 in critically ill patients. Curr Opin Crit Care. 2008;14(3):361–6.

88. Mesquida J, Gruartmoner G, Espinal C. Skeletal muscle oxygen saturation (StO2) measured by near-infrared spectroscopy in the critically ill patients. Biomed Res Int. 2013;2013:502194.
89. Santora RJ, Santora RJ, Moore FA. Monitoring trauma and intensive care unit resuscitation with tissue hemoglobin oxygen saturation. Crit Care. 2009;13(Suppl 5):S10.
90. Wahr JA, Tremper KK, Samra S, Delpy DT. Near-infrared spectroscopy: theory and applications. J Cardiothorac Vasc Anesth. 1996;10:406–18. https://doi.org/10.1016/S1053-0770(96)80107-8.
91. Orbegozo Cortes D, Rahmania L, Irazabal M, et al. Microvascular reactivity is altered early in patients with acute respiratory distress syndrome. Respir Res. 2016;17:59.
92. Baydur A, Behrakis PK, Zin WA, et al. A simple method for assessing the validity of the esophageal balloon technique. Am Rev Respir Dis. 1982;126:788–91.
93. Van de Woestijne KP, Trop D, Clement J. Influence of the mediastinum on the measurement of esophageal pressure and lung compliance in man. Pflugers Arch. 1971;323:323–41.
94. Piquilloud L, Vignaux L, Bialais E, et al. Neurally adjusted ventilatory assist improves patient ventilator interaction. Intensive Care Med. 2011;37:263–71.
95. Mauri T, Bellani G, Grasselli G, et al. Patient-ventilator interaction in ARDS patients with extremely low compliance undergoing ECMO: a novel approach based on diaphragm electrical activity. Intensive Care Med. 2013;39:282–91.
96. Bellani G, Bronco A, Arrigoni Marocco S, et al. Measurement of diaphragmatic electrical activity by surface electromyography in intubated subjects and its relationship with inspiratory effort. Respir Care. 2018;63:1341–9.
97. Owens RL, Campana LM, Hess L, Eckert DJ, Loring SH, Malhotra A. Sitting and supine esophageal pressures in overweight and obese subjects. Obesity (Silver Spring). 2012;20(12):2354–60.
98. Akoumianaki E, Maggiore SM, Valenza F, Bellani G, Jubran A, Loring SH, et al. The application of esophageal pressure measurement in patients with respiratory failure. Am J Respir Crit Care Med. 2014;189(5):520–31.
99. Grieco DL, Chen L, Brochard L. Transpulmonary pressure: importance and limits. Ann Transl Med. 2017;5(14):285.
100. Talmor D, Sarge T, Malhotra A, O'Donnell CR, Ritz R, Lisbon A, et al. Mechanical ventilation guided by esophageal pressure in acute lung injury. N Engl J Med. 2008;359(20):2095–104.

Role of Point-of-Care Ultrasound in the Management of Mechanical Ventilation

Ahmed Tarek Youssef Aboulkheir and Ashraf Al Tayar

Point-of-care ultrasound (POCUS) is considered to be the fifth pillar of physical exam in general {inspection, palpation, percussion, auscultation, and sonation (ultrasound)}. Ultrasound (US) became an essential tool in the hands of intensivists and is now recommended both for procedural guidance and diagnostic purposes. And as ultrasound machines become smaller, indeed reduced to the size of mobile phones, Intensivists in the not-too-distant future may carry transducers next to stethoscopes in their pockets. Point-of-care ultrasound (POCUS) is an immediately available, repeatable and non-irradiating bedside tool integrating the clinical examination.

Recent years were characterized by a growing interest in the fields of lung ultrasound (LUS) and diaphragm ultrasound. The combination of these two ultrasound techniques with echocardiography may integrate the classical approach to mechanically ventilated patients, both for monitoring [1] and diagnostic purposes [2], finally contributing to the titration of mechanical ventilation [3] and to the management of respiratory disease.

A. T. Y. Aboulkheir (✉)
Surgical ICU, Rashid Hospital, Dubai, UAE

A. Al Tayar
ICU/RT Department, Security Forces Hospital, Dammam, Saudi Arabia

J. Hidalgo et al. (eds.), *Personalized Mechanical Ventilation*,
https://doi.org/10.1007/978-3-031-14138-6_19

1 Lung Ultrasound (LUS)

1.1 Equipment and Examination

The selection of the ultrasound probe to perform LUS is important. A simplified approach is to "pair the probe to the potential pathological condition." Select a transducer with a lower frequency (3–5 MHz) (curvilinear or convex probe) to examine deeper structures and pathologies such as pneumonia, atelectasis, effusion, and edema and use one with higher frequencies (5–12 MHz) (linear/vascular probe) to visualize superficial structures and pathologies such as pneumothorax, pleural line, and pulmonary infarct.

Traditionally, the ultrasound probe should be positioned with the indicator marker toward the patient's head, regardless of the probe selected. The patient can be satisfactorily examined in the supine position. The lateral decubitus position offers a better view on dorsal regions of lower lobes. A complete evaluation of both lungs requires a systematic protocol of examination. First, the operator should locate the diaphragm and the lungs. Lung consolidation or pleural effusion is found predominantly in dependent and dorsal lung regions and can be easily distinguished from liver or spleen once the diaphragm has been located [4].

Adhering to standardized protocol for lung ultrasound image acquisition is strongly recommended. Zone schema protocols can include from 4 up to 28 zones depending on the indication (Fig. 1). With this in mind, one must cater the scanning approach to the condition of concern, as in a targeted physical examination; the level of detail required is directed by the clinical pretest probability.

To provide an exhaustive assessment of lung aeration and pleural effusion, the ultrasound examination should cover both lungs, just as for auscultation. To be comprehensive, a chest ultrasound examination should take around 15 min, although with enough knowledge and skills, users can perform lung examination more quickly [4].

1.2 Normal Lung Ultrasound Pattern

Normally, ultrasounds are not transmitted through lung as it is filled with gas and the lung parenchyma would not be normally visible beyond the pleura. When the lung is injured and turned to be non-aerated, tissue-like extending to lung periphery produces ultrasound artifacts resulting from the abnormal gas/tissue interface [4].

For each considered intercostal space, the probe should be positioned perpendicular to the ribs. Using a longitudinal view, the ribs, characterized by a posterior hypoechoic shadowing, should be identified. A hyperechoic and sliding line, moving forward and backward with ventilation, is seen usually 0.5 cm below the rib line and is called the "pleural line (PL)." PL with upper and lower rib shadow forms what looks like a bat and is called bat sign (Fig. 2).

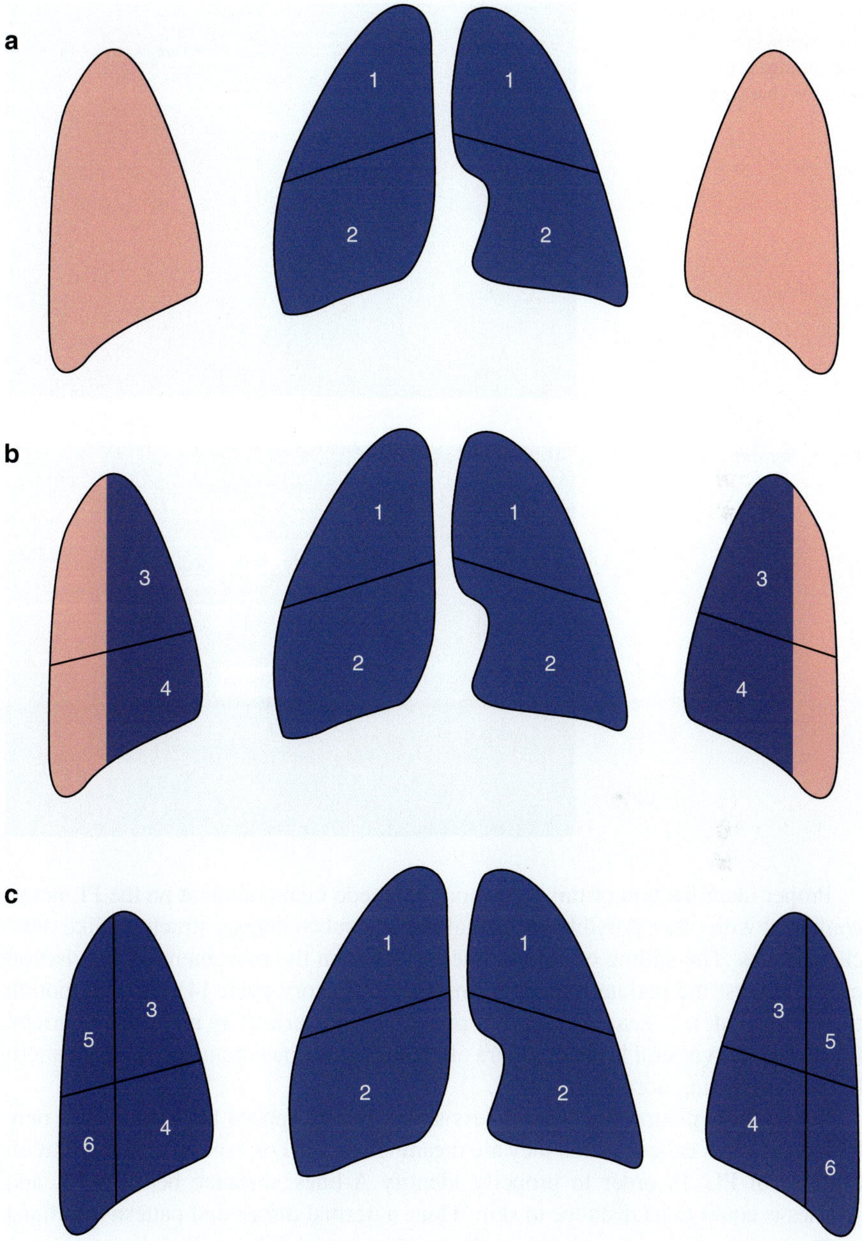

Fig. 1 Lung zone schema: (**a**) 4 zones, (**b**) 8 zones, (**c**) 12 zones

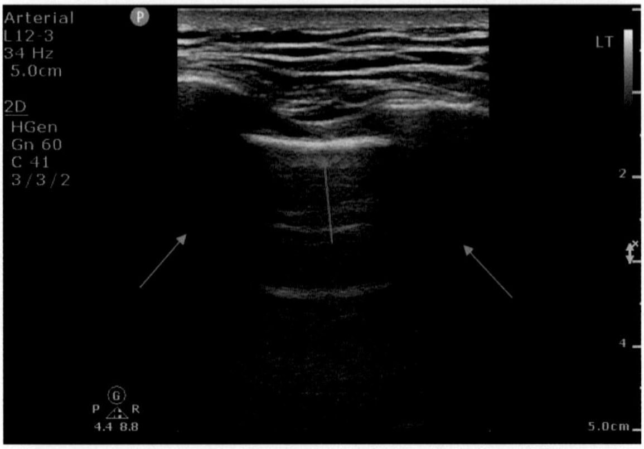

Fig. 2 Two rib shadows (blue arrows) with pleural line (orange arrow) in between (bat sign)

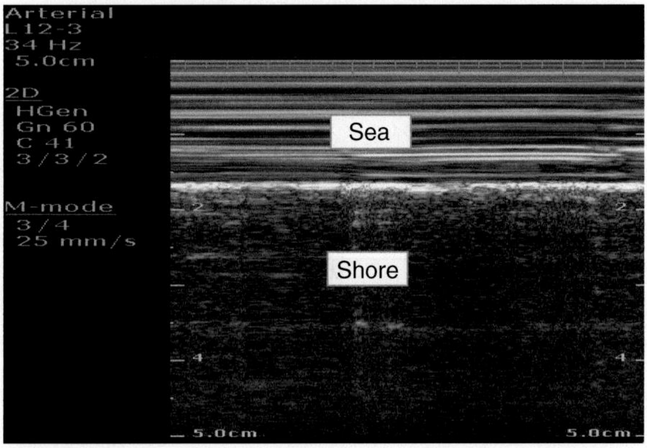

Fig. 3 Seashore sign

Proper identification of this sign should precede final comment on the PL not to confuse it with other possible artifactual lines of subcutaneous structures like muscle capsules .The sliding of pleural line results from the movement of the visceral pleura against the parietal pleura during the respiratory cycle [4]. In time-motion mode (M-mode), a "seashore sign" is present, characterized by motionless parietal layer over the visceral layer of pleura and a homogeneous granular (sandy) pattern below it reflecting normal lung (Fig. 3).

Beyond this pleural line, motionless and regularly spaced horizontal lines may be seen and it is called A-line: they are meaningless and correspond to reverberation artifacts of PL. In order to properly identify A-lines, distance between PL and A-lines is equal to its distance to skin. Thus, a normal ultrasound pattern is defined by "lung sliding" associated with artifactual horizontal A-lines (Fig. 4).

In one-third of patients with normal lungs, however, less than three vertical lines, called B-lines, can be detected in one or more intercostal space (ICS) more in dependent lung regions, and they are artifact reverberation of interstitial septa devoid of any pathological significance. B-lines should start at and move with PL and end by bottom of the screen, and eradicate A-lines [4]. When B-lines are numerous, more than three in one ICS, it will indicate wet interstitium, interstitial lung syndrome, and can be seen as a rocket sign.

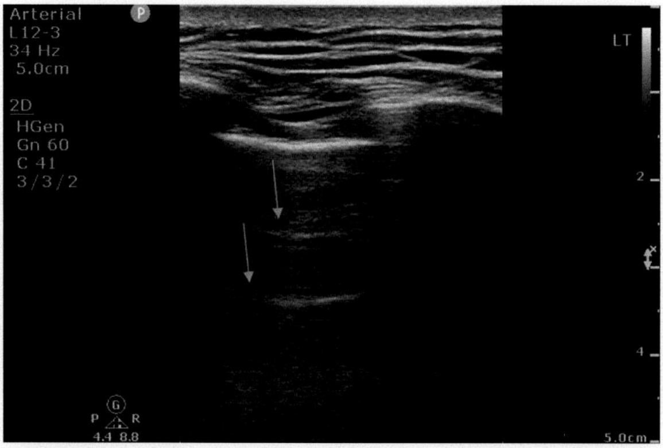

Fig. 4 A-lines (blue arrows)

2 Diaphragmatic Ultrasound

The diaphragm is the main respiratory muscle and is responsible for 60% of inhaled air volume. Evaluating the diaphragm allows the clinician to estimate the patient's respiratory effort, [5] especially because the diaphragm is the final part of the chain of neurological signals that regulate ventilation. It is a thin dome-shaped muscle that inserts into the lower ribs, xiphoid process, and lumbar vertebrae. It runs parallel to the rib cage in the zone of apposition before curving along the inferior pleural surface. Shortening of the diaphragm muscle fibers during inspiration results in a pistonlike action, drawing the lungs downward and forcing the lower chest wall outward. Downward excursion of the diaphragm varies from about 1 cm during normal tidal breathing to over 1–2 cm during deep inspiration. Diaphragmatic dysfunction is frequent in critical care and may worsen the patient's outcome and impair weaning from mechanical ventilation [6].

Ultrasound allows both qualitative and quantitative assessment of the diaphragm [7]. Two techniques to image the diaphragm using ultrasound have been described. First, diaphragm excursion: with a low-frequency probe in a lateral approach, the diaphragmatic dome is visualized as a hyperechoic line that separates abdominal and thoracic cavities. Its movement during inspiratory efforts can be measured by aligning the anatomic M-mode along the main axis of excursion [8] (Fig. 5). Normal values range from 1.5 to 2.5 cm [9], while excursion less than 1.0 cm identifies severe dysfunction.

Second technique is diaphragm thickness and thickening, which illustrate muscular trophism and contractility, respectively. The zone of apposition of the diaphragm to the thoracic wall is visualized with a high-frequency probe as a double-rail image parallel to the probe: diaphragm thickness and thickening fraction [(Tmax – Tmin)/Tmin] can be measured (Fig. 6) with acceptable feasibility and reproducibility [10]. Normal values of diaphragmatic thickness in the zone of apposition are

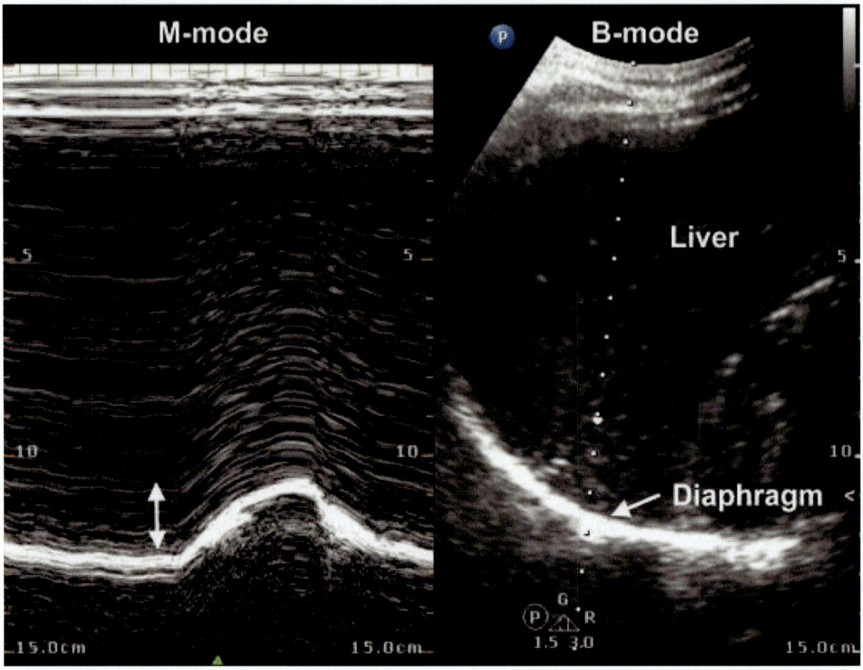

Fig. 5 The diaphragm can be seen as a hyperechogenic line indicated with an arrow. The excursion is measured as the difference between the end of inspiration and the end of expiration (cm)

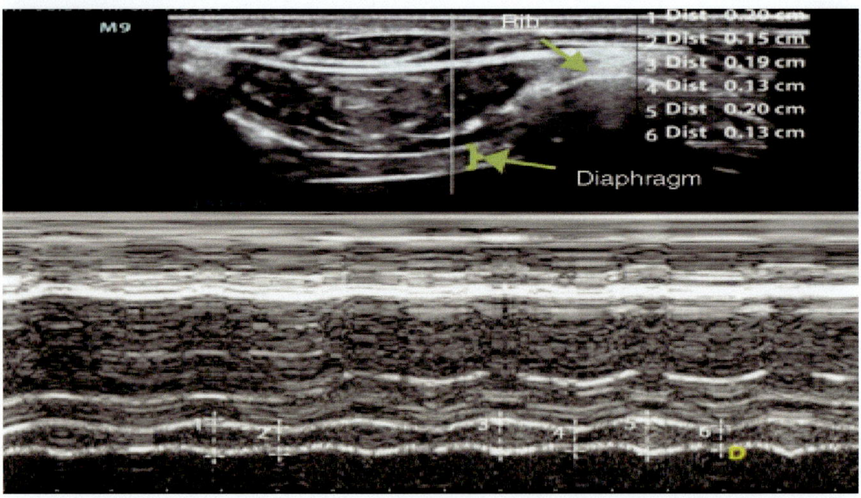

Fig. 6 M-mode measurement of diaphragm thickness variation. The diaphragm is seen as three parallel lines: two hyperechogenic layers and a thicker, central hypoechogenic layer. Numbers 1, 3, and 5 are the inspiratory thickness (Tmax), and numbers 2, 4, and 6 are the expiratory thickness(Tmin)

1.7 ± 0.2 mm when the muscle is relaxed, increasing to 4.5 ± 0.9 mm during a deep inspiration. The thickening fraction is normal if greater than 20% [11].

Mechanical ventilation deeply affects diaphragm thickness, mainly in the first days of mechanical ventilation [12]. A diaphragm that maintains a constant thickness during the course of mechanical ventilation will also preserve a good thickening fraction. Both thinning and thickening can be observed, and both are associated with reduced diaphragmatic performance, presumably due to disuse atrophy and edema associated with muscle damage, respectively. Both thinning and thickening have a significant impact on patient outcomes in terms of duration and complications of mechanical ventilation [13].

3 POCUS-Guided Mechanical Ventilation

3.1 Respiratory Complications in Mechanically Ventilated Patients

3.1.1 Pneumothorax

Pneumothorax is defined by the presence of air between visceral and parietal pleural layers. LUS is superior to chest plain radiography (CXR) and comparable to gold standard CT in the diagnosis of pneumothorax. Sensitivity and specificity of LUS are 78.6% and 98.4% consequently compared to 39.8% and 99.3 for CXR [14]. As a consequence, lung sliding is abolished, ultrasounds cannot be transmitted through the injured lung parenchyma, and comet tails (vertical B-lines) will be no longer visible. Presence of lung sliding and B-lines is 100% against pneumothorax [15]. Only longitudinal reverberations of motionless pleural line (horizontal A-lines) can be seen.

Absence of lung sliding is not 100% specific for pneumothorax as many other causes may lead to that as the presence of an intercostal tube, unilateral lung ventilation, apnea, pleural adherences, bullous emphysema, and advanced chronic obstructive pulmonary disease. The patient should lie strictly supine to allow the location of pleural gas effusion in nondependent lung regions. To confirm the diagnosis of partial pneumothorax, examination should be extended lo lateral regions of the chest wall to localize the point where the normal lung pattern (lung sliding and/or the presence of vertical B-lines) replaces the pneumothorax pattern (absent lung sliding and horizontal A-lines). This point is called the "lung point." Utilization of the time motion mode can facilitate detection of the lung point by presenting barcode sign (Fig. 7).

Lung point is 100% specific but only 60% sensitive in diagnosing pneumothorax [16]. When lung beats with the heart at the site of probe attachment to chest wall, it is called lung pulsation and is considered as a sign against pneumothorax and may indicate the presence of collapse as in the case of right main bronchial stem intubation [17].

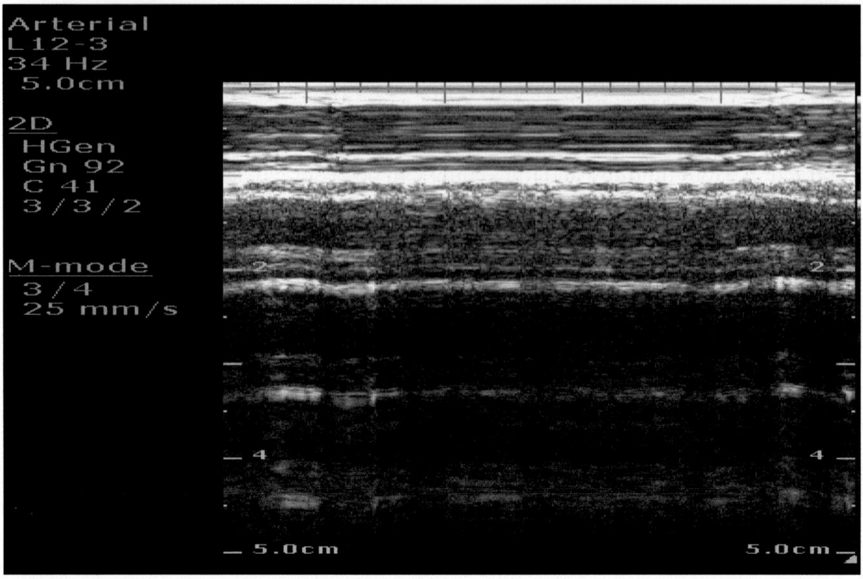

Fig. 7 Barcode sign of pneumothorax

3.1.2 Pleural Effusion

Pleural effusion is found to be common in ventilated patients and is associated with morbidity including difficulty to wean, longer stay in ICU, and increased mortality [18].

LUS was found to be equal to CT chest in diagnosing pleural effusion of whatever volume as even very small amount of more than 20 ml can be detected. Pleural effusion in LUS will appear as hypoechoic fluid like dark-dependent zone that will be located above the diaphragm. When a low-frequency (phased array or curvilinear) probe is placed on a longitudinal view perpendicular to chest wall in seventh to ninth ICS and probe mark is being cephalic. Identification of liver, spleen, and diaphragm has to be clear. Pleural effusion should be sought in dependent lung regions delineated by the chest wall and the diaphragm. It appears as a hypoechoic and homogeneous structure with no gas inside and is present during expiration and inspiration. In other words, it appears as a dependent dark zone free of echo [19] (Fig. 8).

LUS has the advantages of its ability to differentiate simple from complicated pleural effusion when debris, fibrin threads, and cells can be seen in the fluid (Fig. 9). LUS can be used to guide drainage when it is indicated, which can be safer from avoiding injuring lung, diaphragm, liver, spleen, or heart. Guidance of drainage can be static, when image will be frozen; measurement will be done before proceeding the needle so as not to reach the surrounding organs, while dynamic guidance means that the needle will be pushed in under vision to secure it in hypoechoic free space of the effusion [20].

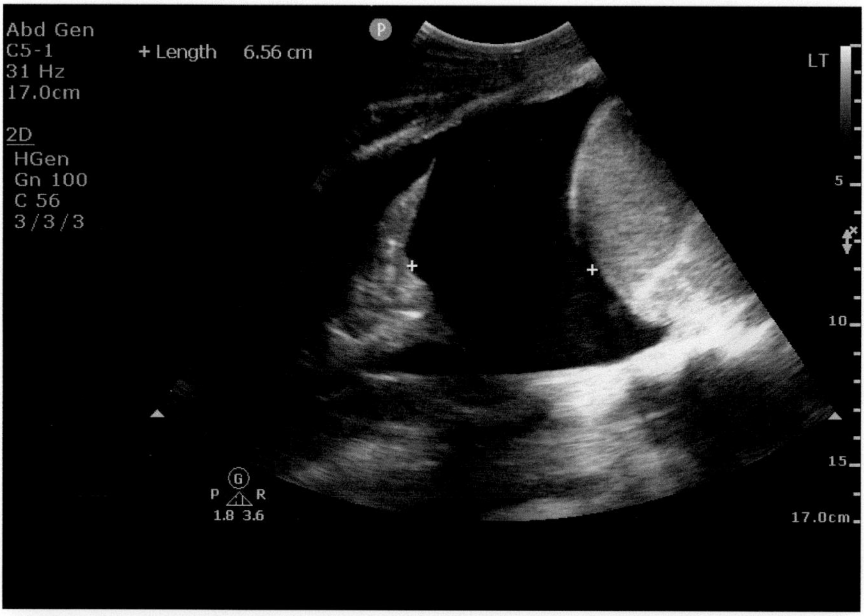

Fig. 8 Clear pleural effusion

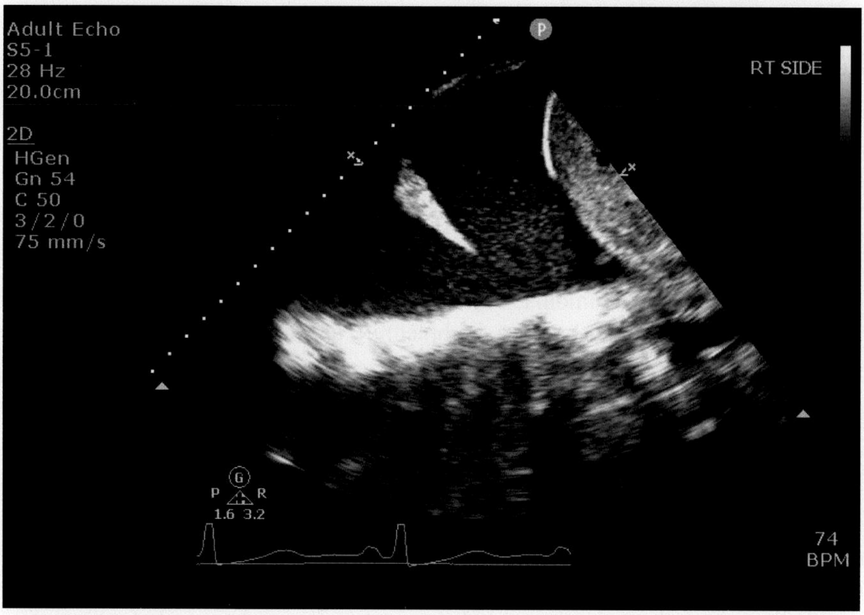

Fig. 9 Turbid pleural effusion

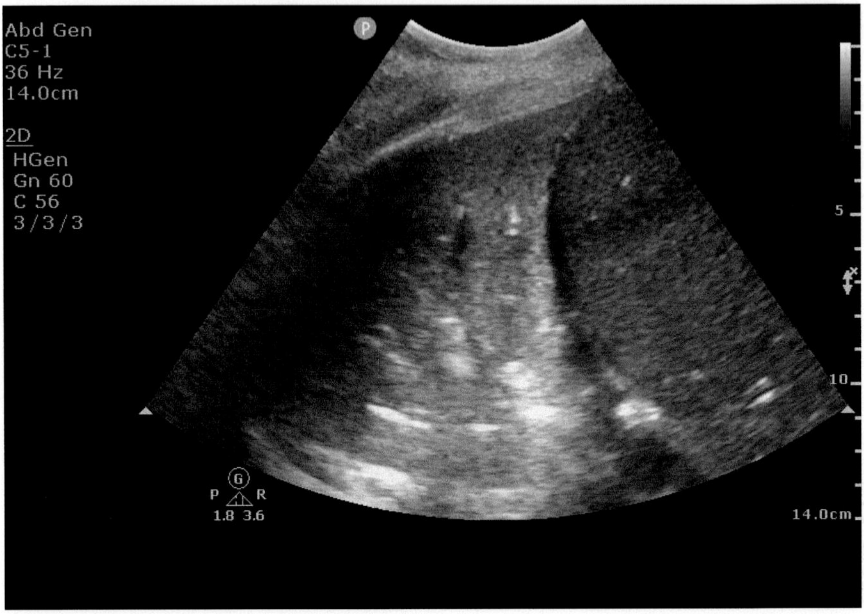

Fig. 10 Consolidation with dynamic air bronchogram

3.1.3 Lung Consolidation/Collapse

When aerated lung is becoming non-aerated, it will be solidified and appears in LUS as echoic texture, tissue-like, or hepatized (liver-like). What differentiates collapse from consolidation is presence of dynamic air bronchogram (hyperechoic puncti form images that reflect air-filled bronchi) that moves in and out in consolidated area with inspiration and expiration consequently, consist with consolidation while static air bronchogram which persist with respiratory phases consist with collapse. Consolidation with dynamic air bronchogram is 95% sensitive and 98% specific for diagnosis of pneumonia (Fig. 10). Consolidation may involve any part of lung, peripherally and under pleura, (subpleural), and will be seen with shred sign (Fig. 11) [21, 22].

3.1.4 Alveolar-Interstitial Lung Syndrome

Presence of numerous B-lines in more than one ICS reflects interstitial lung syndrome, which can be due to cardiogenic pulmonary edema (CPE), non-CPE (ARDS), interstitial lung fibrosis (ILF), and pneumonitis. The number of these vertical B-lines depends on the degree of lung aeration loss and amount of extravascular lung water (EVLW), and their intensity increases with inspiratory movements [23].

It has been demonstrated that multiple B-lines 7 mm apart are considered to be non-confluent and can be due to ILF and may be caused by thickened interlobular

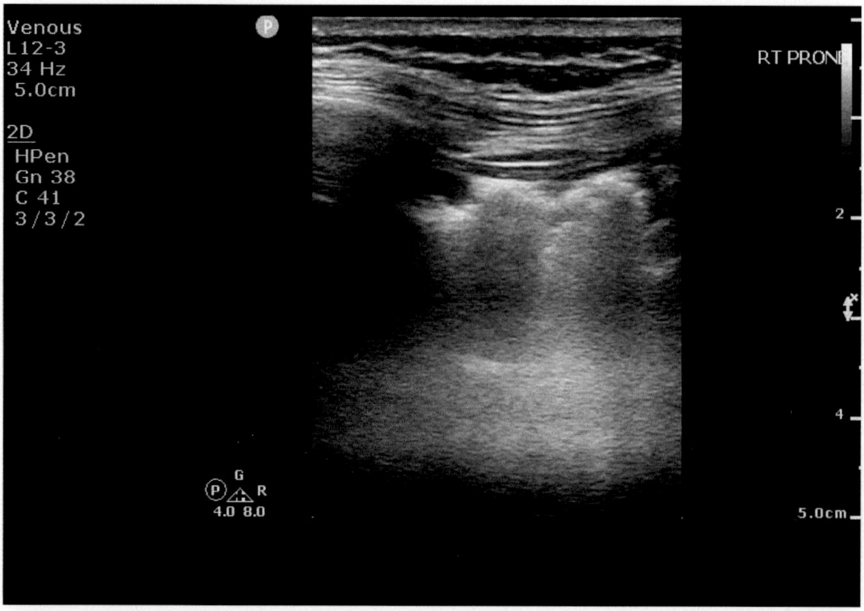

Fig. 11 Subpleural consolidation (shred sign)

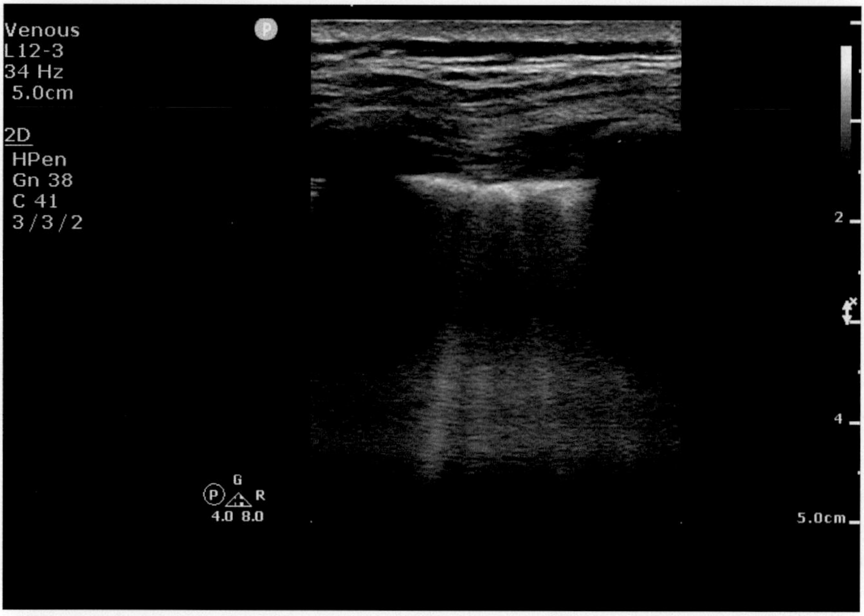

Fig. 12 Non-confluent B-lines

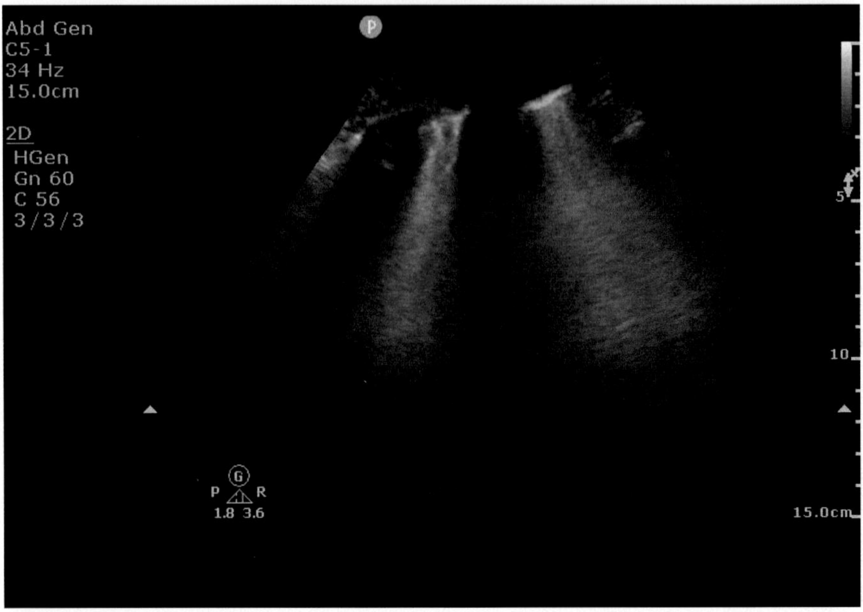

Fig. 13 Confluent B-lines

septa (Fig. 12). In contrast, B-lines 3 mm or less apart are known as confluent and can be caused by ground-glass areas characterizing alveolar-interstitial edema (Fig. 13) [24].

The following items can help to differentiate CPE from non-CPE ARDS:

- Pleura: Healthy thin-looking and good sliding will match more with cardiogenic edema, while thickened, adhered, and not well-sliding pleura will be in favor of non-CPE (ARDS).
- Presence of subpleural consolidation and shred sign and deep areas of consolidation will favor ARDS.
- Bilateral equally distributed confluent B-lines with no spared areas will match cardiogenic PE, while the presence of spared area in the same adjacent ICS matches ARDS.
- Large pleural effusion is found more with CPE.

LUS has a valuable role in detecting EVLW and in deciding to dry lung using diuresis or even fluid removal by dialysis machine; follow-up of such interventions and monitoring using LUS with accuracy comparable to CT was found by Chiumello et al. [25].

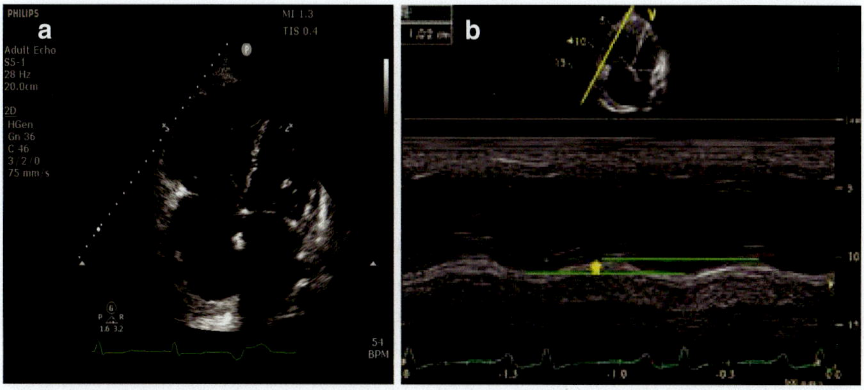

Fig. 14 (**a**) RV dilatation. (**b**) Low TAPSE (10 mm)

3.2 Heart-Lung Interaction

Mechanical ventilation especially with high pressures has some drawbacks: not only does it expose to barotrauma and higher risk of complications, but it may also have a negative impact on gas exchange and hemodynamics due to lung overdistention and right-ventricle (RV) impairment [26].

Overdistention mainly affects anterior fields, impairing both alveolar ventilation and vascularization, favoring perfusion of non-aerated regions (i.e., shunt), thus worsening respiratory acidosis and hypoxemia. Overdistention cannot be formally measured by US; however, a reduction of physiological pleural sliding in anterior regions may be observed while increasing airway pressure [27].

Moreover, an increase of airway pressure may substantially increase RV afterload. This may complicate a scenario already characterized by pulmonary vasoconstriction induced by hypoxemia and respiratory acidosis, eventually leading to a significant worsening of hemodynamics [28]. Incidence of acute cor pulmonale (ACP) in ARDS ranges from 14 to 50% [29]. ACP may be detected by transthoracic echocardiography (TTE) as an enlarged RV (right-to-left ventricle end-diastolic area ratio > 0.6), low TAPSE, and a paradoxical septal motion [26] (Fig. 14).

Pulmonary hypertension secondary to increased airway pressure may lead to a right-to-left shunt through a previously silent patent foramen ovale (PFO), significantly worsening hypoxemia [30]. The gold standard for patent PFO diagnosis is transesophageal echocardiography; however, TTE examination with bubble test presents high specificity and reliably identifies significant shunts [31]. Only rare cases of PFO paradoxical response to PEEP are reported in the literature [32]. Prone position may help in unloading the RV by correcting the factors inducing pulmonary vasoconstriction (i.e., hypoxemia, hypercarbia) with no increase of airway pressure [33].

Therefore, a combination of lung and heart US findings may help in setting the best PEEP level, considering both lung aeration and hemodynamic impact.

3.3 Ultrasound Assessment of Lung Aeration

Lung ultrasound (LUS) signs are mainly composed by artifacts. A normally aerated lung is characterized by **A-lines**: horizontal reverberation artifacts beneath the pleural line. When the ratio between air and tissue is impaired, vertical artifacts called **B-lines** appear: their number and coalescence are proportional to lung density [34] and loss of aeration [35].

LUS scores based on the number and type of visualized artifacts have been proposed in the last years to allow semi-quantification of lung aeration. The most frequently used score in the intensive care unit (ICU) distinguishes six areas per hemithorax: sternum, anterior, and posterior axillary lines identifying anterior, lateral, and posterior regions, each divided into superior and inferior fields [36]. LUS score is counted according to the findings on LUS exam in every area (Table 1).

According to this table, there may be a score from 0 to 36 bilaterally and if LUS score is less than 13, the lung is well aerated and the likelihood of success in weaning from mechanical ventilation (MV) is high, while a score above 17 is indicative of likelihood of failure, while a score in between is indeterminate [36].

LUS can be of value in assessing the effect of PEEP on lung aeration; in case of PEEP-responsive patients when there is diffuse pathology, reaeration can be monitored after applying/increasing PEEP [37]; while LUS is poor to diagnose lung overinflation, presence of abolished lung sliding may reflect it especially in nondependent areas [38] and when sliding reappears after reducing PEEP [39]. Prone position is one of the rescue therapies in severe ARDS; LUS exam is possible during prone position, and it can observe the degree of response to prone and to match this with improvement in oxygenation parameters [40].

Lung ultrasound has been shown to provide the possibility of assessing quantitatively the lung reaeration resulting from antimicrobial therapy of critically ill patients with ventilator-associated pneumonia [41].

Table 1 Lung ultrasound (LUS) assessment

Pattern	LUS finding	Score
A	A-lines or B-lines less than 2	0
B1	Non-confluent B-lines	1
B2	Confluent B-lines	2
C	Consolidation	3

3.4 Lung Recruitment

In patients with ARDS, PEEP keeps lung regions open that would otherwise collapse. Recruitability may be predicted to some extent by a ratio of arterial partial oxygen pressure to the fraction of inspired oxygen of less than 150 and a decrease in dead space with concomitant increase in lung compliance when applying increased PEEP. In patients with minimal recruitable lung, application of higher PEEP is of little benefit and may even be harmful. Lung recruitment has been traditionally evaluated by computed tomography or static pressure-volume curves, which are generally impractical. Alternatively, lung recruitability may be evaluated with LUS.

A direct monitoring of reaeration during recruitment maneuver can be performed bedside by LUS [42]: when a consolidated lung is successfully reaerated by the maneuver, a real-time switch from a tissue-like pattern to an artifact pattern can be visualized, corresponding to the increase of air within the lung area.

A single group studied the assessment of PEEP-induced recruitment by LUS: when compared to pressure-volume (PV) curve, a reaeration score > 8 corresponded to a gain of 600 ml [43]. Moreover, the distribution of US artifacts and therefore of loss of aeration helps in predicting recruitment: as already assessed by CT [44], patients with focal loss of aeration, and thus with normal anterior fields, are classified as non-recruiter; high PEEP and recruitment maneuvers are here contraindicated. On the other hand, patients with diffuse loss of aeration (i.e., affecting also anterior fields) may positively respond to recruitment and an US-monitored PEEP trial is recommended.

When patients are classified as nonresponders to PEEP, they may positively respond to prone position [45]. Patients with focal loss of aeration, compared with those with a diffuse disease, showed in fact a greater improvement of aeration in posterior lung areas during pronation [46]. A significant reaeration of posterior fields during the first cycle of pronation identified "long-term" responders to prone position, defined by a P/F (pO_2/FIO_2) ratio > 300 mmHg after 7 days of 6-h prone position twice daily [47]. In this experience, reaeration assessed by US was associated with the decrease of dead space and also with better outcome, a finding consistent with previous observations [48].

3.5 Weaning from Mechanical Ventilation

The weaning process from mechanical ventilation covers up to 40–50% of total mechanical ventilation time [49]. Weaning failure ranges from 25 to 61% [50], depending on the clinical context; multiple physiopathological mechanisms may be involved; therefore, weaning process remains a significant challenge for the intensivist. Three of the main mechanisms leading to weaning failure can be assessed by US: cardiac dysfunction, lung derecruitment, and diaphragm dysfunction.

While no impact of systolic parameters has been found, diastolic assessment by transmitralic pattern and tissue Doppler of mitral annulus can identify the failing patient with moderate sensitivity and high specificity [51]. The assessment of lung aeration score at the end of a spontaneous breathing trial predicts extubation failure with 0.86 area under curve (AUC) [36]. Finally, respiratory muscle dysfunction as assessed by diaphragm US during a spontaneous breathing trial or low-pressure support ventilation is associated with weaning failure [52].

A combined US approach assessing lung, heart, and diaphragm has been suggested, not only for early identification of the failing patient but also for a better understanding of the underlying mechanism of failure, thus guiding therapeutic management to improve weaning success rate [53].

3.5.1 Weaning Failure of Cardiovascular Origin

Switching a patient from passive to active ventilation is the first step in the transition to reestablish negative inspiratory intrathoracic pressure, thus increasing venous return, central blood volume, and left ventricular (LV) transmural pressure and afterload. The return to inspiratory effort during SBT or pressure support ventilation during the weaning process often represents a stress test for the ICU patient and can induce cardiogenic pulmonary edema in cases of volume overload as well as LV systolic or diastolic dysfunction. An increased LV pressure leads to retrograde pressure transmission into the pulmonary circulation and causes elevation of pressure in the pulmonary microcirculation. To summarize, cardiac-related weaning failure may be due to either a systolic or an isolated diastolic LV dysfunction [54], which can be diagnosed through echocardiography.

So to optimize the weaning process, patients with a high risk of weaning failure of cardiac origin are screened at admission or during their stay in the ICU. Echocardiography should be performed on patients to detect decreased LV ejection fraction due to cardiomyopathy or relevant valvular heart disease. Usually, LV function is found to be normal, and decreased LV ejection fraction is present in less than 20% of weaning patients [55]. Weaning failure occurs more frequently in patients with diastolic dysfunction: up to 80% in patients with moderate (pseudonormal pattern) or severe (restrictive pattern) degree of dysfunction [6]. Thus, an echo should always be performed after weaning or extubation failure in order to rule out significant diastolic dysfunction.

Standard guidelines for the evaluation of LV filling pressures recommend the use of PWD of mitral inflow and TDI of mitral annulus displacement [56]. The pulsed wave Doppler (PWD) study of mitral flow (recorded at the tip of the mitral valve) (Fig. 15) consists of early diastolic E waves and atrial contraction A waves. The pattern of this mitral flow (aspects of E and A waves) depends on LV diastolic function and filling pressure (Fig. 16). The parameters commonly used to characterize this pattern include the peak velocity ratio of E and A waves (E/A ratio) and the deceleration time of E waves (DTE). A restrictive pattern (E/A ratio $\geq$ 2,

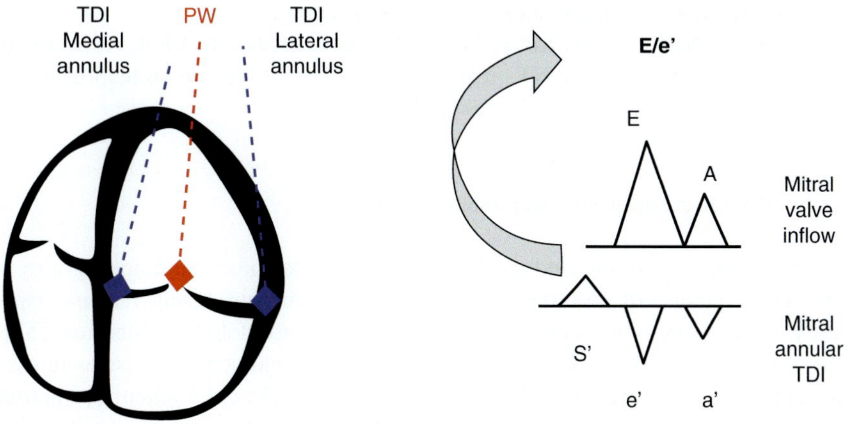

Fig. 15 PWD and TDI

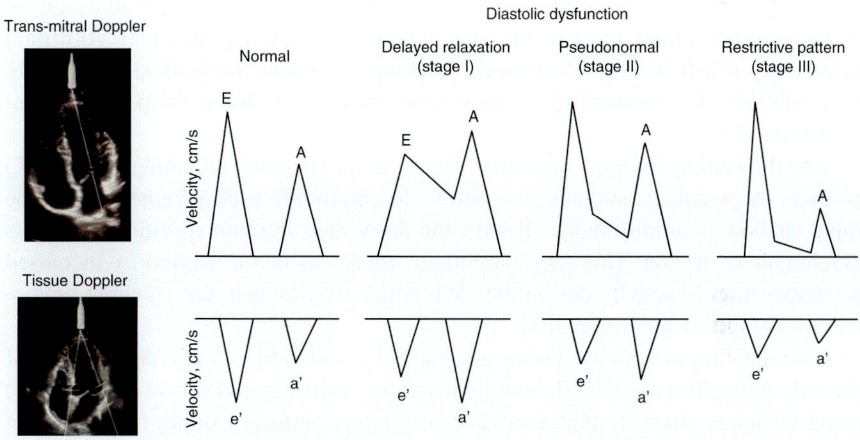

Fig. 16 Grades of diastolic dysfunction

DTE < 120 ms) is highly suggestive of a pulmonary capillary wedge pressure less than 18 mm Hg [56].

Tissue Doppler (TDI) allows measurement of early diastolic mitral annulus velocity (E′ wave). The measurement can be taken at the lateral and septal parts of the mitral annulus; the averaged value should be considered. Theoretically, TDI of the mitral annulus allows evaluation of LV relaxation (E′ wave during early diastole) independently of LV filling pressure, contrary to E. Thus, E′ and LV relaxation is correlated, and the E/E′ ratio is correlated with LV filling pressure (pulmonary capillary wedge pressure) [56].

In previous studies, increases in LV pressure and in the E/E′ ratio were observed during SBT using a T-piece [57] or during a trial of 7 cmH2O pressure-support with zero positive end-expiratory pressure [58]. In these studies, the E/E′ ratio was predictive of weaning failure, and threshold values ranged from 8 to 15, with sensitivity and specificity varying from 75% to 82% and from 91% to 100%, respectively [57]. This may explain why NT-proBNP levels during SBT can be helpful in the prediction of postextubation respiratory distress [58].

3.5.2 Weaning Failure of Diaphragmatic Origin

Diaphragmatic excursion and thickening can help to diagnose diaphragm dysfunction as a cause of weaning failure. Reduced excursion during various inspiratory maneuvers is an established diagnostic criterion for dysfunction [59]. Serial measurements of diaphragm thickness can reveal acute decreases in diaphragm thickness, indicative of rapid muscle atrophy. As the thickening fraction is related to the degree of diaphragmatic shortening during inspiration, it correlates with the changes in lung volume, inspiratory pressure development [60], and work of breathing [61]. As a result, a reduced maximal thickening fraction is a marker for diaphragm weakness. The validity of this technique to diagnose diaphragm weakness is crucially dependent on obtaining maximal volitional inspiratory effort. Using ultrasound to diagnose diaphragm weakness may help to guide the management of patients with difficult weaning from mechanical ventilation [62].

The thickening fraction measured during a spontaneous breathing trial (SBT) predicts the weaning outcome. In contrast to commonly used parameters like the rapid shallow breathing index (RSBI), the thickening fraction specifically reflects diaphragmatic action. This way, diaphragm weakness is not masked by increased accessory muscle activity during the SBT, which may explain the excellent predictive results of this parameter [63].

Also diaphragm activity during mechanical ventilation is a key determinant of the risk of diaphragm injury. Insufficient activity leads to rapid disuse atrophy [13]; some evidence suggests that excessive respiratory muscle loading may result in inflammation, injury, and dysfunction, although it is unclear whether this happens frequently in the clinical setting.

Monitoring diaphragm activity by ultrasound might be used to guide the titration of ventilatory support. By targeting support levels producing relatively normal levels of respiratory effort (thickening fraction in the range of 15–30%), diaphragm atrophy and injury might be prevented. This concept is referred to as diaphragm-protective ventilation [64]. A recent study found that the length of ICU stay, the duration of ventilation, and the risk of complications of respiratory failure (prolonged ventilation, re-intubation, tracheostomy, or death) were minimized when patients' thickening fraction averaged 15–30%—similar to that of healthy subjects breathing at rest—during the first 3 days of ventilation [13]. This may represent the optimal level of spontaneous breathing during mechanical ventilation to protect the diaphragm from injury.

Ultrasound can also be used to diagnose patient-ventilator dyssynchrony [7], as it provides real-time information of contractile activity. Recognizing and treating dyssynchrony may help to improve outcomes, as frequent dyssynchrony strongly predicts poor clinical outcomes [65].

3.5.3 Weaning Failure of Lung Origin

The switch from positive-pressure ventilation to spontaneous breathing is associated with changes in lung aeration. If significant, these changes can be detected by LUS. The best way to quantify the lung loss of aeration is to use a LUS rating system (aeration score). This score is computed in six regions per hemithorax: sternum, anterior, and posterior axillary lines defining anterior, lateral, and posterior areas, each divided into superior and inferior fields. The global LUS score corresponds to the sum of each region's score and ranges from 0 (all regions are well aerated) to 36 (all regions are consolidated) [66].

In patients with acute respiratory distress syndrome, the regional LUS score is strongly correlated with tissue density when assessed by quantitative computed tomography. Each step increase of the score from 0 to 3 is associated with a significant gain in density [66]. This score was successfully used in a trial of positive end-expiratory pressure [46] and has been used to monitor pulmonary infections. Moreover, the global LUS score directly correlates with both extravascular lung water, as assessed by transpulmonary thermodilution [67], and overall lung tissue density, as assessed by quantitative computed tomography [66].

In the context of weaning, the LUS score can help distinguish patients who are at high and low risk of postextubation distress. In patients who pass a 1-h SBT, ultrasound changes of lung aeration are predictive of extubation success or failure: in patients who are definitively weaned, overall lung aeration does not significantly change during SBT, whereas in patients with extubation failure, lung aeration decreases during SBT. A LUS score higher than 17 at the end of the SBT is highly predictive of extubation failure, while a score lower than 13 is highly predictive of successful weaning [36]. Moreover, LUS allows for a regional analysis of aeration changes. It seems that opposite regional changes in aeration occur during SBT and can be highlighted by LUS: posterior and dependent lung regions may increase their aeration due to the active contraction of the diaphragm, whereas lateral and anterior nondependent lung regions may decrease their aeration [36]. An increase in the number of B-lines in anterolateral fields during the SBT seems to allow the diagnosis of weaning-induced pulmonary edema. On the contrary, a simplified approach distinguishing two patterns (with or without a B predominance) in anterior fields only seems not to be accurate enough to identify the failing patients [68].

Pleural effusion can also be easily detected as an anechoic space between the pleura and quantified by measuring the interpleural distance in a transversal scan in supine patients. The impact of pleural effusion on weaning failure is, however, controversial.

3.6 LUS in COVID-19

COVID-19 presented a challenging clinical dilemma for clinicians at the frontline, with its atypical features which are different from the classical presentation of ARDS. Two different phenotypes have been described, at least in a theoretical model [69]. The more frequent phenotype "L" typically presents with normal to mildly reduced lung compliance, albeit with a level of hypoxemia disproportionate to the relatively preserved lung compliance, in which chest CT typically shows predominantly peripheral ground-glass opacifications that worsen with the progression of the disease. On the other hand, the less frequent phenotype "H" is more similar to the classic ARDS presentation with reduced lung compliance and evidence of dense lobar consolidations on chest CT.

LUS is potentially able to distinguish these two phenotypes, based on the different signs and patterns. In COVID-19, we typically see various grades of multiple B-lines with patchy distribution. B-lines can be separated or coalescent, including pictures of sonographic "white lung" (Fig. 17). B-lines are often visible in the context of "spared" areas of good aeration in which we see multiple horizontal A-lines that are reverberations of the pleural line [70]. A recently described finding is observed in most patients in the early phases of COVID-19 pneumonia: it is a shiny "light" beam that is a band-like artifact, often appearing and disappearing with

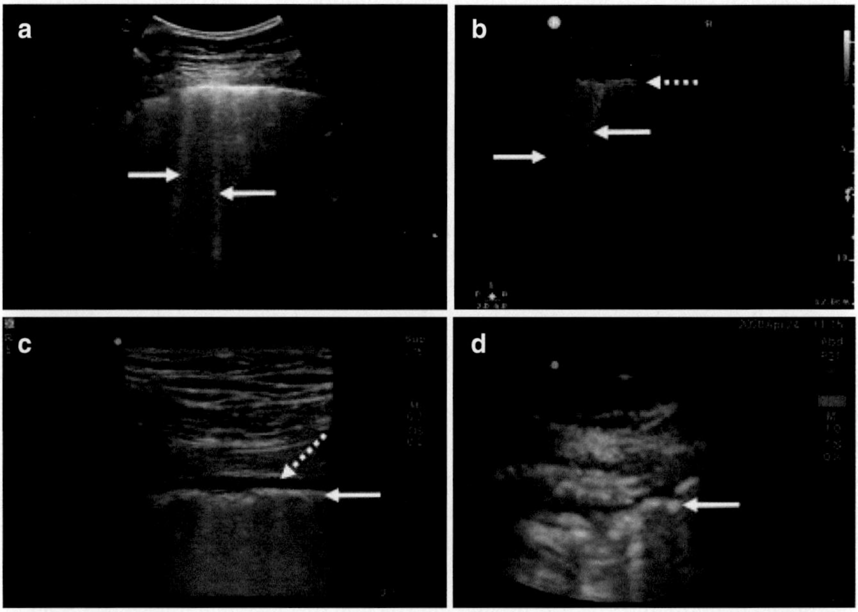

Fig. 17 (**a**) Multiple B-lines (arrows). (**b**) Multiple B-lines (arrows) and a thickened irregular pleural line (dotted arrow). (**c**) Thickened irregular pleura (arrow) and an associated small pleural effusion (dotted arrow). (**d**) Thickened irregular pleura (arrow)

respiration [71]. Other common findings in COVID-19 are an irregular "fragmented" pleural line with small peripheral consolidations. Larger consolidations characterize the phenotype "H" or a superimposed bacterial pneumonia, and it is debated whether they may represent pulmonary infarctions. Large pleural effusions are not commonly seen, whereas trivial localized pleural effusion can be visualized in the context of more deaerated areas [70].

References

1. Bouhemad B, Mongodi S, Via G, et al. Ultrasound for "lung monitoring" of ventilated patients. Anesthesiology. 2015;122:437–47.
2. Riviello E, Kiviri W, Twagirumugabe T, et al. Hospital incidence and outcomes of the acute respiratory distress syndrome using the Kigali modification of the Berlin definition. Am J Respir Crit Care Med. 2016;193(1):1546–56.
3. Luecke T, Corradi F, Pelosi P. Lung imaging for titration of mechanical ventilation. Curr Opin Anaesthesiol. 2012;25(2):131–40.
4. Bouhemad B, Zhang M, Lu Q, Rouby JJ. Bedside lung ultrasound in critical care practice. J Crit Care. 2007;11:205–13.
5. Umbrello M, Formenti P, Longhi D, et al. Diaphragm ultrasound as indicator of respiratory effort in critically ill patients undergoing assisted mechanical ventilation: a pilot clinical study. Crit Care. 2015;19:161.
6. Laghi F, Cattapan SE, Jubran A, et al. Is weaning failure caused by low-frequency fatigue of the diaphragm? Am J Respir Crit Care Med. 2003;167:120–7.
7. Matamis D, Soilemezi E, Tsagourias M, et al. Sonographic evaluation of the diaphragm in critically ill patients. Technique and clinical applications. Intensive Care Med. 2013;39:801–10.
8. Pasero D, Koeltz A, Placido R, et al. Improving ultrasonic measurement of diaphragmatic excursion after cardiac surgery using the anatomical M-mode: a randomized crossover study. Intensive Care Med. 2015;41:650–6.
9. Lerolle N, Guerot E, Dimassi S, et al. Ultrasonographic diagnostic criterion for severe diaphragmatic dysfunction after cardiac surgery. Chest. 2009;135:401–7.
10. Goligher EC, Laghi F, Detsky ME, et al. Measuring diaphragm thickness with ultrasound in mechanically ventilated patients: feasibility, reproducibility and validity. Intensive Care Med. 2015;41:734.
11. Zambon M, Beccaria P, Matsuno J, et al. Mechanical ventilation and diaphragmatic atrophy in critically ill patients: an ultrasound study. Crit Care Med. 2016;44:1347–52.
12. Goligher EC, Fan E, Herridge MS, et al. Evolution of diaphragm thickness during mechanical ventilation: impact of inspiratory effort. Am J Respir Crit Care Med. 2015;192:1080–8.
13. Goligher EC, Dres M, Fan E, et al. Mechanical ventilation-induced diaphragm atrophy strongly impacts clinical outcomes. Am J Respir Crit Care Med. 2018;197:204–13.
14. Alrajab S, Youssef AM, Akkus NI, Caldito G. Pleural ultrasonography versus chest radiography for the diagnosis of pneumothorax: review of the literature and meta-analysis. Crit Care. 2013;17:R208.
15. Lichtenstein D, Meziere G, Biderman P, Gepner A. The comet tail artifact: an ultrasound sign ruling out pneumothorax. Intensive Care Med. 1999;25:383–8.
16. Lichtenstein D, Meziere G, Biderman P, Gepner A. The "lung point": an ultrasound sign specific to pneumothorax. Intensive Care Med. 2000;26:1434–40.
17. Lichtenstein DA, Lascols N, Prin S, Mezière G. The "lung pulse" an early ultrasound sign of complete atelectasis. Intensive Care Med. 2003;29:2187–92.
18. Mattison LE, Coppage L, Alderman DF, Herlong JO, Sahn SA. Pleural effusions in the medical ICU: prevalence, causes, and clinical implications. Chest. 1997;111:1018–23.

19. Doust BD, Baum JK, Maklad NF, Doust VL. Ultrasonic evaluation of pleural opacities. Radiology. 1975;114:135–40.
20. Lichtenstein D, Hulot JS, Rabiller A, Tostivint I, Meziere G. Feasibility and safety of ultrasound-aided thoracentesis in mechanically ventilated patients. Intensive Care Med. 1999;25:955–8.
21. Weinberg B, Diakoumakis EE, Kass EG, Seife B, Zvi ZB. The air bronchogram: sonographic demonstration. Am J Roentgenol. 1986;147:593–5.
22. Yang PC, Luh KT, Chang DB, Yu CJ, Kuo SH, Wu HD. Ultrasonographic evaluation of pulmonary consolidation. Am Rev Respir Dis. 1992;146:757–62.
23. Lichtenstein D, Meziere G. A lung ultrasound sign allowing bedside distinction between pulmonary edema and COPD: the comet-tail artifact. Intensive Care Med. 1998;24:1331–4.
24. Lichtenstein D, Meziere G, Biderman P, Gepner A, Barre O. The comet-tail artifact. An ultrasound sign of alveolar-interstitial syndrome. Am J Respir Crit Care Med. 1997;156:1640–6.
25. Chiumello D, Mongodi S, Algieri I, Vergani GL, Orlando A, Via G, Crimella F, Cressoni M, Mojoli F. Assessment of lung aeration and recruitment by CT scan and ultrasound in ARDS patients. Crit Care Med. 2018;46:1761–8.
26. Repessé X, Charron C, Vieillard-Baron A. Acute cor pulmonale in ARDS: rationale for protecting the right ventricle. Chest. 2015;147(1):259–65.
27. Pesenti A, Musch G, Lichtenstein D, et al. Imaging in acute respiratory distress syndrome. Intensive Care Med. 2016;42(5):686–98.
28. Mongodi S, Orlando A, Tavazzi G, et al. Veno-venous extracorporeal membrane oxygenation for acute respiratory distress syndrome in a patient with acute right heart failure. J Cardiothorac Vasc Anesth. 2017b;31(4):1374–7.
29. Mekontso Dessap A, Boissier F, Charron C, et al. Acute cor pulmonale during protective ventilation for acute respiratory distress syndrome: prevalence, predictors, and clinical impact. Intensive Care Med. 2016;42(5):862–70.
30. Mekontso Dessap A, Boissier F, Leon R, et al. Prevalence and prognosis of shunting across patent foramen ovale during acute respiratory distress syndrome. Crit Care Med. 2010;38(9):1786–92.
31. Mojadidi MK, Winoker JS, Roberts SC, et al. Accuracy of conventional transthoracic echocardiography for the diagnosis of intracardiac right-to-left shunt: a meta-analysis of prospective studies. Echocardiography. 2014;31:1036–48.
32. Tavazzi G, Pozzi M, Via G, et al. Weaning failure for disproportionate hypoxemia caused by paradoxical response to positive end-expiratory pressure in a patient with patent foramen ovale. Am J Respir Crit Care Med. 2016;193(1):e1–2.
33. Vieillard-Baron A, Charron C, Caille V, et al. Prone positioning unloads the right ventricle in severe ARDS. Chest. 2007;132(5):1440–6.
34. Soldati G, Inchingolo R, Smargiassi A, et al. Ex vivo lung sonography: morphologic-ultrasound relationship. Ultrasound Med Biol. 2012;38(7):1169–79.
35. Via G, Lichtenstein D, Mojoli F, et al. Whole lung lavage: a unique model for ultrasound assessment of lung aeration changes. Intensive Care Med. 2010;36(6):999–1007.
36. Soummer A, Perbet S, Brisson H, et al. Ultrasound assessment of lung aeration loss during a successful weaning trial predicts postextubation distress. Crit Care Med. 2012;40(7):2064–72.
37. Bouhemad B, Brisson H, Le-Guen M, Arbelot C, Lu Q, Rouby JJ. Bedside ultrasound assessment of positive end-expiratory pressure-induced lung recruitment. Am J Respir Crit Care Med. 2011;183:341–7.
38. Markota A, Golub J, Stožer A, Fluher J, Prosen G, Bergauer A, Svenšek F, Sinkovič A. Absence of lung sliding is not a reliable sign of pneumothorax in patients with high positive end-expiratory pressure. Am J Emerg Med. 2016;34:2034–6.
39. Pesenti A, Musch G, Lichtenstein D, Mojoli F, Amato MBP, Cinnella G, Gattinoni L, Quintel M. Imaging in acute respiratory distress syndrome. Intensive Care Med. 2016;42:686–98.
40. Wang XT, Ding X, Zhang HM, Chen H, Su LX, Liu DW, Chinese Critical Ultrasound Study Group (CCUSG). Lung ultrasound can be used to predict the potential of prone positioning and assess prognosis in patients with acute respiratory distress syndrome. Crit Care. 2016;20:385.

41. Bouhemad B, Liu ZH, Arbelot C, Zhang M, Ferarri F, Le Guen M, et al. Ultrasound assessment of antibiotic-induced pulmonary reaeration in ventilator-associated pneumonia. Crit Care Med. 2010;38:84–92.
42. Nguyen M, Benkhadra S, Douguet C, et al. Real-time visualization of left lung consolidation relief using lung ultrasound. Am J Respir Crit Care Med. 2016;193(11):e59–60.
43. Bouhemad B, Brisson H, Le-Guen M, et al. Bedside ultrasound assessment of positive end-expiratory pressure-induced lung recruitment. Am J Respir Crit Care Med. 2011;183(3):341–7.
44. Constantin JM, Futier E, Cherprenet AL, et al. A recruitment maneuver increases oxygenation after intubation of hypoxemic intensive care unit patients: a randomized controlled study. Crit Care. 2010;14(2):R76.
45. Prat G, Guinard S, Bizien N, et al. Can lung ultrasonography predict prone positioning response in acute respiratory distress syndrome patients? J Cri Care. 2015;32:36–41.
46. Haddam M, Zieleskiewicz L, Perbet S, et al. Lung ultrasonography for assessment of oxygenation response to prone position ventilation in ARDS. Intensive Care Med. 2016;42(10):1546–56.
47. Wang XT, Ding X, Zhang HM, Chinese Critical Ultrasound Study Group (CCUSG), et al. Lung ultrasound can be used to predict the potential of prone positioning and assess prognosis in patients with acute respiratory distress syndrome. Crit Care. 2016;20(1):385.
48. Gattinoni L, Vagginelli F, Carlesso E, et al. Decrease in PaCO2 with prone position is predictive of improved outcome in acute respiratory distress syndrome. Crit Care Med. 2003;31(12):2727–33.
49. McConville JF, Kress JP. Weaning patients from the ventilator. N Engl J Med. 2012;367(23):2233–9.
50. Esteban A, Alía I, Tobin MJ, et al. Effect of spontaneous breathing trial duration on outcome of attempts to discontinue mechanical ventilation. Spanish Lung Failure Collaborative Group. Am J Respir Crit Care Med. 1999;159(2):512–8.
51. Moschietto S, Doyen D, Grech L, et al. Transthoracic echocardiography with Doppler tissue imaging predicts weaning failure from mechanical ventilation: evolution of the left ventricle relaxation rate during a spontaneous breathing trial is the key factor in weaning outcome. Crit Care. 2012;16(3):R81.
52. Blumhof S, Wheeler D, Thomas K, et al. Change in diaphragmatic thickness during the respiratory cycle predicts extubation success at various levels of pressure support ventilation. Lung. 2016;194(4):519–25.
53. Mayo P, Volpicelli G, Lerolle N, et al. Ultrasonography evaluation during the weaning process: the heart, the diaphragm, the pleura and the lung. Intensive Care Med. 2016;42(7):1107–17.
54. Lemaire F, Teboul JL, Cinotti L, et al. Acute left ventricular dysfunction during unsuccessful weaning from mechanical ventilation. Anesthesiology. 1988;69:171–9.
55. Caille V, Amiel JB, Charron C, et al. Echocardiography: a help in the weaning process. Crit Care. 2010;14:R120.
56. Nagueh SF, Smiseth OA, Appleton CP, et al. Recommendations for the evaluation of left ventricular diastolic function by echocardiography: an update from the American Society of Echocardiography and the European Association of Cardiovascular Imaging. J Am Soc Echocardiogr. 2016;29:277–314.
57. Lamia B, Maizel J, Ochagavia A, et al. Echocardiographic diagnosis of pulmonary artery occlusion pressure elevation during weaning from mechanical ventilation. Crit Care Med. 2009;37:1696–701.
58. Gerbaud E, Erickson M, Grenouillet-Delacre M, et al. Echocardiographic evaluation and N-terminal pro-brain natriuretic peptide measurement of patients hospitalized for heart failure during weaning from mechanical ventilation. Minerva Anestesiol. 2012;78:415–25.
59. Lerolle N, Guérot E, Dimassi S, et al. Ultrasonographic diagnostic criterion for severe diaphragmatic dysfunction after cardiac surgery. Chest. 2009;135(2):401–7.
60. Dubé B-P, Dres M, Mayaux J, et al. Ultrasound evaluation of diaphragm function in mechanically ventilated patients: comparison to phrenic stimulation and prognostic implications. Thorax. 2017;72(9):811–8.

61. Vivier E, Mekontso Dessap A, Dimassi S, et al. Diaphragm ultrasonography to estimate the work of breathing during non-invasive ventilation. Intensive Care Med. 2012;38(5):796–803.
62. Vorona S, Sabatini U, Al-Maqbali S, et al. Inspiratory muscle rehabilitation in critically ill adults. A systematic review and meta-analysis. Annals ATS. 2018;15(6):735–44.
63. DiNino E, Gartman EJ, Sethi JM, et al. Diaphragm ultrasound as a predictor of successful extubation from mechanical ventilation. Thorax. 2014;69(5):423–7.
64. Heunks L, Ottenheijm C. Diaphragm-protective mechanical ventilation to improve outcomes in ICU patients? Am J Respir Crit Care Med. 2018;197(2):150–2.
65. Blanch L, Villagra A, Sales B, et al. Asynchronies during mechanical ventilation are associated with mortality. Intensive Care Med. 2015;41(4):633–41.
66. Chiumello D, Mongodi S, Algieri I, et al. Assessment of lung aeration and recruitment by CT scan and ultrasound in acute respiratory distress syndrome patients. Crit Care Med. 2018;46:1761–8.
67. Zhao Z, Jiang L, Xi X, et al. Prognostic value of extravascular lung water assessed with lung ultrasound score by chest sonography in patients with acute respiratory distress syndrome. BMC Pulm Med. 2015;15:98.
68. Antonio ACP, Knorst MM, Teixeira C. Lung ultrasound prior to spontaneous breathing trial is not helpful in the decision to wean. Respir Care. 2018;63:873–8.
69. Gattinoni L, Chiumello D, Caironi P, Busana M, Romitti F, Brazzi L, Camporota L. COVID-19 pneumonia: different respiratory treatment for different phenotypes? Intensive Care Med. 2020;46:1099.
70. Gargani L, Soliman-Aboumarie H, Volpicelli G, et al. Why, when, and how to use lung ultrasound during the COVID-19 pandemic: enthusiasm and caution. Eur Heart J Cardiovasc Imaging. 2020;21:941–8.
71. Volpicelli G, Gargani L. Sonographic signs and patterns of COVID-19 pneumonia. Ultrasound J. 2020;12:22.

Mechanical Ventilation in ARDS

Shijing Jia and Robert C Hyzy

1 ARDS

Acute respiratory distress syndrome (ARDS) is a form of acute respiratory failure driven by an aggressive inflammatory response either due to direct lung injury or indirectly due to an extrapulmonary insult [1]. The 2012 updated Berlin Definition for ARDS [2] is as follows:

Timing

- Within 1 week of a known clinical insult or new or worsening respiratory symptoms.

Chest Imaging

- Bilateral opacities—not fully explained by effusions, lobar/lung collapse, or nodules.

S. Jia (✉) · R. C Hyzy
Division of Pulmonary and Critical Care Medicine, University of Michigan, Ann Arbor, MI, USA
e-mail: sjia@med.umich.edu; rhyzy@med.umich.edu

J. Hidalgo et al. (eds.), *Personalized Mechanical Ventilation*,
https://doi.org/10.1007/978-3-031-14138-6_20

Origin of Edema

- Respiratory failure not fully explained by cardiac failure or fluid overload.
- Need objective assessment (e.g., echocardiography) to exclude hydrostatic edema if no risk factor present.

Oxygenation

- Mild 200 mmHg < $PaO_2/FIO_2 \leq 300$ mmHg with PEEP or CPAP ≥ 5 cm H_2O.
- Moderate 100 mmHg < $PaO_2/FIO_2 \leq 200$ mmHg with PEEP $\geq$5 cm H_2O.
- Severe $PaO_2/FIO_2 \leq 100$ mmHg with PEEP $\geq$5 cm H_2O.

Although these definitions provide guidance for the diagnosis and severity of ARDS, ARDS is ultimately a clinical diagnosis based on patient presentation and physiology. Underdiagnosis of ARDS leads to underutilization of appropriate lung-protective ventilation and other therapeutic strategies, which may lead to poor patient outcomes [3]. For this reason, it is important to be vigilant about the possibility of ARDS particularly in those with mild disease.

2 Risk Factors for ARDS

Many risk factors for ARDS have been identified and can broadly be categorized as direct and indirect lung injury. The lung injury prediction score (LIPS) [1] was developed to predict the likelihood of ARDS in patients with known risk factors (Table 1).

While the LIPS scoring system is regarded as predictive for the development of ARDS, many patients with multiple risk factors do not progress to ARDS. As such, a LIPS of 4 corresponds to an ~7% rate of ARDS, and a score of 7 predicted an ~20% chance for the development of ARDS. Likewise, there may be other risk factors for ARDS not represented in the table.

ARDS is a clinical syndrome with variable outcomes associated with different underlying risk factors. For example, ARDS due to sepsis is associated with a worse outcome compared with other causes [4, 5]. Likewise, ARDS occurring in hyperinflammatory states is associated with poor outcomes and tends to persist longer than a noninflammatory phenotype [6]. Conversely, ARDS due to trauma is associated with less mortality [7]. A way to classify ARDS phenotypes is by direct versus indirect lung injury (Table 2) [8]. Direct lung injury is associated with more severe ARDS, an epithelial versus endothelial molecular pattern of inflammation, more alveolar collapse and fibrosis pathologically, and less response to positive end-expiratory pressure (PEEP) [9–11].

Indeed, the diagnosis of ARDS encompasses a wide spectrum of pathologies for respiratory failure, with only 45% of patients exhibiting the classic diffuse alveolar damage (DAD) on histopathology associated with ARDS [12]. Not surprisingly, more severe ARDS as graded by PaO_2/FIO_2 of the Berlin Criteria was associated

Table 1 Lung injury prediction score (LIPS). Reprinted with permission of the American Thoracic Society. Copyright © 2022 American Thoracic Society. All rights reserved. Gajic O, Dabbagh O, Park PK, et al. Early identification of patients at risk of acute lung injury: evaluation of lung injury prediction score in a multicenter cohort study. *American journal of respiratory and critical care medicine*. 2011;183(4):462–470. The American Journal of Respiratory and Critical Care Medicine is an official journal of the American Thoracic Society

	LIPS points	Examples
Predisposing conditions		
Shock	2	(1) Patient with a history of alcohol abuse with septic shock from pneumonia requiring $FIO_2 > 0.35$ in the emergency room: Sepsis + shock + pneumonia + alcohol abuse + $FIO_2 > 0.35$ 1 + 2 + 1.5 + 1 + 2 = 7.5
Aspiration	2	
Sepsis	1	
Pneumonia	1.5	
High-risk surgery[a]		
Orthopedic spine	1	
Acute abdomen	2	
Cardiac	2.5	
Aortic vascular	3.5	
High-risk trauma		(2) Motor vehicle accident with traumatic brain injury, lung contusion, and shock requiring $FIO_2 > 0.35$: Traumatic brain injury + lung contusion + shock + $FIO_2 > 0.35$ 2 + 1.5 + 2 + 2 = 7.5
Traumatic brain injury	2	
Smoke inhalation	2	
Near drowning	2	
Lung contusion	1.5	
Multiple fractures	1.5	
Risk modifiers		
Alcohol abuse	1	
Obesity (BMI >30)	1	(3) Patient with a history of diabetes mellitus and urosepsis with shock: Sepsis + shock + diabetes 1 + 2–1 = 2
Hypoalbuminemia	1	
Chemotherapy	1	
$FIO_2 > 0.35$ (> 4 L/min)	2	
Tachypnea (RR >30)	1.5	
$SpO_2 < 95\%$	1	
Acidosis (pH <7.35)	1.5	
Diabetes mellitus[b]	-1	

Definition of abbreviations: *BMI* body mass index, *RR* respiratory rate, SpO_2 oxygen saturation by pulse oximetry

[a] Add 1.5 points if emergency surgery

[b] Only if sepsis

both with higher rates of histopathologic DAD and mortality, 27% for mild, 32% for moderate, and 45% for severe cases of ARDS [2, 12]. When considering ARDS physiologically, it is also not surprising that those with more severe hypoxia have a higher mortality [13]. However, those patients with robust PaO_2/FIO_2 responses to PEEP had better outcomes [14].

Table 2 Common direct and indirect lung injury in ARDS

Direct lung injury	Indirect lung injury
Aspiration	Systemic inflammatory response syndrome (SIRS)
Pulmonary infection	Non-thoracic trauma
Near drowning	Transfusion reaction
Inhalation injury	Cardiopulmonary bypass
Lung contusion	Pancreatitis

3 Noninvasive Modalities for Oxygenation and Ventilation

Noninvasive modalities for oxygenation and ventilation for respiratory failure include the venturi mask, high-flow nasal cannula (HFNC), and noninvasive ventilation (NIV) via facemask, nasal prongs, or helmet. The assessment of these modalities for ARDS is somewhat complex because the diagnosis of ARDS requires a PEEP of at least 5 cm H_2O [2]. Thus, unless patients subsequently progress to noninvasive ventilation with PEEP or intubation and invasive mechanical ventilation, the diagnosis of ARDS is rarely confirmed in this population. However, there is evidence that a significant portion of these patients treated with noninvasive method would be the diagnostic criteria for ARDS [15].

With the advent of HFNC, the increased use in hypoxemic respiratory failure has largely replaced other noninvasive modalities for oxygenation such as the venturi mask, given the favorable evidence in mild ARDS. Meta-analyses of available trial data favor the use of HFNC over other oxygenation methods in more severe cases of acute hypoxemic respiratory failure [16, 17]. In the FLORALI trial, HFNC performed better than both NIV and conventional oxygenation and prevented intubation in a significant subset of patients who would have met the criteria for ARDS [18, 19]. While the strongest data for HFNC remains in those with community-acquired or hospital-acquired pneumonia, a subgroup analysis of the FLORALI trial showed benefit in patients with $PaO_2/FIO_2 \leq 200$ [18].

Traditional NIV in hypoxemic respiratory failure or ARDS has largely fallen out of favor, particularly with data from the Large Observational Study to Understand the Global Impact of Severe Acute Respiratory Failure (LUNG-SAFE) showing increased mortality with the use of NIV in patients with severe ARDS with $PaO_2/FIO_2 \leq 150$ [20]. Speculation for worse outcomes has largely surrounded the inability to control tidal volumes in NIV [21]. Despite these data, NIV likely performs better than conventional oxygen modalities such as the venturi mask in specific populations [22]. Another development in NIV therapy is the use of the helmet interface, which showed promising results in ventilator-free days, ICU stay, and mortality as compared with the traditional facemask interface [23]. Network meta-analyses suggest that helmet interface NIV may be superior to HFNC, although currently there are no studies that directly compare these two modalities [24, 25]. Due to the high mortality rate of 35–45% in ARDS [3], it is prudent to frequently assess patient status and operate with a low threshold for intubation and mechanical ventilation.

4 Lung-Protective Ventilation

4.1 Low Tidal Volume Ventilation

The most influential change in the philosophy of the ventilator management of ARDS stemmed from the realization that mechanical ventilation can cause increased harm in patients, such as in the case of excessive volume or pressure leading to volutrauma or barotrauma. From this, studies examined ways to reduce ventilator-induced lung injury (VILI) [26]. The single intervention with a definite clinical benefit is the utilization of low tidal volume ventilation (LTVV), a term sometimes used interchangeably with lung-protective ventilation (LPV) [27].

This was largely due to the landmark ARDS Network low tidal volume trial (ARMA) showing that using an assist control (AC) mode of mechanical ventilation (MV) with a tidal volume of 6 mL/kg of the ideal body weight (IBW) significantly reduced mortality in ARDS patients compared with higher volumes of 12 mL/kg [28]. In the study, LTVV targeted V_T ranging from 4 to 8 mL/kg while maintaining plateau pressures (P_{plat}) <30, compared to a traditional ventilation strategy of targeting V_T of 12 mL/kg while maintaining P_{plat} < 50 cm H_2O. Positive end-expiratory pressure (PEEP) and fraction of inspired oxygen (FiO_2) strategy were the same in both groups. Resulting mean ± standard deviation (SD) V_T and P_{plat} in the LTVV versus standard ventilation groups were 6.2 ± 0.8 mL/kg and 25 ± 6 cm H_2O versus 11.8 ± 0.8 mL/kg and 33 ± 8 cm H_2O. The trial was stopped early due to a significant mortality difference of 31.0% in the LTVV group versus 39.8% in the conventional ventilation group after 861 subjects, which translates to an absolute risk reduction of 8.8% and a number needed to treat (NNT) of 11. Follow-up meta-analyses repeatedly demonstrate the importance of low tidal volume ventilation in clinical outcomes [29–31].

Female ideal body weight (IBW) = 45.5 kg + 2.3 kg × (height, in – 60)
Male ideal body weight (IBW) = 50 kg + 2.3 kg × (height, in – 60) [32]

It is important to note that the protective benefit for a low V_T and P_{plat} is not a threshold effect, but rather likely a dose effect. Though P_{plat} was a set parameter in the ARMA trial, follow-up studies show that there is no safe upper limit. But rather, the mortality risk trends with increasing pressures (Fig. 1) [33]. Likewise, meta-analyses of data from multiple ARDS trials show a similar dose affect for V_T [34,

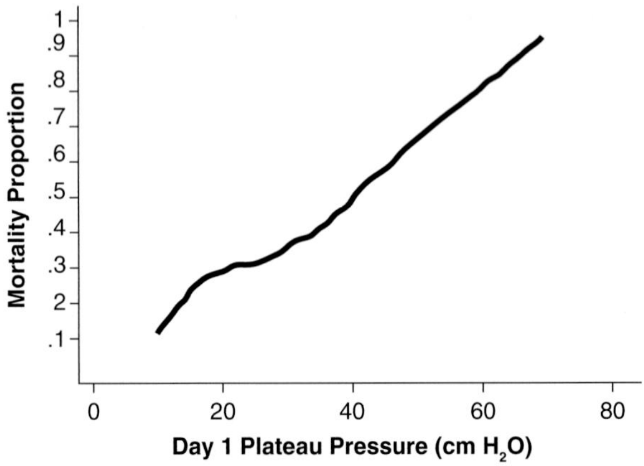

Fig. 1 Mortality as related to plateau pressure and tidal volumes in mechanical ventilation. Reprinted with permission of the American Thoracic Society. Copyright © 2021 American Thoracic Society. All rights reserved. Hager DN, Krishnan JA, Hayden DL, Brower RG. Tidal volume reduction in patients with acute lung injury when plateau pressures are not high. *American journal of respiratory and critical care medicine.* 2005;172 (10):1241–1245. The American Journal of Respiratory and Critical Care Medicine is an official journal of the American Thoracic Society

35]. The limiting factor of very low V_T in ARDS ventilation is the disproportional increase of dead-space ventilation with each decrease in V_T, particularly since physiologic dead space increases with increased ARDS severity [36]. While respiratory rate can be increased to compensate for the ventilatory needs with lowering the V_T, there is a limit to this approach particularly with the onset of auto-PEEP. Since ARDS patients also tend to have low lung compliance, this typically allows for slightly higher limits to respiratory rate without the occurrence of auto-PEEP.

LTVV attenuates the volutrauma induced by overdistention of the alveolar with inappropriately high volumes delivered by mechanical ventilation. This is likely due to the heterogeneous nature of the ARDS lung composition, consisting of normal lung, diseased but recruitable, and diseased and not recruitable [37]. As such, the portion of the lungs participating in ventilation and gas exchange is reduced compared to the normal state. Thus, a reduced V_T need in ARDS is physiologically logical compared to the typical volumes in the healthy state.

Due to the strong evidence for LTVV, it is important to recognize ARDS and utilize appropriate ventilator strategies. Unfortunately, an international cohort study of 3022 patients revealed that clinicians only recognized ARDS 60% of the time. As a result, only 65% of ARDS patients received V_T of $\leq$8 mL/kg IBW [3]. This lapse may be mitigated by a protocolized approach to mechanical ventilation in the ICU [38].

4.2 Alternative Targets for Lung-Protective Ventilation

The P_{plat} measured given a set V_T is reflective of the static compliance of the lung and chest wall. In groups of patients with a disproportionately low chest wall compliance (such as abdominal compartment syndrome, obesity, circumferential burns), the transpulmonary pressures (P_L) may be quite low despite a high P_{plat}. In these cases, the consideration of transesophageal pressure (P_{es}) may be helpful in targeting goals in LPV:

$$P_L = P_{plat} - P_{es}$$

P_{es} can be measured by placing an esophageal balloon and is considered a surrogate for pleural pressure (P_{pl}). V_T and PEEP can then be adjusted to ensure a P_L of <25 cm H_2O at end inspiration to avoid barotrauma and 0–5 cm H_2O at end expiration to avoid atelectrauma and alveolar derecruitment. The first single-center randomized clinical trial (EPVent1) of using this approach showed improved oxygenation and a trend towards mortality benefit in 61 patients, though the study group was enriched for patients at risk for increased abdominal pressure in this surgical ICU population as compared to the typical ARDS patient [39]. However, a subsequent larger multicenter trial (EPVent2) did not confirm the same clinical benefit [40]. While the two studies had some minor differences and limitations to interpretation and applicability, the conclusion is that routine use of P_{es} is likely not appropriate for all patients with ARDS [41]. However, a small, carefully selected subset of patients may benefit from this approach.

More recently, driving pressure (ΔP) has emerged as a potential target in lung-protective ventilation. A review of data from 3562 patients of nine clinical trials revealed ΔP as the strongest correlate of clinical outcomes in ARDS patients undergoing mechanical ventilation, as compared to other ventilator variables (V_T, Pplat, PEEP) [42]. For each 7 cm H_2O increase in ΔP, there was a 1.36 relative risk increase for mortality. This association has been confirmed in follow-up studies [43–45]. However, it is important to note that this data is entirely retrospective. This variable has not been manipulated in a randomized clinical trial to determine a more direct relationship to clinical outcomes. Additionally, the interdependency of the various ventilator parameters and the physiology of the ARDS lung are complex. Thus, ΔP may well be a marker of disease severity. Physiologically, ΔP reflects the recruitability of the ARDS lung since it is a marker of static respiratory system compliance (C_{RS}). An overdistended lung will have a proportionally high increase in ΔP per incremental V_T as compared to an under-recruited lung [37]. In clinical practice, a ΔP target of <15 mg H_2O in patients receiving LTVV is generally reasonable: [44, 46]

$$\Delta P = \text{Ventilator-measured } P_{plat} - \text{PEEP} = V_T / C_{RS}$$

Despite consideration of these clinical targets, our assessment of the true stress on the mechanically ventilated lung is likely very rudimentary. Partly, this is because these conveniently monitored variables with robust clinical data are static in nature, while ventilation is a dynamic process. Other variables accounting for the dynamic respiratory process are flow, inspiratory contour, and inspiratory time, among others. The energy applied over time is the mechanical power applied to the lung [47]. While each individual perimeter is difficult to manipulate and monitor in an experimental model in human subjects [48], animal data suggests that many of these dynamic variables may be associated with clinical outcomes [49–51]. When taking into account the heterogeneous nature of the ARDS lung, it becomes easy to recognize how crude our current ventilator targets are in predicting lung injury at the alveolar level.

5 Open-Lung Ventilation

5.1 Optimal PEEP

Open-lung ventilation (OLV) employs a high PEEP in combination with recruitment maneuvers to theoretically reduce the incidence of atelectrauma. The first large multicenter randomized trial of PEEP in ARDS was the ALVEOLI study, which was conducted out of concern for potential harms of higher PEEP in patients [52]. When comparing an average low PEEP of 8.3 cm H_2O versus high PEEP of 13.2 cm H_2O in ARDS patients receiving LTVV, there were no differences in clinical outcomes (Table 3). A follow-up study, the Expiratory Pressure Study (ExPress), showed no difference in mortality, but reduced mechanical ventilation duration when higher PEEP was used [53]. The Lung Open Ventilation Study (LOVS) found no difference in mortality, but did show improved oxygenation using high PEEP (average 14.6 cm H_2O) compared to low PEEP (9.8 cm H_2O) (Table 3) [54].

Several meta-analyses of individual trial data have been published. One such study showed that a higher PEEP strategy is associated with improved mortality in patients with moderate or severe ARDS with PaO_2/FiO_2 ratio of 200 mm Hg or less [55]. Another secondary analysis again showed mortality benefit in ARDS patients

Table 3 High versus low PEEP ladders in two clinical trials

FiO_2	0.3	0.4	0.5	0.6	0.7	0.8	0.9	1.0
ALVEOLI [52]								
Low PEEP	5	5–8	8–10	10	10–14	14	14–18	18–24
High PEEP	12–14	14–16	16–20	20	20	22	22	22–24
LOVS [54]								
Low PEEP	5	5–8	8–10	10	10–14	14	14–18	18–24
High PEEP	5–10	10–18	18–20	20	20	20–22	22	22–24

with severe hypoxemia ($PaO_2/FiO_2 \leq 150$ mm Hg) [14]. However, the most comprehensive meta-analysis of eight trails showed no difference in mortality or ventilator-free days in an unselected ARDS population [56]. These results likely stem from the heterogeneity of ARDS patients at the inter-individual level as well as at the alveolar level [37]. Some patients have highly recruitable lungs or segments of the lung, while others do not. This recruitability also seems to change as ARDS evolves through the course of disease, with the early ARDS lung being more recruitable than later in disease [57]. These and other factors make it impossible to propose a one-size-fits-all approach to a PEEP to FiO_2 recommendation in all cases of ARDS. Rather, PEEP optimization per the individual patient [58] and a constant reassessment through the progression of disease are important in the management of mechanical ventilation for ARDS. It is important to note the ranges of PEEP utilized even in low-PEEP ladders when caring for ARDS patients, as sufficient PEEP is key in preventing atelectrauma. Additionally, select patients with more severe disease or those with increased extrapulmonary pressures likely benefit from higher levels of PEEP [59].

5.2 *Recruitment Maneuvers*

While recruitment maneuvers are more regarded as a salvage therapy in cases of refractory hypoxemia, it logically follows the discussion regarding PEEP in OLV. The concept of OLV pairs recruitment maneuvers to open areas of recruitable lung followed by increased PEEP to keep those recruited segments open for improved alveolar oxygen diffusion. The clinical benefit of recruitment maneuvers has been assessed in multiple clinical trials over the years and remains undefined. While small early studies showed mixed results [54, 60, 61], the largest multicenter interventional study of recruitment maneuvers paired with increased PEEP (Alveolar Recruitment for ARDS Trial [ART]) showed increased mortality [62]. In this study, 1013 patients with at least moderate ARDS ($PaO_2/FiO_2 < 200$ mg Hg) were randomized to an aggressive OLV strategy of progressively increased PEEP up to 35–45 cm H_2O versus control. The OLV arm had increased 28-day mortality (55.3% vs. 49.3%; $P = 0.041$), increased 6-month mortality (65.3% vs. 59.9%; $P = 0.04$), and decreased ventilator-free days (5.3 vs. 6.4; $P = 0.03$), likely due to increased barotrauma events noted in the study. These results may be explained again by the heterogeneous nature of the ARDS lung [63]. It is also important to note that the recruitment protocol in ART was quite aggressive compared to more reasonable recruit maneuvers such as a 30-s inspiratory hold not exceeding a pressure of 30 cm H_2O.

Follow-up meta-analyses also present conflicted results [64–66]. Thus despite some recommendations for recruitment maneuvers based on weak evidence [59], these interventions are generally limited to severe ARDS patients with refractory hypoxemia who would benefit from a temporary improvement in oxygenation.

6 COVID-19 Pandemic

The coronavirus disease 2019 (COVID-19) pandemic, caused by the severe acute respiratory syndrome coronavirus 2 (SARS-CoV-2), contributed to significant morbidity and mortality globally with 170+ million confirmed cases and almost 4 million deaths [67]. A majority of deaths were due to acute respiratory failure, with large portions of patients meeting clinical diagnostic and histopathologic criteria for ARDS [68, 69]. As such, the airway and respiratory management of these patients mirrors that of other ARDS patients. Since patients can deteriorate rapidly, experts advocate for a low threshold for intubation and mechanical ventilation [70]. However, noninvasive modalities such as HFNC and NIV are readily employed for those with milder forms of respiratory failure [71, 72]. Though data is sparse, the overall rate of HFNC and NIV usage and outcomes likely does not deviate from other forms of ARDS [73, 74].

Management of mechanical ventilation follows conventional practice for LPV with LTVV [70]. Care should be taken to adhere to low V_T and P_{plat} due to some modest evidence for increased risk for barotrauma in COVID-19 [75]. However, because of the high degree of hypoxemia associated with COVID-19 pneumonia, increased levels of PEEP may need to be utilized [71]. In patients with refractory disease, advanced techniques such as prone ventilation, OLV, inhaled vasodilators, neuromuscular blockade, and extracorporeal membrane oxygenation (ECMO) should be employed [70, 76, 77].

7 Modes of Ventilation

7.1 Volume- Versus Pressure-Limited Mechanical Ventilation

The assist control (AC) mode of mechanical ventilation has two main sub-modes depending on whether each assisted breath is volume limited or pressure limited. The main distinction is that the volume-limited AC ventilation requires a set flow rate, with the inspiratory breath cycled to the exhalation phase once the targeted volume per breath is achieved. However, in pressure-limited AC ventilation, the inspiratory flow is variable depending on the respiratory effort of the patient in combination with the set inspiratory pressure. The inspiratory breath terminates or is cycled once the set inspiratory time has elapsed. Due to the allowance of variable flow in pressure-limited AC ventilation, there is an argument for better patient tolerance due to improved comfort [78, 79]. However, this has not firmly borne out in studies.

Since almost all ARDS evidence has been built on volume-limited AC ventilation, most experts continue to use this mode for this patient population. Furthermore, large meta-analyses of the available literature have not shown any benefit of pressure control over volume control [80, 81]. The variable volumes delivered per breath as well as the dynamic nature of the evolving compliance in the ARDS lung give cause for concern over the limitations of this mode to consistently deliver lung-protective ventilation at or below 6 mL/kg IBW [82]. Thus, the first approach for mechanical ventilation in ARDS patients should start with volume-limited AC ventilation.

Pressure-regulated volume control (PRVC) is a form of pressure-limited MV where the breath is cycled once inspiratory time has been achieved. The main distinction between this mode of MV and the classic AC modes is that it is an adaptive form of MV in which each breath is variable and is adapted to the changing interactions between the ventilator and the patient. In PRVC, a goal VT is set. Then, depending on the VT achieved on the last breath based on variable pressure and inspiratory time selected by the ventilator, the ensuing breath is adjusted based on the goal VT. While the set goal is a volume, the mechanics of each ventilated breath is inherently pressure limited. Because this is a newer mode of MV, there is a paucity of evidence to either support or refute its use in ARDS.

Proponents of PRVC ventilation argue that it provides the theoretical patient comfort associated with pressure-limited assist control ventilation with a relative assurance of staying within the goals of a set VT. Unfortunately, as the clinical status evolves, patients may receive inadequate or excessive ventilator support without frequent clinical assessments [83]. Moreover, the predictive algorithm to achieve VT may not consistently assure LTVV from breath to breath, and the variability of breaths may be difficult for some patients to tolerate. Because of these reasons, PRVC is not typically recommended as a first-line MV approach for patients with ARDS, but is rather reserved for those who may benefit from a trial of pressure-limited MV.

7.2 Spontaneous Ventilation

Spontaneous modes of ventilation include pressure support ventilation (PSV) in its most basic form, but may also include synchronized intermittent mandatory ventilation (SIMV) and airway pressure release ventilation (APRV). Some consider the latter two modes to be spontaneous ventilation modes due to the intermittently unsupported, spontaneous breaths in the case of SIMV and the ability of the patient to spontaneously ventilate without synchrony to the set pressures in APRV. However, discussion of spontaneous ventilation in this section mostly pertains to PSV, with further discussion of APRV and SIMV in the following sections.

While theoretical benefits to spontaneous ventilation during MV in ARDS may include preventing the disuse atrophy associated with diaphragmatic inactivity in prolonged MV [84], there is emerging evidence of the increasing harm associated with spontaneous ventilation, particularly in more severe ARDS [85]. The physiologic underpinnings for this are likely multifaceted. First, VT is more difficult to regulate in spontaneous ventilation, with patient effort dictating much of each supported breath [86]. Additionally, when there is spontaneous effort during MV, the phenomenon of pendelluft, the exchange of air from one region of the lung to another without changes in the overall lung volumes, occurs due to diaphragmatic effort and may cause regional VILI [87, 88]. Increased transpleural negative pressures during spontaneous inspiratory effort will lead to increased lung perfusion and interstitial and alveolar edema, possibly worsening the local inflammatory response [89]. For these reasons and others, spontaneous modes of ventilation are not recommended in ARDS. Rather, the spontaneous modes of PSV or CPAP are reserved for MV weaning and assessment for extubation readiness in those patients who are improving from ARDS [90].

8 Advanced Techniques and Rescue Therapies

8.1 Airway Pressure Release Ventilation, Biphasic Ventilation, and Inverse Ratio

Airway pressure release ventilation (APRV) was first described in the late 1980s as a novel mode of MV [91]. It is a pressure-limited form of MV that allows spontaneous ventilation throughout the ventilator-delivered breath and is thus an asynchronous form of MV. However, when patients are heavily sedated or paralyzed, the spontaneous breaths ebb. Classically, an inspiratory pressure and time are set so that the expiratory time is quite short, and the expiratory pressure is set at 0–5 cm H_2O, allowing for maximum "airway pressure release" within a short duration. The PEEP detected on the ventilator at the end of expiration in excess of set PEEP is attributable to auto-PEEP. In this way, APRV employs both biphasic ventilation and inverse ratio strategies for MV. Biphasic ventilation, sometimes referred to as bilevel ventilation (though this term is more frequently associated with NIV), describes an asynchronous pressure-limited mode of MV, which allows for spontaneous patient-driven breaths, in which inspiratory pressure and time and a nonzero PEEP are set [92]. Inverse ratio ventilation (IRV) refers to a strategy where the inspiratory time is greater than the expiratory time during a ventilator-delivered breath [93]. This strategy can actually be employed in both pressure-limited and volume-limited modes of MV. The key benefit to IRV is increased mean airway pressure (Paw) by spending more time at the higher inspiratory pressure rather than the PEEP, thus allowing more time for gas exchange in those patients with refractory hypoxemia [94]. However, IRV is regarded as difficult to tolerate in a non-paralyzed or heavily sedated patient since physiologic expiration is longer than inhalation. By maximizing Paw through maximizing the time in inspiration, APRV is a rescue MV mode, which can improve oxygenation in severe ARDS patients.

However, despite several observational and smaller studies showing benefit in oxygenation, APRV in its purest form has not been shown to improve clinical outcomes in larger trials [95]. In the earliest randomized trial of APRV of 30 patients, those in the APRV group had more ventilator-free days [96]. However, the study control group underwent pressure-limited assist control (AC) ventilation with neuromuscular blockade. PEEP was not different in either group. Thus, the true evaluation of the study was the spontaneous breathing associated with APRV and not the mode as compared to volume-limited LTVV. Furthermore, patients in the control arm were sicker, with more ARDS than the APRV group. In the largest and single trial of APRV compared to volume-limited LTVV, out of 138 patients, those ventilated early with APRV had more ventilator-free days [97]. However, the control group again had sicker patients [98], and mortality benefit was not definitive. It is important to note that this trial of APRA set a maximum inspiratory pressure of 30 cm H_2O and a PEEP of 5 cm H_2O. Perhaps, the reason behind the indeterminate value of APRV in ARDS is due to the potential harms of spontaneous breaths in ARDS, or the potential for decruitment of the lung during the low PEEP exhalation phase, or more importantly VILI secondary to the heterogeneous nature of the ARDS lung and the high potential for auto-PEEP. When airway pressures are completely or near-completely released in exhalation, the potential for air trapping and thus auto-PEEP is high. Thus, areas of lung can become overdistended and fail to adequately participate in gas exchange due to airway collapse during the exhalation phase, while other areas of the lung may completely collapse, derecruit, and suffer from atelectrauma. Regardless of the reasons, current guidelines do not recommend APRV as a routine mode of MV in ARDS, but it can be used as a rescue modality in a subset of patients [99].

8.2 *High-Frequency Oscillatory Ventilation (HFOV)*

Theoretically, high-frequency oscillatory ventilation (HFOV) minimized the difference between inspiratory and expiratory pressures in mechanically ventilated ARDS patients and is the closest interventional manipulation of minimizing the driving pressure (ΔP). While this in principle should decrease the incidence of barotrauma, volutrauma, and atelectrauma, clinical trials show no clinical benefit. The Oscillation for ARDS Treated Early (OSCILLATE) trial compared HFOV with LTVV in 548 patients with at least moderate ARDS and was stopped early due to increased mortality with the use of HFOV (47% vs. 35%, RR 1.33, 95% CI 1.12–1.79, $p = 0.004$) [100]. The Oscillation in ARDS (OSCAR) trial, also comparing HFOV to LTVV in moderate-to-severe ARDS, showed no benefit with HFOV in 789 patients (30-day mortality 42% vs. 41%, $p = 0.85$) [101]. However, average VT in the OSCAR trial control arm was significantly higher than that in OSCILLATE (8.3 ± 2.9 mL/kg IBW vs. 6.1 ± 1.3 mL/kg IBW), which may contribute to these results. Follow-up meta-analyses of these and prior smaller studies show increased harm in ARDS patients [102, 103]. Due to these data, HFOV is not used in adults with ARDS.

9 Non-ventilator Treatment Strategies in ARDS

9.1 Prone Positioning

There have been several major clinical trials aimed at examining the clinical benefit of prone positioning in mechanically ventilated patients with ARDS [104]. However, the most recent and well-designed study, PROSEVA, showed a significant mortality benefit in severe ARDS patients with $PaO_2/FiO_2 < 150$ mm Hg who underwent prone ventilation for 18 h per day (28-day mortality 16.0% vs. 32.8%, $p < 0.001$, 90-day mortality 23.6% vs. 41.0%, $p < 0.001$) [105]. Since the publication of this trial, prone positioning has been widely adopted in ARDS patients undergoing MV.

9.2 Neuromuscular Blockade

The ACURASYS trial showed a significant mortality benefit when patients with severe ARDS ($PaO_2/FiO_2 < 150$) received neuromuscular blockade with cisatracurium besylate for 48 h within 48 h of ARDS onset [106]. The follow-up confirmatory Prevention and Early Treatment of Acute Lung Injury (PETAL) network study, the Reevaluation of Systemic Early Neuromuscular Blockade (ROSE) trial, was stopped early after the second interim analysis due to futility [107]. Early paralysis with cisatracurium for 48 hours failed to show a mortality benefit (42% vs. 43% control, $p = 0.93$) or secondary in-hospital clinical outcomes in 1006 subjects with severe ARDS with $PaO_2/FiO_2 < 150$. Because of these results and concern for heavy sedation required for paralysis in ICU patients, routine neuromuscular blockade is not used early in ARDS.

9.3 Fluid Management

The Fluids and Catheters Treatment Trial (FACCT) compared a conservative fluid management strategy targeting CVP <4 mmHg with a liberal strategy targeting CVP 10–14 mmHg and showed that, while there was no morality difference, a conservative fluid strategy in ARDS was associated with more ventilator-free days (14.6 vs. 12.1, $p < 0.001$) [108]. However, a follow-up study raised concerns for increased neurocognitive dysfunction with conservative fluid management [109]. Based on this, it is more prudent to assess volume status on a case-by-case basis as opposed to employing an aggressive conservation fluid management strategy for all patients with ARDS.

9.4 Inhaled Vasodilators

Neither inhaled nitric oxide nor nebulized prostacyclin has been shown to improve mortality in ARDS, despite evidence for transient improvements in oxygenation [110, 111]. As such, use of these agents is not recommended routinely in ARDS, but may have a role in those patients with refractory hypoxemia, particularly with right-heart dysfunction.

9.5 Extracorporeal Membrane Oxygenation

Extracorporeal membrane oxygenation (ECMO) has been shown to be lifesaving in patients with severe refractory ARDS. The pragmatic CESAR trial randomized patients with ARDS to be transported to specialty ECMO centers and showed significant mortality benefit [112]. However, concerns were raised regarding the usual care of specialty hospitals confounding the results. The follow-up crossover design trial, EOLIA, sought to eliminate this concern and showed a 60-day mortality benefit for ECMO (35% vs. 46%, $p = 0.09$) [113]. Statistical significance was not achieved due to early stoppage of the trial for failure to meet an ambitious stoppage rule to detect a 20% mortality difference. Post hoc Bayesian analysis of the data provided more statistical reassurance of the value of ECMO in ARDS [114]. ECMO should be offered for patients with severe ARDS unresponsive to less invasive therapies.

10 Liberation from Ventilator

For patients who are improving, weaning from the ventilator is achieved on a personalized basis, with some patients needing dramatically less MV support over hours or days, while others may need weeks. In ARDS patients, liberation from the ventilator should follow the same guidelines as for all mechanically ventilated patients. Daily spontaneous breathing trials (SBTs) have the strongest evidence for rapid liberation from the ventilator and should be used over other modalities like SIMV [90, 115].

11 Conclusion

In patients with ARDS who need MV, the initial ventilator strategy should be LTVV using the volume-limited AC mode. In the event of ventilator asynchrony or patient intolerance, a trial of pressure-limited AC ventilation such as traditional

Table 4 Suggested targets for mechanical ventilation in patients with ARDS

PaO_2	55–80 mm Hg (SpO_2 88–95%)
$PaCO_2$	40 mm Hg if possible
pH	7.20–7.40
VT	<6 mL/kg IBW
P_{plat}	<30 cm H_2O
ΔP	<15 cm H_2O
FiO_2	Lowest to achieve PaO_2 target in combination with PEEP
PEEP	According to PEEP/FiO_2 ladder

pressure-limited AC or PRVC may be attempted. PEEP is important for maintenance of Paw and should be titrated as FiO_2 requirements change over the clinical course. Some targets for MV are listed in Table 4. The data supporting advanced techniques such as APRV, inverse ratio ventilation, and open-lung ventilation with high PEEP and recruitment maneuvers are mixed and should be reserved for patients with refractory hypoxemia. Data shows harm with HFOV; thus, this mode of MV should not be used in adults with respiratory failure. Non-MV adjunctive measures such as prone positioning and ECMO offer mortality benefit in ARDS patients requiring MV. Other measures may be used in carefully selected patients.

References

1. Gajic O, Dabbagh O, Park PK, et al. Early identification of patients at risk of acute lung injury: evaluation of lung injury prediction score in a multicenter cohort study. Am J Respir Crit Care Med. 2011;183(4):462–70.
2. Ranieri VM, Rubenfeld GD, Thompson BT, et al. Acute respiratory distress syndrome: the Berlin definition. JAMA. 2012;307(23):2526–33.
3. Bellani G, Laffey JG, Pham T, et al. Epidemiology, patterns of care, and mortality for patients with acute respiratory distress syndrome in intensive care units in 50 countries. JAMA. 2016;315(8):788–800.
4. Sheu CC, Gong MN, Zhai R, et al. Clinical characteristics and outcomes of sepsis-related vs non-sepsis-related ARDS. Chest. 2010;138(3):559–67.
5. Sevransky JE, Martin GS, Shanholtz C, et al. Mortality in sepsis versus non-sepsis induced acute lung injury. Crit Care. 2009;13(5):R150.
6. Calfee CS, Delucchi K, Parsons PE, Thompson BT, Ware LB, Matthay MA. Subphenotypes in acute respiratory distress syndrome: latent class analysis of data from two randomised controlled trials. Lancet Respir Med. 2014;2(8):611–20.
7. Calfee CS, Eisner MD, Ware LB, et al. Trauma-associated lung injury differs clinically and biologically from acute lung injury due to other clinical disorders. Crit Care Med. 2007;35(10):2243–50.
8. Bernard GR, Artigas A, Brigham KL, et al. The American-European Consensus Conference on ARDS. Definitions, mechanisms, relevant outcomes, and clinical trial coordination. Am J Respir Crit Care Med. 1994;149(3 Pt 1):818–24.
9. Calfee CS, Janz DR, Bernard GR, et al. Distinct molecular phenotypes of direct vs indirect ARDS in single-center and multicenter studies. Chest. 2015;147(6):1539–48.

10. Hoelz C, Negri EM, Lichtenfels AJ, et al. Morphometric differences in pulmonary lesions in primary and secondary ARDS. A preliminary study in autopsies. Pathol Res Pract. 2001;197(8):521–30.
11. Albaiceta GM, Taboada F, Parra D, Blanco A, Escudero D, Otero J. Differences in the deflation limb of the pressure-volume curves in acute respiratory distress syndrome from pulmonary and extrapulmonary origin. Intensive Care Med. 2003;29(11):1943–9.
12. Thille AW, Esteban A, Fernández-Segoviano P, et al. Comparison of the Berlin definition for acute respiratory distress syndrome with autopsy. Am J Respir Crit Care Med. 2013;187(7):761–7.
13. Madotto F, Pham T, Bellani G, et al. Resolved versus confirmed ARDS after 24 h: insights from the LUNG SAFE study. Intensive Care Med. 2018;44(5):564–77.
14. Goligher EC, Kavanagh BP, Rubenfeld GD, et al. Oxygenation response to positive end-expiratory pressure predicts mortality in acute respiratory distress syndrome. A secondary analysis of the LOVS and express trials. Am J Respir Crit Care Med. 2014;190(1):70–6.
15. Coudroy R, Frat JP, Boissier F, Contou D, Robert R, Thille AW. Early identification of acute respiratory distress syndrome in the absence of positive pressure ventilation: implications for revision of the Berlin criteria for acute respiratory distress syndrome. Crit Care Med. 2018;46(4):540–6.
16. Ou X, Hua Y, Liu J, Gong C, Zhao W. Effect of high-flow nasal cannula oxygen therapy in adults with acute hypoxemic respiratory failure: a meta-analysis of randomized controlled trials. CMAJ. 2017;189(7):E260–e267.
17. Rochwerg B, Granton D, Wang DX, et al. High flow nasal cannula compared with conventional oxygen therapy for acute hypoxemic respiratory failure: a systematic review and meta-analysis. Intensive Care Med. 2019;45(5):563–72.
18. Frat JP, Thille AW, Mercat A, et al. High-flow oxygen through nasal cannula in acute hypoxemic respiratory failure. N Engl J Med. 2015;372(23):2185–96.
19. Frat JP, Ragot S, Girault C, et al. Effect of non-invasive oxygenation strategies in immunocompromised patients with severe acute respiratory failure: a post-hoc analysis of a randomised trial. Lancet Respir Med. 2016;4(8):646–52.
20. Bellani G, Laffey JG, Pham T, et al. Noninvasive ventilation of patients with acute respiratory distress syndrome. Insights from the LUNG SAFE study. Am J Respir Crit Care Med. 2017;195(1):67–77.
21. Carteaux G, Millán-Guilarte T, De Prost N, et al. Failure of noninvasive ventilation for de novo acute hypoxemic respiratory failure: role of tidal volume. Crit Care Med. 2016;44(2):282–90.
22. Zhan Q, Sun B, Liang L, et al. Early use of noninvasive positive pressure ventilation for acute lung injury: a multicenter randomized controlled trial. Crit Care Med. 2012;40(2):455–60.
23. Patel BK, Wolfe KS, Pohlman AS, Hall JB, Kress JP. Effect of noninvasive ventilation delivered by helmet vs face mask on the rate of endotracheal intubation in patients with acute respiratory distress syndrome: a randomized clinical trial. JAMA. 2016;315(22):2435–41.
24. Sud S, Friedrich JO, Adhikari NKJ, et al. Comparative effectiveness of protective ventilation strategies for moderate and severe acute respiratory distress syndrome. A network meta-analysis. Am J Respir Crit Care Med. 2021;203(11):1366–77.
25. Ferreyro BL, Angriman F, Munshi L, et al. Association of noninvasive oxygenation strategies with all-cause mortality in adults with acute hypoxemic respiratory failure: a systematic review and meta-analysis. JAMA. 2020;324(1):57–67.
26. Slutsky AS, Ranieri VM. Ventilator-induced lung injury. N Engl J Med. 2013;369(22):2126–36.
27. Tonelli AR, Zein J, Adams J, Ioannidis JP. Effects of interventions on survival in acute respiratory distress syndrome: an umbrella review of 159 published randomized trials and 29 meta-analyses. Intensive Care Med. 2014;40(6):769–87.
28. Brower RG, Matthay MA, Morris A, Schoenfeld D, Thompson BT, Wheeler A. Ventilation with lower tidal volumes as compared with traditional tidal volumes for acute lung injury and the acute respiratory distress syndrome. N Engl J Med. 2000;342(18):1301–8.

29. Walkey AJ, Goligher EC, Del Sorbo L, et al. Low tidal volume versus non-volume-limited strategies for patients with acute respiratory distress syndrome. A systematic review and meta-analysis. Ann Am Thorac Soc. 2017;14(Supplement_4):S271–s279.
30. Putensen C, Theuerkauf N, Zinserling J, Wrigge H, Pelosi P. Meta-analysis: ventilation strategies and outcomes of the acute respiratory distress syndrome and acute lung injury. Ann Intern Med. 2009;151(8):566–76.
31. Petrucci N, De Feo C. Lung protective ventilation strategy for the acute respiratory distress syndrome. Cochrane Database Syst Rev. 2013;2013(2):CD003844.
32. Pai MP, Paloucek FP. The origin of the "ideal" body weight equations. Ann Pharmacother. 2000;34(9):1066–9.
33. Hager DN, Krishnan JA, Hayden DL, Brower RG. Tidal volume reduction in patients with acute lung injury when plateau pressures are not high. Am J Respir Crit Care Med. 2005;172(10):1241–5.
34. Needham DM, Colantuoni E, Mendez-Tellez PA, et al. Lung protective mechanical ventilation and two year survival in patients with acute lung injury: prospective cohort study. BMJ. 2012;344:e2124.
35. Needham DM, Yang T, Dinglas VD, et al. Timing of low tidal volume ventilation and intensive care unit mortality in acute respiratory distress syndrome. A prospective cohort study. Am J Respir Crit Care Med. 2015;191(2):177–85.
36. Nuckton TJ, Alonso JA, Kallet RH, et al. Pulmonary dead-space fraction as a risk factor for death in the acute respiratory distress syndrome. N Engl J Med. 2002;346(17):1281–6.
37. Gattinoni L, Caironi P, Cressoni M, et al. Lung recruitment in patients with the acute respiratory distress syndrome. N Engl J Med. 2006;354(17):1775–86.
38. Umoh NJ, Fan E, Mendez-Tellez PA, et al. Patient and intensive care unit organizational factors associated with low tidal volume ventilation in acute lung injury. Crit Care Med. 2008;36(5):1463–8.
39. Talmor D, Sarge T, Malhotra A, et al. Mechanical ventilation guided by esophageal pressure in acute lung injury. N Engl J Med. 2008;359(20):2095–104.
40. Beitler JR, Sarge T, Banner-Goodspeed VM, et al. Effect of titrating positive end-expiratory pressure (PEEP) with an esophageal pressure-guided strategy vs an empirical high PEEP-Fio2 strategy on death and days free from mechanical ventilation among patients with acute respiratory distress syndrome: a randomized clinical trial. JAMA. 2019;321(9):846–57.
41. Turbil E, Galerneau LM, Terzi N, Schwebel C, Argaud L, Guérin C. Positive-end expiratory pressure titration and transpulmonary pressure: the EPVENT 2 trial. J Thorac Dis. 2019;11(Suppl 15):S2012–s2017.
42. Amato MB, Meade MO, Slutsky AS, et al. Driving pressure and survival in the acute respiratory distress syndrome. N Engl J Med. 2015;372(8):747–55.
43. Guérin C, Papazian L, Reignier J, Ayzac L, Loundou A, Forel JM. Effect of driving pressure on mortality in ARDS patients during lung protective mechanical ventilation in two randomized controlled trials. Crit Care. 2016;20(1):384.
44. Villar J, Martín-Rodríguez C, Domínguez-Berrot AM, et al. A quantile analysis of plateau and driving pressures: effects on mortality in patients with acute respiratory distress syndrome receiving lung-protective ventilation. Crit Care Med. 2017;45(5):843–50.
45. Schmidt MFS, Amaral A, Fan E, Rubenfeld GD. Driving pressure and hospital mortality in patients without ARDS: a cohort study. Chest. 2018;153(1):46–54.
46. Goligher EC, Costa ELV. Reply to: the dethroning of 6 ml per kg as the "go-to" setting in ARDS. Am J Respir Crit Care Med. 2021;204(7):868–9.
47. Marini JJ, Rocco PRM, Gattinoni L. Static and dynamic contributors to ventilator-induced lung injury in clinical practice. Pressure, energy, and power. Am J Respir Crit Care Med. 2020;201(7):767–74.
48. Serpa Neto A, Deliberato RO, Johnson AEW, et al. Mechanical power of ventilation is associated with mortality in critically ill patients: an analysis of patients in two observational cohorts. Intensive Care Med. 2018;44(11):1914–22.

49. Vaporidi K, Voloudakis G, Priniannakis G, et al. Effects of respiratory rate on ventilator-induced lung injury at a constant PaCO2 in a mouse model of normal lung. Crit Care Med. 2008;36(4):1277–83.
50. Spieth PM, Silva PL, Garcia CS, et al. Modulation of stress versus time product during mechanical ventilation influences inflammation as well as alveolar epithelial and endothelial response in rats. Anesthesiology. 2015;122(1):106–16.
51. Cressoni M, Gotti M, Chiurazzi C, et al. Mechanical power and development of ventilator-induced lung injury. Anesthesiology. 2016;124(5):1100–8.
52. Brower RG, Lanken PN, MacIntyre N, et al. Higher versus lower positive end-expiratory pressures in patients with the acute respiratory distress syndrome. N Engl J Med. 2004;351(4):327–36.
53. Mercat A, Richard JC, Vielle B, et al. Positive end-expiratory pressure setting in adults with acute lung injury and acute respiratory distress syndrome: a randomized controlled trial. JAMA. 2008;299(6):646–55.
54. Meade MO, Cook DJ, Guyatt GH, et al. Ventilation strategy using low tidal volumes, recruitment maneuvers, and high positive end-expiratory pressure for acute lung injury and acute respiratory distress syndrome: a randomized controlled trial. JAMA. 2008;299(6):637–45.
55. Briel M, Meade M, Mercat A, et al. Higher vs lower positive end-expiratory pressure in patients with acute lung injury and acute respiratory distress syndrome: systematic review and meta-analysis. JAMA. 2010;303(9):865–73.
56. Walkey AJ, Del Sorbo L, Hodgson CL, et al. Higher PEEP versus lower PEEP strategies for patients with acute respiratory distress syndrome. A systematic review and meta-analysis. Ann Am Thorac Soc. 2017;14(Supplement_4):S297–s303.
57. Coppola S, Froio S, Marino A, et al. Respiratory mechanics, lung recruitability, and gas exchange in pulmonary and Extrapulmonary acute respiratory distress syndrome. Crit Care Med. 2019;47(6):792–9.
58. McKown AC, Semler MW, Rice TW. Best PEEP trials are dependent on tidal volume. Crit Care. 2018;22(1):115.
59. Fan E, Del Sorbo L, Goligher EC, et al. An Official American Thoracic Society/European Society of Intensive Care Medicine/Society of Critical Care Medicine Clinical Practice Guideline: Mechanical Ventilation in Adult Patients with Acute Respiratory Distress Syndrome. Am J Respir Crit Care Med. 2017;195(9):1253–63.
60. Amato MB, Barbas CS, Medeiros DM, et al. Beneficial effects of the "open lung approach" with low distending pressures in acute respiratory distress syndrome. A prospective randomized study on mechanical ventilation. Am J Respir Crit Care Med. 1995;152(6 Pt 1):1835–46.
61. Brower RG, Morris A, MacIntyre N, et al. Effects of recruitment maneuvers in patients with acute lung injury and acute respiratory distress syndrome ventilated with high positive end-expiratory pressure. Crit Care Med. 2003;31(11):2592–7.
62. Cavalcanti AB, Suzumura ÉA, Laranjeira LN, et al. Effect of lung recruitment and titrated positive end-expiratory pressure (PEEP) vs low PEEP on mortality in patients with acute respiratory distress syndrome: a randomized clinical trial. JAMA. 2017;318(14):1335–45.
63. Zampieri FG, Costa EL, Iwashyna TJ, et al. Heterogeneous effects of alveolar recruitment in acute respiratory distress syndrome: a machine learning reanalysis of the alveolar recruitment for acute respiratory distress syndrome trial. Br J Anaesth. 2019;123(1):88–95.
64. Fan E, Wilcox ME, Brower RG, et al. Recruitment maneuvers for acute lung injury: a systematic review. Am J Respir Crit Care Med. 2008;178(11):1156–63.
65. Goligher EC, Hodgson CL, Adhikari NKJ, et al. Lung recruitment maneuvers for adult patients with acute respiratory distress syndrome. A systematic review and meta-analysis. Ann Am Thorac Soc. 2017;14(Supplement_4):S304–s311.
66. Lu J, Wang X, Chen M, et al. An open lung strategy in the management of acute respiratory distress syndrome: a systematic review and meta-analysis. Shock (Augusta, Ga). 2017;48(1):43–53.

67. World Health Organization. WHO Coronavirus (COVID-19) Dashboard; 2021. https://covid19.who.int/. Accessed 30 June 2021.
68. Tzotzos SJ, Fischer B, Fischer H, Zeitlinger M. Incidence of ARDS and outcomes in hospitalized patients with COVID-19: a global literature survey. Crit Care. 2020;24(1):516.
69. Hariri LP, North CM, Shih AR, et al. Lung histopathology in coronavirus disease 2019 as compared with severe acute respiratory sydrome and H1N1 influenza: a systematic review. Chest. 2021;159(1):73–84.
70. Alhazzani W, Møller MH, Arabi YM, et al. Surviving sepsis campaign: guidelines on the management of critically ill adults with coronavirus disease 2019 (COVID-19). Crit Care Med. 2020;48(6):e440–69.
71. Grasselli G, Zangrillo A, Zanella A, et al. Baseline characteristics and outcomes of 1591 patients infected with SARS-CoV-2 admitted to ICUs of the Lombardy region, Italy. JAMA. 2020;323(16):1574–81.
72. Wu C, Chen X, Cai Y, et al. Risk factors associated with acute respiratory distress syndrome and death in patients with coronavirus disease 2019 pneumonia in Wuhan, China. JAMA Intern Med. 2020;180(7):934–43.
73. Menzella F, Barbieri C, Fontana M, et al. Effectiveness of noninvasive ventilation in COVID-19 related-acute respiratory distress syndrome. Clin Respir J. 2021;15:779.
74. Bertaina M, Nuñez-Gil IJ, Franchin L, et al. Non-invasive ventilation for SARS-CoV-2 acute respiratory failure: a subanalysis from the HOPE COVID-19 registry. Emerg Med J. 2021;38:359.
75. McGuinness G, Zhan C, Rosenberg N, et al. Increased incidence of barotrauma in patients with COVID-19 on invasive mechanical ventilation. Radiology. 2020;297(2):E252–e262.
76. Shelhamer MC, Wesson PD, Solari IL, et al. Prone positioning in moderate to severe acute respiratory distress syndrome due to COVID-19: a cohort study and analysis of physiology. J Intensive Care Med. 2021;36(2):241–52.
77. Bartlett RH, Ogino MT, Brodie D, et al. Initial ELSO guidance document: ECMO for COVID-19 patients with severe cardiopulmonary failure. ASAIO J. 2020;66(5):472–4.
78. Marini JJ. Point: is pressure assist-control preferred over volume assist-control mode for lung protective ventilation in patients with ARDS? Yes Chest. 2011;140(2):286–90.
79. MacIntyre N. Counterpoint: is pressure assist-control preferred over volume assist-control mode for lung protective ventilation in patients with ARDS? No Chest. 2011;140(2):290–2.
80. Rittayamai N, Katsios CM, Beloncle F, Friedrich JO, Mancebo J, Brochard L. Pressure-controlled vs volume-controlled ventilation in acute respiratory failure: a physiology-based narrative and systematic review. Chest. 2015;148(2):340–55.
81. Rittayamai N, Beloncle F, Goligher EC, et al. Effect of inspiratory synchronization during pressure-controlled ventilation on lung distension and inspiratory effort. Ann Intensive Care. 2017;7(1):100.
82. Kallet RH, Campbell AR, Dicker RA, Katz JA, Mackersie RC. Work of breathing during lung-protective ventilation in patients with acute lung injury and acute respiratory distress syndrome: a comparison between volume and pressure-regulated breathing modes. Respir Care. 2005;50(12):1623–31.
83. Singh G, Chien C, Patel S. Pressure regulated volume control (PRVC): set it and forget it? Respir Med Case Rep. 2020;29:100822.
84. Levine S, Nguyen T, Taylor N, et al. Rapid disuse atrophy of diaphragm fibers in mechanically ventilated humans. N Engl J Med. 2008;358(13):1327–35.
85. Yoshida T, Fujino Y, Amato MB, Kavanagh BP. Fifty years of research in ARDS. Spontaneous breathing during mechanical ventilation. Risks, mechanisms, and management. Am J Respir Crit Care Med. 2017;195(8):985–92.
86. Sasidhar M, Chatburn RL. Tidal volume variability during airway pressure release ventilation: case summary and theoretical analysis. Respir Care. 2012;57(8):1325–33.
87. Yoshida T, Torsani V, Gomes S, et al. Spontaneous effort causes occult pendelluft during mechanical ventilation. Am J Respir Crit Care Med. 2013;188(12):1420–7.

88. Yoshida T, Roldan R, Beraldo MA, et al. Spontaneous effort during mechanical ventilation: maximal injury with less positive end-expiratory pressure. Crit Care Med. 2016;44(8):e678–88.
89. Mauri T, Yoshida T, Bellani G, et al. Esophageal and transpulmonary pressure in the clinical setting: meaning, usefulness and perspectives. Intensive Care Med. 2016;42(9):1360–73.
90. Blackwood B, Burns KE, Cardwell CR, O'Halloran P. Protocolized versus non-protocolized weaning for reducing the duration of mechanical ventilation in critically ill adult patients. Cochrane Database Syst Rev. 2014;2014(11):Cd006904.
91. Stock MC, Downs JB, Frolicher DA. Airway pressure release ventilation. Crit Care Med. 1987;15(5):462–6.
92. Baum M, Benzer H, Putensen C, Koller W, Putz G. Biphasic positive airway pressure (BIPAP)—a new form of augmented ventilation. Anaesthesist. 1989;38(9):452–8.
93. Marcy TW, Marini JJ. Inverse ratio ventilation in ARDS. Rationale and implementation. Chest. 1991;100(2):494–504.
94. Prince R, Ballantine TV. Formula for calculating mean airway pressure. J Pediatr. 1983;102(1):164–5.
95. Daoud EG, Farag HL, Chatburn RL. Airway pressure release ventilation: what do we know? Respir Care. 2012;57(2):282–92.
96. Putensen C, Zech S, Wrigge H, et al. Long-term effects of spontaneous breathing during ventilatory support in patients with acute lung injury. Am J Respir Crit Care Med. 2001;164(1):43–9.
97. Zhou Y, Jin X, Lv Y, et al. Early application of airway pressure release ventilation may reduce the duration of mechanical ventilation in acute respiratory distress syndrome. Intensive Care Med. 2017;43(11):1648–59.
98. Mireles-Cabodevila E, Dugar S, Chatburn RL. APRV for ARDS: the complexities of a mode and how it affects even the best trials. J Thorac Dis. 2018;10(Suppl 9):S1058–s1063.
99. Papazian L, Aubron C, Brochard L, et al. Formal guidelines: management of acute respiratory distress syndrome. Ann Intensive Care. 2019;9(1):69.
100. Ferguson ND, Cook DJ, Guyatt GH, et al. High-frequency oscillation in early acute respiratory distress syndrome. N Engl J Med. 2013;368(9):795–805.
101. Young D, Lamb SE, Shah S, et al. High-frequency oscillation for acute respiratory distress syndrome. N Engl J Med. 2013;368(9):806–13.
102. Goligher EC, Munshi L, Adhikari NKJ, et al. High-frequency oscillation for adult patients with acute respiratory distress syndrome. A systematic review and meta-analysis. Ann Am Thorac Soc. 2017;14(Supplement_4):S289–s296.
103. Meade MO, Young D, Hanna S, et al. Severity of hypoxemia and effect of high-frequency oscillatory ventilation in acute respiratory distress syndrome. Am J Respir Crit Care Med. 2017;196(6):727–33.
104. Gattinoni L, Busana M, Giosa L, Macrì MM, Quintel M. Prone positioning in acute respiratory distress syndrome. Semin Respir Crit Care Med. 2019;40(1):94–100.
105. Guérin C, Reignier J, Richard JC, et al. Prone positioning in severe acute respiratory distress syndrome. N Engl J Med. 2013;368(23):2159–68.
106. Papazian L, Forel JM, Gacouin A, et al. Neuromuscular blockers in early acute respiratory distress syndrome. N Engl J Med. 2010;363(12):1107–16.
107. Moss M, Huang DT, Brower RG, et al. Early neuromuscular blockade in the acute respiratory distress syndrome. N Engl J Med. 2019;380(21):1997–2008.
108. Wiedemann HP, Wheeler AP, Bernard GR, et al. Comparison of two fluid-management strategies in acute lung injury. N Engl J Med. 2006;354(24):2564–75.
109. Mikkelsen ME, Christie JD, Lanken PN, et al. The adult respiratory distress syndrome cognitive outcomes study: long-term neuropsychological function in survivors of acute lung injury. Am J Respir Crit Care Med. 2012;185(12):1307–15.
110. Adhikari NK, Dellinger RP, Lundin S, et al. Inhaled nitric oxide does not reduce mortality in patients with acute respiratory distress syndrome regardless of severity: systematic review and meta-analysis. Crit Care Med. 2014;42(2):404–12.

111. Fuller BM, Mohr NM, Skrupky L, Fowler S, Kollef MH, Carpenter CR. The use of inhaled prostaglandins in patients with ARDS: a systematic review and meta-analysis. Chest. 2015;147(6):1510–22.
112. Peek GJ, Mugford M, Tiruvoipati R, et al. Efficacy and economic assessment of conventional ventilatory support versus extracorporeal membrane oxygenation for severe adult respiratory failure (CESAR): a multicentre randomised controlled trial. Lancet (London, England). 2009;374(9698):1351–63.
113. Combes A, Hajage D, Capellier G, et al. Extracorporeal membrane oxygenation for severe acute respiratory distress syndrome. N Engl J Med. 2018;378(21):1965–75.
114. Goligher EC, Tomlinson G, Hajage D, et al. Extracorporeal membrane oxygenation for severe acute respiratory distress syndrome and posterior probability of mortality benefit in a post hoc Bayesian analysis of a randomized clinical trial. JAMA. 2018;320(21):2251–9.
115. Kallet RH, Zhuo H, Yip V, Gomez A, Lipnick MS. Spontaneous breathing trials and conservative sedation practices reduce mechanical ventilation duration in subjects with ARDS. Respir Care. 2018;63(1):1–10.

Patient-Ventilator Dyssynchrony

Bruno De Oliveira and Jihad Mallat

Abbreviations

EAdi	Electrical activity of the diaphragm
NAVA	Neurally adjusted ventilatory assist
PAV	Proportional assist ventilation
PEEPi	Intrinsic positive end-expiratory pressure
Pes	Esophageal pressure
T_I	Inspiratory time

1 Introduction

Mechanical ventilation is the most common procedure used in the intensive care unit (ICU) [1]. Mechanical ventilatory support can be fully controlled by the ventilator and can suppress the patient's respiratory load (controlled ventilation) or can interact with patient breathing efforts (assisted/supported ventilation), depending on the severity and timing of the insult [2]. A perfect mechanical ventilation

B. De Oliveira
Critical Care Institute, Cleveland Clinic Abu Dhabi, Abu Dhabi, UAE

J. Mallat (✉)
Critical Care Institute, Cleveland Clinic Abu Dhabi, Abu Dhabi, UAE

Cleveland Clinic Lerner College of Medicine of Case Western Reserve University, Cleveland, OH, USA

Normandy University, UNICAEN, ED, Caen, France

J. Hidalgo et al. (eds.), *Personalized Mechanical Ventilation*,
https://doi.org/10.1007/978-3-031-14138-6_21

delivery would diminish respiratory distress by minimizing excessive respiratory load while preserving a suitable level of spontaneous effort (limiting diaphragm muscle atrophy) with appropriate patient-ventilator interaction. However, this balance is fragile, and patient-ventilator dyssynchrony occurs when this situation is not fulfilled.

1.1 What Is Patient-Ventilator Dyssynchrony?

In positive-pressure ventilation, the clinician faces two possibilities: either the machine controls all phases of ventilation or there are interactions between the ventilator and the patient who remains able to develop respiratory efforts [3].

In the first case, the patient is usually being given sedatives or neuromuscular blockers that have been shown to have deleterious effects, namely delirium [4], weakness [5], and prolonged ICU length of stay [6].

In the second case, the clinician would face the challenge of recognizing and managing noneffective and possibly harmful interactions between the ventilator and patient breaths. This inappropriate interaction is called patient-ventilator dyssynchrony. Thus, dyssynchrony is defined as a mismatch between the patients' own inspiratory and expiratory times and the mechanical ventilator delivery times [7]. This mismatch usually unveils a discrepancy between the patients' requirements and the machine's amount of support. Dyssynchrony detection needs a rigorous examination of flow and airway pressure waveforms displayed on the ventilator screen [8], together with a clinical examination of the patients' breathing pattern. Dyssynchronies can easily be missed by clinicians who may not recognize them.

1.2 Why Should we Care about Patient-Ventilator Dyssynchrony?

It is approximately estimated that at least one-third of patients manifest frequent dyssynchrony during mechanical ventilation [9–12]. Dyssynchronies, among other effects, overload respiratory muscles, increase alveolar distension with the risk of lung injury, and compromise sleep quality resulting in more sedation and delirium. Indeed, observational studies have consistently found dyssynchrony to be associated with poor outcomes, such as longer duration of ventilatory support and higher mortality [10, 13].

Decreasing dyssynchrony by adjusting ventilatory settings is often doable [14, 15]. An adequately synchronized interaction between patient and ventilator is desirable due to lower sedation requirements, progressive improvement in respiratory muscle function, and, consequently, shortened ventilation time, fewer complications, and earlier liberation from mechanical ventilation [16].

This review aims to define the different types of dyssynchrony and then discuss the evidence for their relationship with patient outcomes and address their potential management. Only dyssynchronies in adult patients during invasive mechanical ventilation will be reviewed.

2 Classification of Patient-Ventilator Dyssynchrony

There are multiple ways to classify patient-ventilator dyssynchrony as one can take different approaches to the problem: either considering foremost the primary condition that leads to the mismatch between patient and mechanical systems or considering first the phase of the respiratory cycle when they occur.

For the first classification, the two main groups are dyssynchronies arising from insufficient assistance in high-respiratory-drive patients and over-assistance in low-respiratory-drive patients [17]. The respiratory phase classification includes trigger dyssynchrony, flow dyssynchrony, and cycling dyssynchrony [18]. In this review, we describe only the dyssynchrony by respiratory phases.

3 Dyssynchrony by Respiratory Phases

3.1 Dyssynchrony of the Trigger Phase

Trigger dyssynchrony discussed here is delayed triggering/ineffective efforts, and auto-triggering.

3.1.1 Delayed Triggering and Ineffective Efforts

When a patient triggers the ventilator, the patient increases intrathoracic volume, which results in a drop in airway pressure and a rise in airflow. If the pressure (called pressure triggering) or airflow (called flow triggering) reaches the threshold set by the clinician, then the ventilator delivers a breath.

There are cases where a patient wants (or attempts) to start a breath and trigger the ventilator, and this fails. This can relate to the ventilator's inability to detect the patient's effort and start the inspiratory phase of the mechanically delivered breath. This is known as ineffective efforts. Ineffective efforts are the most common type of dyssynchrony in patients under invasive mechanical ventilation, both early in the course of the disease and during prolonged mechanical ventilation. A quarter to 38% of invasive mechanically ventilated patients experience ineffective triggering [10, 11, 13, 19]. The incidence is higher in patients with chronic obstructive pulmonary disease (COPD) [14].

Clinical evidence of inspiratory efforts by the expansion of the patient's thoracic volume (that may be subtle, such as a small retraction above the suprasternal notch) without accompanied mechanical insufflation is specific for the diagnosis [9] but not very sensitive. The gold standard for their recognition is a negative deflection in esophageal pressure (Pes) or a significant increase in the electrical activity of the diaphragm (EAdi) not followed by a mechanical breath (Fig. 1) [8]. However, both methods are invasive and require the insertion of specified catheters. In most cases, ineffective efforts can be recognized noninvasively by scrutinizing the flow-time and airway pressure-time waveforms on the ventilator screen. Ineffective triggering is manifested by a decrease in airway pressure waveform along with an increase in airflow tracing during expiration (Fig. 1) [8, 9, 16–19]. Triggering delay is the time interval between the start of the neural and mechanical inspiration [11, 18]. If Pes or EAdi monitoring is available, it is recognized as the time elapsed between the decrease in Pes or rise in EAdi (commencement of neural inspiration) and the sudden increase of airflow or airway pressure (beginning of mechanical inspiration) (Fig. 1) [8].

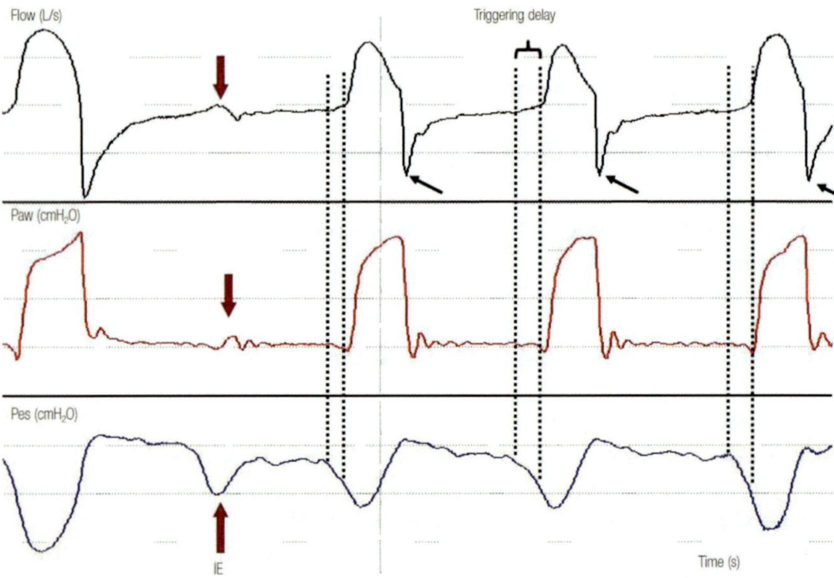

Fig. 1 Example of a tracing with ineffective efforts and delayed triggering in pressure-support ventilation mode. Note that the second decrease in esophageal pressure (Pes) (red arrow), which represents ineffective effort (IE) of the patient, is not followed by a ventilator breath. At the time of the missed effort, a positive deflection in the airway flow waveform (black arrow) and a negative deflection in the airway pressure (Paw) (red arrow) can be noted. Observe that in every ventilator breath, there is a time gap (delayed triggering) between the start of neural inspiration (first dotted line) and the start of ventilator inspiration (second dotted line). Notice the spike early in expiratory flow (black arrows) after each breath that suggests high airway resistance causing incomplete exhalation and delayed triggering [18]

Ineffective efforts and delayed triggering can be due to ventilator settings and/or patients' issues [10, 14, 20, 21]. Indeed, low triggering sensitivity and delayed opening of the expiratory valve result in ineffective or delayed triggering. These factors are set up by the clinician. The most important cause of ineffective efforts and delayed triggering related to patient disease (COPD) is the presence of dynamic hyperinflation that generates intrinsic positive end-expiratory pressure (PEEPi). This happens because the patient's ventilatory muscles must first counterbalance the PEEPi in the alveoli before the ventilator senses any variation in flow or pressure and then triggers the next breath: this is the "threshold load" [22–25]. This produces a delay between the start of inspiratory effort and ventilator triggering, and in severe cases of dynamic hyperinflation, the patient might fail to trigger the ventilator (ineffective triggering). This can be recognized by noticing abrupt expiratory flow end before a triggered breath (Fig. 1). A spike in expiratory flow can also be appreciated at the early expiratory phase, suggesting increased airway resistance (Fig. 1).

Patients with a low respiratory drive (sedation, central nervous diseases, etc.) and weak inspiratory muscles (critical illness polyneuromyopathy, myasthenia, etc.) can also have ineffective respiratory efforts that do not translate to mechanically delivered efforts. This is suggested by a decrease in pressure and increase in airway flow that is not followed by a typical breath.

3.1.2 Auto-Triggering

There are situations where the patient makes no attempt at breathing, and the ventilator will trigger a breath on its own. This is called auto-triggering [26, 27] and is caused by a sensed change in pressure or flow by the ventilator that is unrelated to the patient's efforts, namely in cases of leaks in the patient-ventilator circuit at any level or very sensitive trigger settings that will activate following thoracic pressure fluctuations derived from the cardiac cycle. A leak will cause auto-triggering in one of the two ways: (1) for flow-triggered mechanical breaths, the trigger is a sensed decrease in airflow in the expiratory limb of the ventilator circuit, and (2) for pressure-triggered breaths, the trigger is a sufficient drop in pressure caused by the leak. The lack of a drop in Pes or airway pressure before the delivery phase, particularly in the presence of a zero flow long enough before the mechanical breath, indicates that the breath is not triggered by the patient (Fig. 2).

3.2 Dyssynchrony of the Flow Phase

Insufficient flow delivery results in patient discomfort and increased inspiratory effort [19, 28, 29]. This effort from the patient produces a decrease in the pressure-time ventilator curve. It more commonly occurs in ventilation modalities of flow-targeted breaths than in pressure-targeted breaths where the flow is not a set variable [30, 31]. In volume-controlled breaths, the inspiratory flow cannot be increased by

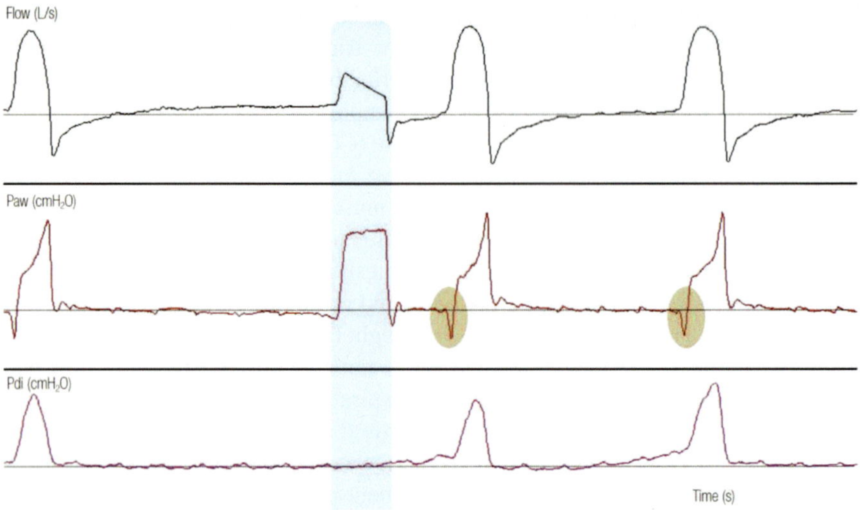

Fig. 2 Example of a tracing with auto-triggering in pressure-support ventilation mode. Note the absence of transdiaphragmatic pressure (Pdi) increase, indicating no inspiratory effort, before the second ventilator breath (blue shaded area). Observe that, in comparison to patient-triggered breaths, where a decrease in airway pressure (Paw) is noticed before the start of ventilator inflation (gray shaded areas), there is no twisting in the Paw (no decrease in Paw) in the auto-triggered breath [18]

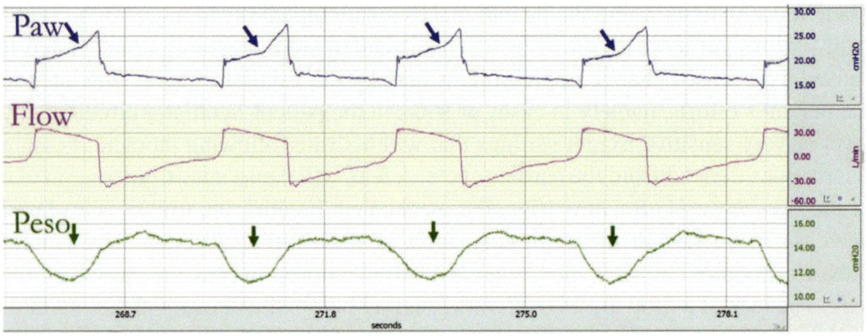

Fig. 3 Example of a tracing with relative flow starvation. The ventilator is in a volume assist-control mode with decelerating flow. The flow delivered by the ventilator does not meet the patient's need. During the inspiration phase, there is a concave deflection of the airway pressure (Paw) (blue arrow), whereas the esophageal pressure (Peso) displays a negative deflection indicating the patient's effort (green arrow). Reprinted by permission from reference [17]

the patient's efforts, and as this effort increases, the airway pressure consequently falls, giving the pressure-time curve the characteristic "scooped-out" look that may be severe enough to decrease peak airway pressure [10, 32] (Fig. 3). Marini et al. were the first to report relative flow hunger and to raise the significance of appropriately setting inspiratory flow during assist-control ventilation [28].

3.3 *Dyssynchrony of the Cycling Phase*

The ventilator cycles or stops the flow to terminate the mechanical inspiratory phase and begin mechanical expiration based on different criteria depending on mode settings. Specifically, in flow-targeted modes, delivered tidal volume and cycle time are set by the physician and cannot change with patients' efforts. In pressure-targeted modes, the cycling criteria are either a set inspiratory time (T_I) in pressure assist-control ventilation or a flow cycle setting in pressure-support ventilation.

Cycling dyssynchrony happens when the neural T_I and the ventilator T_I are mismatched [21, 33].

3.3.1 Premature Cycling Off

Short cycling dyssynchrony occurs when the mechanical T_I is shorter than the neural T_I. This can leave the patient uncomfortable (air hungry) as activation of inspiratory muscles during mechanical expiration (lengthening) results in an eccentric contraction of the diaphragm, which is potentially injurious for the respiratory muscles [34, 35]. When the inspiratory muscle contraction is strong enough, it can overcome the respiratory system's elastic recoil pressure and trigger a second mechanical breath, known as double triggering, before full deflation of the first one, leading to an increased total tidal volume. This phenomenon is also named breath stacking [36] because of the occurrence of a new breath on top of the previous one. Breath stacking is common during low tidal volume ventilation in patients with acute respiratory distress syndrome not receiving neuromuscular blocking agents [36]. Double triggering was one of the most common ventilator dyssynchronies, and it seems to increase in incidence in patients with worse lung injury and high respiratory drive [8].

Premature cycling was associated with particular ventilator settings, such as a set of low tidal volume [36], a shorter set of inflation time [37], and being ventilated with assist-control ventilation [10].

Premature cycling off can be appreciated on the ventilator screen by observing, in the flow-time curve, an abrupt drop from the peak expiratory flow, which lasts for a few milliseconds followed by an increase and then decreases gradually to zero toward the end of expiration (Fig. 4) [18].

3.3.2 Delayed Cycling Off

Dyssynchrony in this phase is usually related to a longer ventilator T_I set than patient neural T_I, which means that mechanical insufflation continues after neural inspiration has stopped or even during neural expiration. This can lead to an increase in work of breathing as the patient is actively using his or her expiratory muscles, struggling to terminate the mechanical inspiration. Additionally, excessive

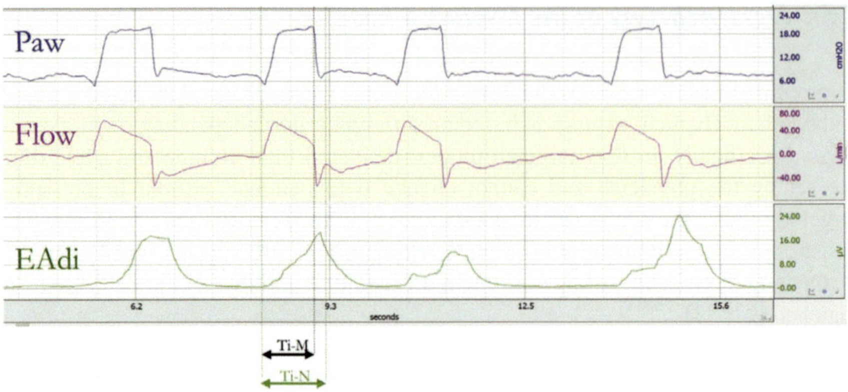

Fig. 4 Example of premature cycling in a pressure-support ventilation. The patient's neural inspiration time (Ti-N), which is from triggering to the moment the electrical activity of the diaphragm (EAdi) drops to 70% of its maximal value, is longer than the breath delivered by the ventilator (Ti-M). Reprinted by permission from reference [17]

ventilator T_I results in a larger tidal volume that can lead to overdistension that may further shorten the neural T_I [38], contributing more to the mismatch between a long mechanical insufflation and a short neural T_I. This can be particularly problematic in COPD or asthma patients ventilated with pressure-support ventilation. Under these circumstances, the increased airway resistance causes the delivered inspiratory airflow to decrease slowly, which results in insufficient expiratory time since during pressure-support ventilation, the ventilator switches to expiration when flow declines to a set percentage of peak inspiratory flow. These effects may contribute to worsening dynamic hyperinflation (higher PEEPi) [39] and consequent trigger dyssynchronies (ineffective triggering, delayed triggering).

Delayed cycling can be recognized by an abrupt spike of the airway pressure near the end of mechanical inspiration on the pressure-time waveform (Fig. 5). High pressure support and low rise time are predisposing factors for this asynchrony [40]. High tidal volume, increased T_I, low insufflation airflow, and inspiratory pause may result in delayed cycling in assisted volume-control mode [40].

3.4 *Reverse Triggering*

In heavily sedated patients, the mechanical breath delivered by the ventilator can trigger a muscular effort. This was called reverse triggering, first described by Akoumianaki et al. [41], who observed, in deeply sedated patients under controlled mechanical ventilation, the occurrence of patient inspiratory efforts (inspiratory activity of the respiratory muscles) that were triggered by the ventilator insufflations. In the absence of Pes or EAdi monitoring, a rise in expiratory flow or decline in inspiratory airway pressure that occurs later in the respiratory cycle can point out to this asynchrony (Fig. 6). Furthermore, if the inspiratory effort is sufficiently

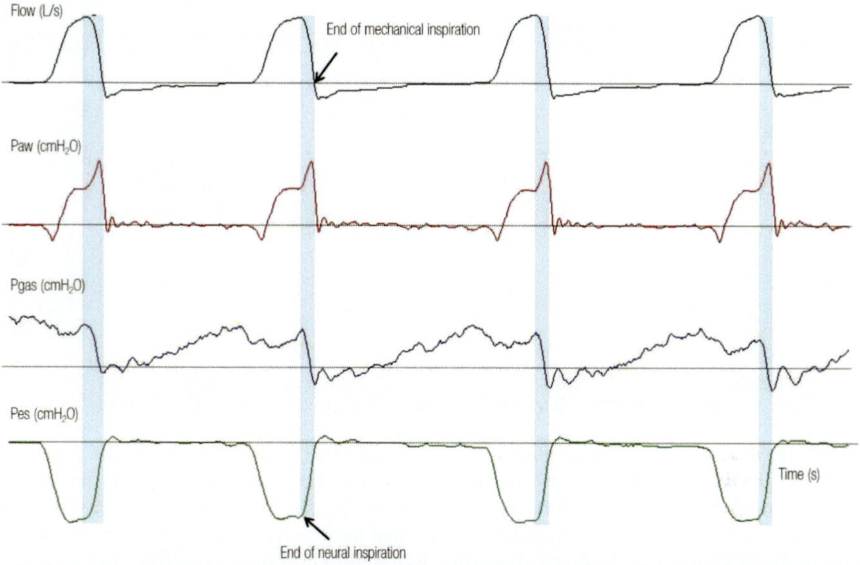

Fig. 5 Example of delayed cycling in a pressure-support ventilation. There is a significant time delay (blue shaded area) between the end of neural inspiration, depicted by a rapid increase in esophageal pressure (Pes), and the end of mechanical inspiration, indicated by the termination of inspiratory flow (inspiratory flow equals zero). Notice the rapid upsurge of Paw near the end of mechanical inspiration, indicating inspiratory muscle relaxation [18]

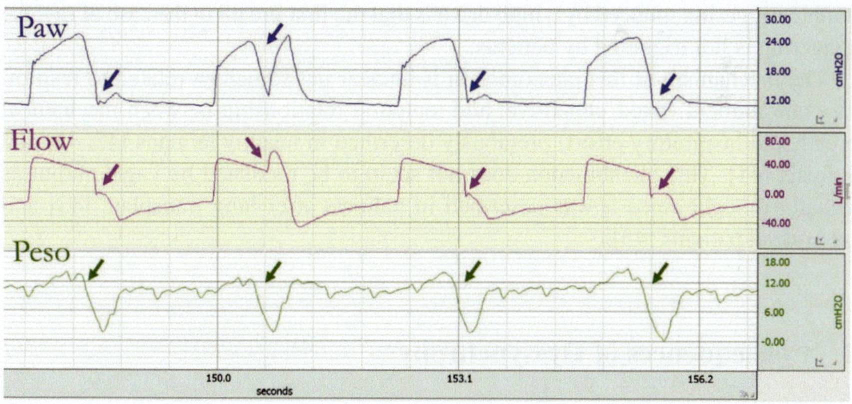

Fig. 6 Reverse triggering in volume assist control with decelerating flow. Each insufflation is triggered by the ventilator; in the middle (breath 2) or at the end of the inspiration phase (breaths 1, 3, and 4), a negative deflection of the esophageal pressure (Peso) happens (green arrow), leading to a negative deflection of the airway pressure (Paw) (blue arrow) and increasing flow during the ventilator insufflation phase or reducing it during the ventilator expiratory phase (pink arrows). Reprinted by permission from reference [17]

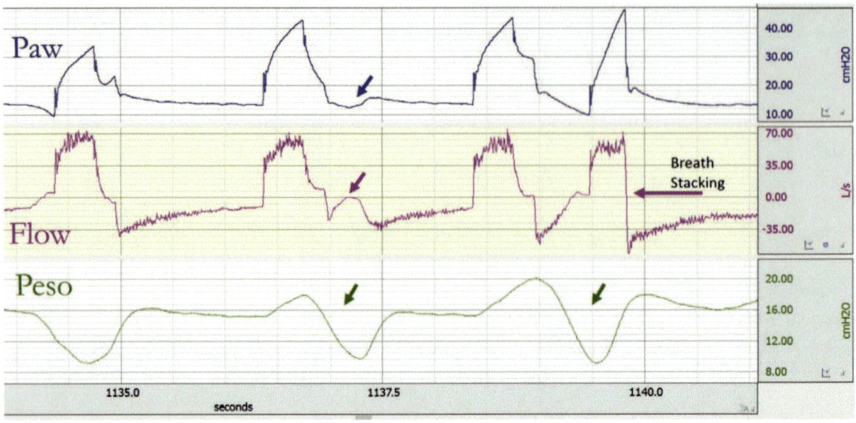

Fig. 7 Reverse triggering and breath stacking in volume assist control. The first breath is patient triggered, the second is triggered by the ventilator, followed by a reverse triggering (first green arrow) starting in the late phase of ventilator insufflation and continuing during the early phase of ventilator exsufflation, leading to a positive deflection of the flow [pink arrow] not triggering a new breath; the third breath is ventilator triggering, followed by a reverse triggering (second green arrow). This reverse triggering leads to a fourth breath before complete exhalation of the previous one (breath stacking). Reprinted by permission from reference [17]

strong, the ventilator can generate a second breath, resulting in breath stacking (Fig. 7) like in patients with a high respiratory drive. However, the difference with double triggering induced by a high drive is that the first breath in the case of reverse triggering is not triggered by patients.

The mechanism of this phenomenon is unclear but somehow related to respiratory entrainment (fixed, repetitive, and temporal relationship between mechanical breath and inspiratory effort) previously described in healthy humans [42, 43] and animals [44]. This phenomenon does not seem to be mediated by vagal output as initially thought since it was described in patients after lung transplant [43] and brain-dead patients [45].

4 Consequences of Dyssynchrony

It is hard to establish the true prevalence of dyssynchronies mainly due to different definitions and criteria, methods of detection, ventilatory modes, and duration and timing of observation [10, 20, 25, 46, 47]. In any case, triggering dyssynchrony is by far the most well studied, and delayed/missed triggering dyssynchronies are the most commonly reported in 26–82% of mechanically ventilated patients depending on the studied population, ventilator settings, and measurement methods used [46]. As expected, trigger dyssynchronies were more prevalent in patients with COPD and asthma that are more prone to develop dynamic hyperinflation [20, 46]. However, trigger dyssynchronies can go undetected in about 20% without the use of invasive monitoring tools such as Pes and EAdi [46]. The incidence of other types of dyssynchrony (double triggering, flow dyssynchrony, and cycle dyssynchrony) has not been as well investigated, with a reported incidence of about 10% [36, 46, 48]. However, the reported incidence is likely underestimated.

Experienced physicians in the ICU would probably agree that every mechanically ventilated patient would present at some point some minor form of patient-ventilator dyssynchrony, and it must be emphasized that dyssynchrony is not always benign. Indeed, many reports suggest an association between dyssynchrony and poor outcomes, including higher mortality and increased duration of mechanical ventilation and ICU length of stay [9, 10, 13, 47, 49]. Ineffective efforts were shown to be associated with a longer mechanical ventilation duration and a lower rate of weaning success [9]. Thille et al., in awake patients under assist-control ventilation or pressure-support ventilation modes, demonstrated that dyssynchrony index (ratio defined by the number of dyssynchronous breaths over the total number of breaths) greater than 10% was associated with increased duration of mechanical ventilation and increased rate of tracheostomy [10]. Other authors confirmed the link between dyssynchrony index ≥10 and outcomes (longer durations of mechanical ventilation, ICU, and hospital length of stay) [13, 47]. Dyssynchronous breathing has been shown to result in episodic increases in transpulmonary pressure, possibly causing ventilation-associated lung injury [50]. Whether the association between adverse outcomes and patient-ventilatory dyssynchrony implies causation or only depicts a common association of a poor prognosis remains unclear.

5 How to Improve Synchrony

5.1 Trigger Synchrony

Both cases of untriggered efforts and extra triggering can be managed in most situations at the bedside.

Firstly, the clinician must be aware of the mode and setting of the ventilator's trigger sensor: either pressure, flow, or both. The trigger sensitivity requires individual patient adjustment and should be set at a level that all patient inspiratory efforts translate into a cycle start.

In cases of untriggered efforts, special attention should be brought to the possibility of intrinsic PEEP (PEEPi) development and an increasing pressure gradient that the patient's efforts fail to overcome. The first step should be to try and minimize PEEPi (usually by decreasing minute ventilation or the global need for increased ventilation that is driving the patient's respiratory drive). The second step would be to reduce the triggering load by approximating the circuit PEEP to the total PEEPi to a level of about 75% of the total PEEPi. This should result in reduced work of breathing, increases in triggered breaths, and also increased patient comfort [9, 22, 51]. However, excessive applied PEEP above the PEEPi will either increase the end-inspiratory pressure in volume-controlled ventilation mode or reduce the generated tidal volume in pressure-targeted ventilation. As long as the external PEEP is lower than the PEEPi, the relationship between inspiratory pressure and tidal volume would not change [52, 53]. Thille et al. showed that the most effective way to reduce ineffective efforts was to decrease over-assistance by reducing the pressure support level in patients ventilated with pressure-support ventilation mode [14]. Adjusting T_I to allow smaller tidal volume was also an effective method to reduce ineffective efforts [54].

For auto-triggering, one should evaluate possible reversible causes like leaks or water in the circuit and/or increase the trigger sensitivity level [55].

5.2 Flow Synchrony

Firstly, in the case of using flow-targeted breaths, the flow cannot vary with patients' efforts and can lead to synchrony issues. This can be somewhat mitigated by adjusting the flow and its shape (sinusoidal, square, decelerating) [56].

Pressure-targeted modes offer advantages in this regard since the set pressure target will allow for the ventilator to variate the flow until a certain pressure is obtained. This has been shown to increase synchrony [30, 31, 52, 56]. Also, the slope (pressure rise time) can be adjusted, and patients producing higher degrees of effort will synchronize better using low rise times [57, 58].

5.3 Cycling Synchrony

Attaining breath cycling synchrony requires delivering an adequate tidal volume in accordance with patient requirements and balancing neural and ventilator T_I.

Premature cycling can be addressed by increasing machine T_I, inspiratory flow, or applying end-inspiratory pause in control modes [8, 32]. A higher support level, slower rising time, and lower flow threshold for cycling can help to minimize premature dyssynchrony in pressure-support ventilation mode [8, 58]. When increasing volume is not an option, usually in cases where strict low-volume protective ventilation is required, a higher level of sedation will be necessary.

Delayed cycling can be minimized by decreasing the machine T_I, increasing the flow threshold of cycling off, decreasing the support level, and increasing the rise pressure time in case of pressure-support ventilation.

6 Newer Ventilator Modes and Patient-Ventilator Synchrony

6.1 *Neurally Adjusted Ventilatory Assist (NAVA)*

NAVA requires inserting a special esophageal catheter with an array of electrodes that sense EAdi [59]. These sensors detect the start, strength, and end of inspiratory efforts directly. In this mode, the ventilator breath is triggered and cycled off by the EAdi signal. The ventilator assistance can vary with the esophageal-diaphragmatic signal's amplitude detected according to a physician's preset gain.

Several clinical studies with NAVA showed a significant reduction in the number of asynchronies in patients than conventional modes [60–63]. The obvious caveat is that this mode requires an intact respiratory drive of the patient. Thus, NAVA must be used cautiously in patients with unpredictable ventilatory drives from either disease or drugs. Also, in patients with high respiratory drive and extremely low respiratory compliance, premature cycling and double triggering can still occur [64].

6.2 *Proportional Assist Ventilation (PAV)*

In PAV, the ventilator regularly estimates the patient's muscular effort based on measured airway pressure, lung compliance, flow, and resistance to determine the pressure of each individual breath in proportion to the desired reduction in the patient's work of breathing [65]. The physician presets the level (as a percentage) of ventilator assistance in proportion to the patients' muscular effort. Contrary to NAVA, PAV has no effects on triggering of the breath but improves patient-ventilator synchrony during inspiration by matching the patient's inspiratory demand and cycling since the ventilator cycles breath when sensed flow demand has stopped. Most clinical studies showed that patients on PAV have less ineffective triggering and other dyssynchronies than patients on pressure-support ventilation [66, 67]. However, data regarding the association between PAV and outcomes (duration of mechanical ventilation, sedation requirements, ICU length of stay, and mortality) are lacking. Also, it is not obvious what the ideal PAV adjustments (gain) should be in different clinical situations. Same as with NAVA, there is no minimum pressure or flow supplied; thus, PAV must be used cautiously in patients with unpredictable ventilatory drives from either disease or drugs.

7 Conclusions

Assisted mechanical ventilation modes offer significant advantages over controlled modes in terms of ventilator-induced diaphragmatic dysfunction and sedation needs. However, patient-ventilator dyssynchrony is a common and polymorphic event that may happen at any phase throughout the respiratory cycle. Various types of asynchrony have diverse physiologic causes and need different management. Dyssynchrony inflicts high loads on respiratory muscles, inducing muscle fatigue. An association between dyssynchrony and outcomes was found in observational studies; however, it is not clear if this link was confounded by the patients' severity or it was a causal association. Also, it is not clear if all dyssynchronies are harmful and if reducing dyssynchrony would result in improving patient outcomes. Clinicians must know how to depict patient-ventilator dyssynchronies by understanding airway pressure and flow waveforms.

Acknowledgments None.

Competing Interest The authors declare that they have no competing interests related to the subject of the study.

Funding None.

Author's Contributions JM and BDO participated in and wrote the manuscript. All authors read and approved the final manuscript.

References

1. Mehta AB, Syeda SN, Wiener RS, et al. Epidemiological trends in invasive mechanical ventilation in the United States: a population-based study. J Crit Care. 2015;30:1217–21.
2. MacIntyre NR. Principles of mechanical ventilation. In: Murray J, Nadel J, Mason R, Boushey H, editors. Textbook of respiratory medicine. 3rd ed. Philadelphia, PA: WB Saunders; 2004.
3. Mora Carpio AL, Mora JI. Ventilator management. [Updated 2020 May 17]. In: StatPearls [Internet]. Treasure Island, FL: StatPearls Publishing; 2020. https://www.ncbi.nlm.nih.gov/books/NBK448186/
4. Kalabalik J, Brunetti L, El-Srougy R. Intensive care unit delirium: a review of the literature. J Pharm Pract. 2014;27(2):195–207. https://doi.org/10.1177/0897190013513804. Epub 2013 Dec 10. PMID: 24326408
5. Hermans G, Van den Berghe G. Clinical review: intensive care unit acquired weakness. Crit Care. 2015;19:274. https://doi.org/10.1186/s13054-015-0993-7.
6. Strom T, Martinussen T, Toft P. A protocol of no sedation for critically ill patients receiving mechanical ventilation: a randomised trial. Lancet. 2010;375:475–80.
7. Mauri T, Yoshida T, Bellani G, et al. PLeUral pressure working Group (PLUG—acute respiratory failure section of the European Society of intensive care Dyssynchrony Consequences and Management 337 medicine). Esophageal and transpulmonary pressure in the clinical setting: meaning, usefulness and perspectives. Intensive Care Med. 2016;42:1360–73.
8. Georgopoulos D, Prinianakis G, Kondili E. Bedside waveforms interpretation as a tool to identify patient-ventilator asynchronies. Intensive Care Med. 2006;32:34–47.
9. Chao DC, Scheinhorn DJ, Stearn-Hassenpflug M. Patient-ventilator trigger asynchrony in prolonged mechanical ventilation. Chest. 1997;112:1592–9.
10. Thille AW, Rodriguez P, Cabello B, et al. Patient-ventilator asynchrony during assisted mechanical ventilation. Intensive Care Med. 2006;32:1515–22.

11. de Wit M, Pedram S, Best AM, et al. Observational study of patient-ventilator asynchrony and relationship to sedation level. J Crit Care. 2009;24:74–80.
12. Colombo D, Cammarota G, Alemani M, et al. Efficacy of ventilator waveforms observation in detecting patient-ventilator asynchrony. Crit Care Med. 2011;39:2452–7.
13. Blanch L, Villagra A, Sales B, et al. Asynchronies during mechanical ventilation are associated with mortality. Intensive Care Med. 2015;41:633–41.
14. Thille AW, Cabello B, Galia F, et al. Reduction of patient-ventilator asynchrony by reducing tidal volume during pressure-support ventilation. Intensive Care Med. 2008;34:1477–86.
15. Chanques G, Kress JP, Pohlman A, et al. Impact of ventilator adjustment and sedation-analgesia practices on severe asynchrony in patients ventilated in assist-control mode. Crit Care Med. 2013;41:2177–87.
16. Gilstrap D, MacIntyre N. Patient-ventilator interactions. Implications for clinical management. Am J Respir Crit Care Med. 2013;188:1058–68.
17. Pham T, Telias I, Piraino T, Yoshida T, Brochard LJ. Asynchrony consequences and management. Crit Care Clin. 2018 Jul;34(3):325–41.
18. Antonogiannaki EM, Georgopoulos D, Akoumianaki E. Patient-ventilator dyssynchrony. Korean J Crit Care Med. 2017;32(4):307–22.
19. de Wit M. Monitoring of patient-ventilator interaction at the bedside. Respir Care. 2011 Jan;56(1):61–72.
20. Leung P, Jubran A, Tobin MJ. Comparison of assisted ventilator modes on triggering, patient effort, and dyspnea. Am J Respir Crit Care Med. 1997;155:1940–8.
21. Younes M, Kun J, Webster K, Roberts D. Response of ventilator-dependent patients to delayed opening of exhalation valve. Am J Respir Crit Care Med. 2002;166:21–30.
22. MacIntyre NR, Cheng KC, McConnell R. Applied PEEP during pressure support reduces the inspiratory threshold load of intrinsic PEEP. Chest. 1997;111(1):188–93.
23. Nava S, Bruschi C, Rubini F, Palo A, Iotti G, Braschi A. Respiratory response and inspiratory effort during pressure support ventilation in COPD patients. Intensive Care Med. 1995;21:871–9.
24. Rossi A, Polese G, Brandi G, Conti G. Intrinsic positive end-expiratory pressure (PEEPi). Intensive Care Med. 1995;21:522–36.
25. Fabry B, Guttmann J, Eberhard L, Bauer T, Haberthür C, Wolff G. An analysis of desynchronization between the spontaneously breathing patient and ventilator during inspiratory pressure support. Chest. 1995;107:1387–94.
26. Imanaka H, Nishimura M, Takeuchi M, Kimball WR, Yahagi N, Kumon K. Autotriggering caused by cardiogenic oscillation during flow-triggered mechanical ventilation. Crit Care Med. 2000;28:402–7.
27. Hill LL, Pearl RG. Flow triggering, pressure triggering, and autotriggering during mechanical ventilation. Crit Care Med. 2000;28:579–81.
28. Marini JJ, Capps JS, Culver BH. The inspiratory work of breathing during assisted mechanical ventilation. Chest. 1985;87:612–8.
29. Marini JJ, Rodriguez RM, Lamb V. The inspiratory workload of patient initiated mechanical ventilation. Am Rev Respir Dis. 1986;134:902–9.
30. Yang LY, Huang YC, Macintyre NR. Patient–ventilator synchrony during pressure-targeted versus flow-targeted small tidal volume assisted ventilation. J Crit Care. 2007;22:252–7.
31. Kallet RH, Campbell AR, Alonso JA, Morabito DJ, Mackersie RC. The effects of pressure control versus volume control assisted ventilation on patient work of breathing in acute lung injury and acute respiratory distress syndrome. Respir Care. 2000;45:1085–96.
32. Kondili E, Xirouchaki N, Georgopoulos D. Modulation and treatment of patient-ventilator dyssynchrony. Curr Opin Crit Care. 2007;13:84–9.
33. Gentile MA. Cycling of the mechanical ventilator breath. Respir Care. 2011;56:52–60.
34. Pierson DJ. Patient–ventilator interaction. Respir Care. 2011;56:214–28.
35. Gea J, Zhu E, Gáldiz JB, et al. Functional consequences of eccentric contractions of the diaphragm. Arch Bronconeumol. 2009;45:68–74.

36. Pohlman MC, McCallister KE, Schweickert WD, et al. Excessive tidal volume from breath stacking during lung-protective ventilation for acute lung injury. Crit Care Med. 2008;36:3019–23.
37. Tokioka H, Tanaka T, Ishizu T, et al. The effect of breath termination criterion on breathing patterns and the work of breathing during pressure support ventilation. Anesth Analg. 2001;92:161–5.
38. Fernandez R, Mendez M, Younes M. Effect of ventilator flow rate on respiratory timing in normal humans. Am J Respir Crit Care Med. 1999;159:710–9.
39. Chiumello D, Polli F, Tallarini F, et al. Effect of different cycling-off criteria and positive end-expiratory pressure during pressure support ventilation in patients with chronic obstructive pulmonary disease. Crit Care Med. 2007;35:2547–52.
40. Kondili E, Prinianakis G, Georgopoulos D. Patient-ventilator interaction. Br J Anaesth. 2003;91:106–19.
41. Akoumianaki E, Lyazidi A, Rey N, Matamis D, Perez-Martinez N, Giraud R, et al. Mechanical ventilation-induced reverse-triggered breaths: a frequently unrecognized form of neuromechanical coupling. Chest. 2013;143:927–38.
42. Graves C, Glass L, Laporta D, et al. Respiratory phase locking during mechanical ventilation in anesthetized human subjects. Am J Phys. 1986;250:R902–9.
43. Simon PM, Habel AM, Daubenspeck JA, et al. Vagal feedback in the entrainment of respiration to mechanical ventilation in sleeping humans. J Appl Physiol. 1985;2000(89):760–9.
44. Muzzin S, Baconnier P, Benchetrit G. Entrainment of respiratory rhythm by periodic lung inflation: effect of airflow rate and duration. Am J Phys. 1992;263:R292–300.
45. Delisle S, Charbonney E, Albert M, et al. Patient-ventilator asynchrony due to reverse triggering occurring in brain-dead patients: clinical implications and physiological meaning. Am J Respir Crit Care Med. 2016;194:1166–8.
46. Epstein SK. How often does patient–ventilator asynchrony occur and what are the consequences? Respir Care. 2011;56:25–38.
47. de Wit M, Miller KB, Green DA, Ostman HE, Gennings C, Epstein SK. Ineffective triggering predicts increased duration of mechanical ventilation. Crit Care Med. 2009;37:2740–5.
48. Kahn JM, Andersson L, Karir V, Polissar NL, Neff MJ, Rubenfeld GD. Low tidal volume ventilation does not increase sedation use in patients with acute lung injury. Crit Care Med. 2005;33:766–71.
49. Vaporidi K, Babalis D, Chytas A, et al. Clusters of ineffective efforts during mechanical ventilation: impact on outcome. Intensive Care Med. 2017;43:184–91.
50. Yoshida T, Fujino Y, Amato MBP, et al. Fifty years of research in ARDS. Spontaneous breathing during mechanical ventilation. Risks, mechanisms, and management. Am J Respir Crit Care Med. 2017;195:985–92.
51. Nava S, Bruschi C, Rubini F, et al. Respiratory response and inspiratory effort during pressure support ventilation in COPD patients. Intensive Care Med. 1995;21:871–9.
52. Imsand C, Feihl F, Perret C, Fitting JW. Regulation of inspiratory neuromuscular output during synchronized intermittent mechanical ventilation. Anesthesiology. 1994;80:13–22.
53. Jubran A, Van de Graaff WB, Tobin MJ. Variability of patient– ventilator interaction with pressure support ventilation in patients with chronic obstructive pulmonary disease. Am J Respir Crit Care Med. 1995;152:129–36.
54. Tassaux D, Gainnier M, Battisti A, et al. Impact of expiratory trigger setting on delayed cycling and inspiratory muscle workload. Am J Respir Crit Care Med. 2005;172:1283–9.
55. Sassoon CS. Triggering of the ventilator in patient–ventilator interactions. Respir Care. 2011;56:39–51.
56. MacIntyre NR. Patient–ventilator interactions: optimizing conventional ventilation modes. Respir Care. 2011;56(73–84):discussion 81–84.
57. MacIntyre NR, Ho LI. Effects of initial flow rate and breath termination criteria on pressure support ventilation. Chest. 1991;99:134–8.

58. Chiumello D, Pelosi P, Croci M, Bigatello LM, Gattinoni L. The effects of pressurization rate on breathing pattern, work of breathing, gas exchange and patient comfort in pressure support ventilation. Eur Respir J. 2001;18:107–14.
59. Sinderby C, Beck J. Proportional assist ventilation and neurally adjusted ventilatory assist—better approaches to patient ventilator synchrony? Clin Chest Med. 2008;29:329–42, vii
60. Colombo D, Cammarota G, Alemani M, Carenzo L, Barra FL, Vaschetto R, Slutsky AS, Della Corte F, Navalesi P. Efficacy of ventilator waveforms observation in detecting patient–ventilator asynchrony. Crit Care Med. 2011;39:2452–7.
61. Spahija J, de Marchie M, Albert M, Bellemare P, Delisle S, Beck J, Sinderby C. Patient–ventilator interaction during pressure support ventilation and neurally adjusted ventilatory assist. Crit Care Med. 2010;38:518–26.
62. Spahija J, de Marchie M, Albert M, et al. Patient-ventilator interaction during pressure support ventilation and neurally adjusted ventilatory assist. Crit Care Med. 2010;38:518–26.
63. Piquilloud L, Vignaux L, Bialais E, et al. Neurally adjusted ventilatory assist improves patient-ventilator interaction. Intensive Care Med. 2011;37:263–71.
64. Mauri T, Bellani G, Grasselli G, et al. Patient-ventilator interaction in ARDS patients with extremely low compliance undergoing ECMO: a novel approach based on diaphragm electrical activity. Intensive Care Med. 2013;39:282–91.
65. Younes M. Proportional assist ventilation, a new approach to ventilatory support. Theory Am Rev Respir Dis. 1992 Jan;145(1):114–20.
66. Alexopoulou C, Kondili E, Plataki M, et al. Patient-ventilator synchrony and sleep quality with proportional assist and pressure support ventilation. Intensive Care Med. 2013;39:1040–7.
67. Xirouchaki N, Kondili E, Vaporidi K, et al. Proportional assist ventilation with load adjustable gain factors in critically ill patients: comparison with pressure support. Intensive Care Med. 2008;34:2026–34.

Unilateral Lung Diseases and Differential Lung Ventilation

Jorge E. Sinclair Ávila, Jorge E. Sinclair De Frías, and Allyson Hidalgo

1 Introduction

Unilateral lung diseases (ULD) can be produced by a variety of processes that lead to changes in the mechanical properties of the involved lung [1–18] (Table 1). Most patients with ULD can be managed successfully with conventional ventilatory support. However, when there is a significant difference in the mechanical properties of both lungs, conventional ventilatory support may fail to maintain adequate gas exchange and may injure the noninvolved lung. When conventional support fails, unconventional therapies, such as lateral decubitus and independent lung ventilation, could be considered.

ILV, also known as differential lung ventilation, was first described in 1931, but it was not until 1976 when it was first reported in an intensive care unit [1, 19, 20]. ILV can be a technically demanding procedure with potential complications. It involves anatomical as well as physiological separation of each lung. Different methods are available for lung separation including endobronchial blockers (EB), Univent tube (UT), coaxial tubes, and double-lumen endotracheal tubes (DLTs). Nowadays, DLTs have become the method of choice for independent lung ventilation in the operating room and in intensive care units.

Literature addressing ventilatory management of ULD with ILV mostly consists of case reports and case series. There are no controlled trials; thus, indications for

J. E. Sinclair Ávila
Critical Medicine, UCI Hospital Pacifica Salud/Johns Hopkins Medicine, Panama City, Panama

J. E. Sinclair De Frías (✉)
Faculty of Medicine, University of Panama, Panama City, Panama

A. Hidalgo
Biochemistry, Arizona State University, Phoenix, AZ, USA

J. Hidalgo et al. (eds.), *Personalized Mechanical Ventilation*,
https://doi.org/10.1007/978-3-031-14138-6_22

Table 1 Unilateral lung diseases

Unilateral lung disease with decreased compliance of involved lung
Massive hemorrhage
Refractory atelectasis
Unilateral pneumonia
Pulmonary contusion
Re-expansion edema
Reperfusion edema
ALI/ARDS
Unilateral lung disease with increased compliance of involved lung
Bronchopleural fistula
Single-lung transplant
Unilateral hyperinflation

Abbreviation: *ALI/ARDS* acute lung injury/acute respiratory distress syndrome

ILV use in critical care setting are poorly defined as compared with its use in thoracic anesthesia [21]. Therefore, decision must be individualized based on the patient's condition, underlying pathology, and clinical expertise.

2 Pathophysiology of Unilateral Lung Diseases

ULDs can be classified based on the underlying pathophysiology and the difference in mechanical properties of the two lungs, whether it increases or decreases the compliance of the involved lung [22]. Understanding these mechanisms may help guide the therapeutic approach of different ULDs.

2.1 Unilateral Lung Diseases with Decreased Compliance of the Involved Lung

In unilateral lung diseases with decreased compliance, changes in lung mechanics results from alveolar filling, interstitial edema, or atelectasis. In the presence of a poorly compliant diseased lung, conventional positive-pressure ventilation may result in preferential distribution of volume to the noninvolved lung [23]. Pulmonary perfusion is less affected and more equally distributed between the two lungs. Nonetheless, physiologic hypoxemic vasoconstriction attempts to redirect blood flow from low and poorly to well-ventilated lung regions. However, in complicated cases, hypoxic vasoconstriction appears to be ineffective resulting in both intrapulmonary shunt and ventilation-perfusion (V/Q) mismatch [23–26].

Application of positive end-expiratory pressure (PEEP) and increasing of minute ventilation may lead to overdistention of the noninvolved lung resulting in redistribution of blood flow to the involved lung, thereby worsening V/Q mismatch and shunt [27]. Other complications reported with the use of conventional ventilation included baro/volutrauma and reduction of cardiac output and blood pressure [23–25, 28, 29].

Therefore, in the setting of a ULD managed with conventional mechanical ventilation, hypoxemia refractory to supplemental oxygen and paradoxical deterioration with increased PEEP levels may suggest severe unilateral lung injuries.

2.2 *Unilateral Lung Diseases with Increased Compliance of the Involved Lung*

In these patients, tidal volume is distributed to the more compliant, involved lung, rather than to the noninvolved lung. ULDs presenting with increased lung compliance include bronchopleural fistula (BPF), single-lung transplant (SLT), and unilateral lung hyperinflation.

BPF is a persistent communication between the bronchial tree and the pleural space. It is usually related to surgical procedures, but can also be caused by chest trauma, necrotizing pneumonia, tuberculosis, lung abscess, empyema, and procedures associated to critical care management such as central line placement and mechanical ventilation [30].

Air leak through the fistula may lead to inadequate alveolar ventilation, pneumothorax, and respiratory insufficiency. Efforts to improve gas exchange with increased minute ventilation and PEEP may increase pressure gradient through the fistula, increasing air leakage and interfering with closure of the defect [30, 31]. Inversely, reducing minute ventilation, PEEP, and inspiratory time to reduce air leak through the fistula may affect ventilation and oxygenation.

In SLT, there is asymmetry in mechanical properties and vascular resistance of the two lungs. The native lung could be more or less compliant than the transplanted lung, depending on the underlying pathology and how compliant the transplanted lung is.

In patients with underlying pulmonary obstructive disease, gas exchange alterations arise when ventilation is preferentially distributed to the native lung and perfusion to the transplanted lung as a result of increased compliance and vascular resistance in the native lung. Mechanical ventilation could also lead to hyperinflation of the native lung with further increase of the already elevated vascular resistance, worsening the V/Q mismatch and intrapulmonary shunt [32]. In addition, postoperative complications, such as reperfusion edema and acute lung rejection, may decrease the compliance of the transplanted lung, enhancing the already increased differences in mechanical properties of both lungs, thus exacerbating gas exchange alterations.

In the setting of pulmonary fibrosis, the transplanted lung may be more or less compliant [33]. In either case, if there is a significant difference in lung mechanics, mechanical ventilation may fail because of preferential ventilation to the more compliant lung.

Unilateral lung hyperinflation may be encountered in the setting of mechanical ventilation in a patient with underlying obstructive disease and a concomitant disease in the contralateral lung, which decreases compliance of the diseased lung [1, 34–36].

3 Independent Lung Ventilation

In most patients with ULD and respiratory insufficiency, general management and conventional ventilatory strategies would provide adequate ventilation and oxygenation [26, 31]. Criteria for initiating conventional mechanical ventilation in these patients are the same as for patients with more equally distributed pulmonary processes. When conventional ventilatory support fails to maintain an adequate ventilation and oxygenation, alternative therapies, such as lateral decubitus position or ILV, must be considered.

ILV is a technically demanding procedure that allows the application of adequate volume and pressure to each lung according to their mechanical properties. It may prevent volume trauma to the noninvolved lung, reduce shunting, and improve alveolar recruitment in the involved lung. Clear indications are not well defined. Some criteria for ILV have been proposed (Table 2).

Table 2 Criteria for independent lung ventilation in unilateral lung disease and bronchopleural fistula

Ventilated patients who have unilateral lung disease
Radiographically apparent unilateral or asymmetrical lung disease with one of the following:
1. Hypoxemia refractory to high FiO_2 and generalized PEEP
2. PEEP-induced deterioration in oxygenation or shunt fraction
3. Overinflation of the noninvolved lung with or without collapse of the involved lung
4. Significant deterioration in circulatory status in response to PEEP
Ventilated patients who have bronchopleural fistula
Any of the following that are unresponsive to usual maneuvers during conventional ventilation:
1. Air leak exceeding 50% of the delivered tidal volume
2. Hypercapnic respiratory acidosis (pH < 7.30)
3. Refractory hypoxemia, particularly in patients in whom PEEP increases exacerbated air leak
4. Persistent lung collapse despite optimum catheter drainage

Abbreviations: *PEEP* positive end-expiratory pressure
Data from [22]

4 Classification

ILV can be classified as synchronous or asynchronous based on the presence or absence of coordination between ventilated breaths provided to each lung. Ventilatory support can be performed either synchronously or asynchronously with similar safety and outcome [2, 21, 37].

4.1 Synchronous

Respiratory rate of both lungs is similar, but respiratory cycle can be in phase or 180 degrees out of phase. Tidal volume, inspiratory flow, PEEP, and FiO_2 are selectively titrated to optimize ventilation and oxygenation while minimizing the risk of lung injury in each lung.

It can be instituted by using either one or two ventilator systems. When using two ventilators, they are synchronized using an external cable [38]. When one ventilator is used, a Y connector with separate PEEP valve is employed [7, 39]; however, this approach has some limitations. The presence of PEEP valves may interfere with accurate measurement of airway pressure, and generation of auto-PEEP might not be detected. In addition, other ventilator parameters cannot be altered independently.

4.2 Asynchronous

Compared to synchronous, asynchronous ventilation is less complicated and offers more flexibility. Respiratory rate, tidal volume, inspiratory flow, PEEP, FiO_2, and mode support can differ between lungs.

5 Ventilator Strategy

Selection of ventilator strategy should be guided by the underlying pathology of each lung and based on the principles of lung-protective ventilation. Hemodynamic parameters should be monitored during titration of ventilator settings, as they can affect cardiac output and shunt fraction.

5.1 PEEP

Optimal PEEP for each lung should be determined separately based on a best PEEP titration trial. Best PEEP trial in the involved lung should be guided by compliance rather than oxygenation, as the diseased lung functions as a shunt and has minimal contribution to gas exchange. For the noninvolved lung, optimal PEEP should be based on oxygenation and compliance, rather than compliance alone. Best PEEP trial in noninvolved lung should also take into account chronic underlying pathologies such as asthma, emphysema, or pulmonary fibrosis.

5.2 *Tidal Volume*

A low tidal volume strategy, 3–5 cc/kg of predicted body weight (PBW), should be applied separately for each lung. Overall, the additive tidal volume delivered to both lungs should not exceed 6–8 cc/kg PBW while maintaining plateau and driving pressure below 30 and 15 cm H_2O, respectively, in each lung [40, 41].

5.3 *Fraction of Inspired Oxygen (FiO_2)*

In the noninvolved lung, FiO_2 should be determined by systemic oxygenation. It should be titrated to maintain partial pressure of arterial oxygen between 55 and 80 mmHg and oxygen saturation (SpO_2) between 88% and 94%.

In the involved lung, a lower FiO_2 may result in poorer oxygenation of the blood circulating the diseased lung, thereby worsening intrapulmonary shunt. In contrast, higher FiO_2 increases the risk of hyperoxic lung injury and may attenuate the hypoxic pulmonary vasoconstriction, thus exacerbating the shunt. Therefore, when titrating FiO_2 in the involved lung, all these factors must be taken into account. When there is minimal contribution to oxygenation by the involved lung, maintaining FiO_2 between 40% and 60% may be favorable.

5.4 *Mode of Ventilation*

Many modes of ventilation have been reported including assist-control volume or pressure ventilation, pressure-support ventilation, continuous positive airway pressure (CPAP), high-frequency oscillatory ventilation (HFOV), and airway pressure release ventilation (APRV) [9, 11, 12, 22, 42–45].

6 Techniques for Lung Separation

6.1 *Endobronchial Blockers*

A variety of endobronchial blocking techniques have been described including Fogarty embolectomy balloons, pulmonary artery catheters, urinary catheters, and Arndt and Cohen blockers [2, 46–49]. Endobronchial blockers (EB) are relatively easy to introduce, offering advantages when intubating difficult upper airways. However, final placement may be more complicated than when using DLTs, especially when bronchoscopic visualization is limited by massive hemoptysis [50, 51]. Moreover, EBs limit monitoring of bleeding and secretion and cannot be used when the site of bleeding is unknown. Displacement and malpositioning are more common than with DLTs [52]. The lack of central lumen prevents ventilation or suctioning of the lung; thus, when ILV is intended, other techniques are more appropriate [2].

6.2 Univent Tube

It was first described in 1982 [53] and consists of a single-lumen endotracheal tube with an anterior channel containing a low-volume high-pressure balloon catheter which acts as a blocker [54]. UTs have some advantages over other EBs [2]. It is attached to the endotracheal tube, consequently decreasing the risk of displacement. The central lumen of the catheter allows some ventilation, suctioning, and pulmonary lavage of the non-ventilated lung. At last, the blocker can be deflated and withdrawn, allowing to initiate conventional ventilation without having to reintubate the patient.

Although UTs offer some advantages, the presence of high-pressure cuffs may increase the risk of adverse events such as bronchial rupture, mucosal ischemia, and pneumothorax [55]. Finally, despite having a central lumen, UTs are most useful for one-lung ventilation, due to its small lumen that limits its usefulness during ILV.

6.3 Double-Lumen Tubes

DLTs are considered the method of choice when ILV is required in the critical care unit. It consists of a bifurcated tube with both an endotracheal and endobronchial lumen, with the latter being either left sided or right sided [56]. Both lumens have separate cuff, the proximal cuff at the tracheal lumen and the distal cuff at the bronchial lumen.

When using DLTs, it is important to consider the tube's design, placement techniques, confirming position and functional separation of the lungs, monitoring of tube position, and potential complications.

6.3.1 Design

Carlens Tube

All DLTs' design is based on the original Carlens tube introduced in 1949 [2]. The Carlens tube is made of firm red rubber with a carinal hook to secure the DLT and prevent distal displacement. Although effective for ILV, Carlens tube has several limitations. The carinal hook is difficult to pass through the larynx and may result in laryngeal trauma. The small lumen size increases airflow resistance, and difficult suctioning and secretion mobilization. The low-volume high-pressure cuffs may lead to tracheal and bronchial injuries.

Right upper lobe bronchus originates 1.5–2 cm from the carina. In consequence, endobronchial cuffs on right-sided tubes often occlude the right upper lobe orifice resulting in right upper lobe atelectasis. Therefore, left-sided Carlens tube was preferred.

Robertshaw Tube

Robertshaw tube is a modification of Carlens tube. Its larger lumen diameter provides easier suctioning and lower airflow resistance. Elimination of carinal hook leads to less traumatic complications. Finally, the presence of a slot on the endobronchial cuff in right-sided tubes allows ventilation of the right upper lobe obstruction.

Polyvinyl Chloride Tubes (PVC)

Polyvinyl chloride tubes (PVCs) are improved versions of Robertshaw tubes. The tube is transparent allowing visualization of the blue endobronchial cuff and tracheobronchial mucosa with the bronchoscope. They have even larger internal to external diameter ratio, reducing more airway resistance. PVCs are less irritative, suppler, and have low-pressure high-volume cuffs, therefore reducing the incidence of airway trauma [2, 52].

6.3.2 Size Selection

Appropriate DLT size must be selected. Using a larger DLT may result in airway trauma, while placing a smaller DLT may fail to provide lung separation requiring a large endotracheal cuff volume, which might increase the incidence of malposition, trauma, and ischemia of the airway. In addition, smaller DLTs might present more resistance to airflow and greater risk of auto-PEEP compared to larger DLTs. The smallest available size is 26 French, followed by 28, 32, 35, 37, 39, and 41 French. In most adults, 39 or 41 French would be adequate (Table 3).

Table 3 Double-lumen tube size

Tube size (French)	Circumference (mm)	Lumen diameter (mm)	Indications
35	38	5	Large children (>40 kg)
37	40	5.5	Small adults
39	44	6	Medium adults/usual female size
41	45	6.5	Large adults/usual male size

Data from Tuxen [1], Thomas and Bryce [22], Ost and Corbridge [2], Burton et al. [57]

6.3.3 Placement Techniques

Transient interruption of ventilation during tube placement may worsen hypoxemia, especially in a critical ill patient with limited reserve. Thus, DLT placement should be performed by individuals experienced in airway management, with difficult airway equipment and bedside bronchoscope.

Right-sided placement is associated with increased risk of bronchial cuff herniation resulting in obstruction of the right upper lobe and/or left mainstem [1, 2, 58, 59]. Therefore, left-sided DLTs are usually preferred over right-sided. Right-sided tubes are reserved for specific situations such as left mainstem bronchus stenosis, tumors, or tracheobronchial lesions [60–62].

DLTs are inserted similarly to single-lumen tubes. Intubation is usually orotracheal, but in some cases, specially designed short DLTs can be used with tracheotomies [63, 64]. Two techniques are commonly used when inserting and placing a DLT: the blind technique and the fiber-optic bronchoscopy (FOB)-guided technique. Placement and positioning of a left-sided DLT can be accomplished by either technique. However, FOB guidance technique is preferred when using right-sided tubes.

In the blind technique, the tube is passed through the larynx with the distal curvature pointing anteriorly via direct laryngoscopy. Then, the tube is rotated 90° toward the side of placement and is advanced until mild resistance is felt. Maintaining stylet in position after intubation increases positioning accuracy [65]. Once intubation is achieved, both cuffs are inflated and correct positioning should be confirmed with FOB [66].

The second technique employs FOB; once the DLT has passed the vocal cords under direct laryngoscopy, the FOB is advanced through the endobronchial lumen. Before advancing the DLT, the tracheal carina and the right or left mainstem bronchus should be identified. Then the tube is rotated 90° right or left and is advanced with the aid of FOB.

6.3.4 Confirming Position

Confirming accurate anatomical position and functional separation of the lungs is required. The two methods for confirming the position of DLTs are auscultation methods and the use of FOB. Before the advent of FOB, auscultation techniques were the primary method for determining correct tube placement. Unfortunately, this method is not reliable as in up to 61% of the left-sided DLTs and 87% of the right-sided DLTs, patients required repositioning when assessed with bronchoscopy [66–68]. However, auscultation maneuvers must be routinely applied prior to the use of FOB.

Correct positioning of DLT with FOB is easier, faster, and more reliable than auscultation alone. Pediatric bronchoscope is used for DLTs smaller than 39 French, while smaller adult bronchoscopes are used for 39 French or larger DLTs.

When using either left-sided or right-sided tubes, the bronchoscope is initially passed through the tracheal lumen to ensure that the tracheal port is positioned proximal to the carina and to rule out bronchial cuff herniation around the carina. If present, herniations of the bronchial cuff should be corrected by deflating the cuff and advancing it under direct visualization.

In left-sided tube placements, the left bronchial cuff should be visualized distal to the carina. Right main bronchus should also be visible; if not, the tube should be withdrawn until both the right bronchial lumen and the left bronchial cuff are visualized. After the correct position is confirmed, bronchoscope should be passed through the bronchial cuff to assess for excess narrowing of the lumen caused by overinflation. At the distal end of the endobronchial tube, left upper and lower lobe bronchus should be visualized.

In right-sided tube placements, confirmation is more complicated. When the bronchoscope is passed through the bronchial lumen, the right upper lobe orifice should be aligned with the opening slot of the endobronchial tube, and distally a clear view of bronchus intermedius and right lower lobe bronchus should be seen from the endobronchial lumen [69].

6.3.5 Confirming Functional Separation

Classically, two methods were used to assess functional separation of the lungs: the "water bubble" and the balloon inflation techniques [70, 71]. The tracheal port is placed under water or in a balloon, respectively, while maintaining a plateau pressure of 40 cm of H_2O through the bronchial port. The appearance of bubbles or balloon inflation at the tracheal port identifies air leak and loss of functional separation of the lungs [70, 71]. However, these techniques require temporary interruption of ventilation and might not be a feasible strategy.

Currently, functional separation can be assessed with modern ventilators by measuring the inspired and expired tidal volumes. Any loss or gain of tidal volume would suggest air leak; however, in patients with BPF, interpretation may be difficult.

6.3.6 Monitoring DLT Placement

DLTs are susceptible to displacement [72]; even movements as small as 16 to 19 mm for left-sided tubes and 1–8 mm for right-sided tubes could result in inadequate ventilation [59, 61]. Displacement may occur with any patient movement or routine changes of patient's position [72]. Therefore, measures to prevent DLT displacement should be always considered, including sedation and neuromuscular paralysis.

Malpositioning should be suspected with sudden changes in volume return, airway pressure, and/or compliance. When displacement is suspected, bronchoscopic assessment should be performed promptly. Although noninvasive monitoring methods, such as dual monitoring of end-tidal carbon dioxide, monitoring of peak inspiratory pressure, and continuous spirometry, may be helpful for the detection of a displaced DLT [73, 74], none should replace bronchoscopy [10, 75, 76].

6.3.7 Complications

Reported complications associated to DLT include laryngeal trauma, bronchial ischemia and stenosis, and bronchial rupture resulting in pneumothorax, pneumomediastinum, and subcutaneous emphysema [9, 77]. Although newer DLTs are safer, they are not exempt of complications.

Laryngeal trauma is more frequent when carinal hooks are used. With the removal of the carinal hook and the use of more flexible PVC catheters, the incidence of these complications has decreased [57, 78].

Bronchial injuries are usually related to the use of high-pressure low-volume bronchial cuffs [79, 80]. The effects of prolonged use of bronchial cuff on bronchial mucosal blood flow are unknown. Risk factors for bronchial trauma and rupture include underlying malignancy, infection, tracheobronchial surgery, chronic steroid use, traumatic intubation, cuff overinflation, oversized DLT, and prolonged intubation [52].

Other complications include inadequate ventilation due to malpositioning of the tube, difficult secretion clearance, and increased inspiratory and expiratory flow resistance caused by the small lumen diameter.

7 Classification of Lung Separation

7.1 Anatomic Separation

Its main goal is to isolate one lung from the other, to prevent cross contamination with lavage fluids, blood, or purulent secretion. It is used mainly in patients with pulmonary alveolar proteinosis, massive hemoptysis, and airway protection from interbronchial aspiration [2, 81]. Anatomic separation provides limited respiratory support and is considered a short-term measure to maintain oxygenation and ventilation until definitive management can be performed.

7.1.1 Massive Hemoptysis

Anatomic separation protects the nonbleeding side from aspiration of blood. Intubation in these patients may be difficult due to poor visibility. If the site of bleeding is localized to one lung, any previously described lung separation technique can be used to isolate the bleeding site; however, endobronchial blockers are preferred. If the site of bleeding is unknown, DLTs are preferred over EB, as they allow bronchoscopy of the bleeding side while maintaining lung separation [2]. It is considered a temporary maneuver until definitive treatment is achieved. Once the bleeding has been contained, lungs can be ventilated with conventional volumes and pressure.

7.1.2 Pulmonary Alveolar Proteinosis

Sequential lung lavage is considered the treatment of choice in patients with pulmonary alveolar proteinosis. Anatomic separation is necessary for this procedure. A DLT is usually used for absolute lung separation. The more affected lung is lavaged first while maintaining ventilation to the other lung to prevent or minimize hypoxemia. Around 40–50 L is lavaged in 3 h until the efflux is clear. The lavage is repeated in the other lung after 2–3 days. Complications related to this procedure may be recognized by desaturation, visualization of fluid in the ventilated lung, or air bubbles in the efflux.

7.1.3 Interbronchial Aspiration

Anatomic separation is also used to prevent interbronchial spread of purulent material. It can be used particularly in patients with tuberculous cavities, bronchiectatic areas of the lung, and lung abscess, including those patients waiting for a definitive surgical procedure [23].

7.2 Physiologic

Both lungs are isolated, allowing different ventilator strategies to each lung. This is most beneficial when there is an important difference in lung mechanics between both lungs or when it is desirable to minimize airway pressure in one lung.

7.2.1 Asymmetrical Parenchymal Lung Diseases

In asymmetrical parenchymal lung diseases, such as pulmonary contusion, atelectasis (Fig. 1), hemorrhage, and pneumonia (Fig. 2) [82–84], lung compliance is lower in the involved side compared with the less involved or noninvolved side. If resistance and compliance are significantly different among both lungs, there may be unequal distribution of ventilation and PEEP. As discussed before, during conventional ventilation, most of the tidal volume is distributed to the more compliant lung resulting in increased risk of hyperinflation and lung injury, and redirection of perfusion toward the affected lung [23–25, 27, 85]. In addition, bilateral PEEP may be insufficient for alveolar recruitment in the involved lung, but excessive in the uninvolved lung. However, the majority of the patients with ULD can be managed successfully with conventional mechanical ventilation. ILV would be reserved for patients in which conventional measures fail to provide adequate support.

ILV allows different ventilator strategies for each lung improving ventilation and oxygenation and reducing the risk of barotrauma. Tidal volume can be initially set

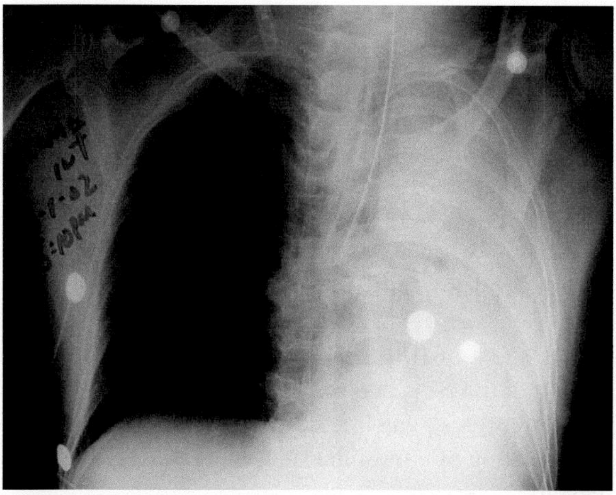

Fig. 1 Chest radiograph of a patient with a left refractory pulmonary atelectasis

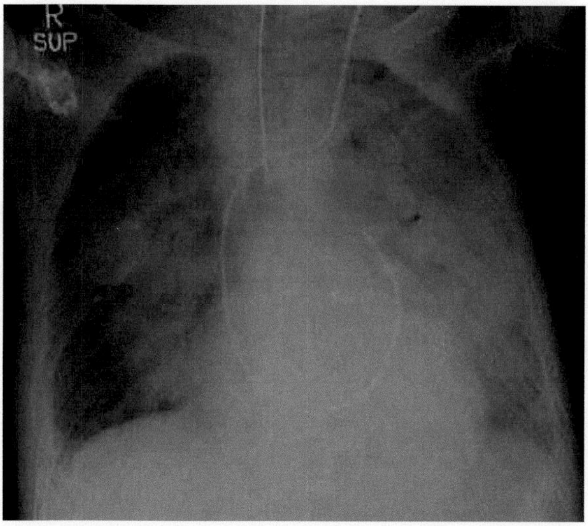

Fig. 2 Chest radiograph of a patient with a predominantly left-sided pneumonia, further complicated with ARDS

at 4–5 ml/kg per lung and adjusted depending on the target plateau pressures [10]. In addition, PEEP can be adjusted according to gas exchange parameters and mean airway pressures on each lung.

7.2.2 Single-Lung Transplant

The relative compliance of both lungs will depend on the underlying pulmonary pathology and injuries to the transplanted lungs. ILV can be useful in the management of postoperative complications including pulmonary graft dysfunction, surgical pulmonary contusion, acute rejection, and acute distress respiratory syndrome

[86]. ILV strategies would be similar to the strategies used in asymmetrical parenchymal lung diseases. Physicians should aim for a plateau pressure of less than 35 mmHg to avoid overdistention. PEEP and FiO_2 levels should be determined by arterial oxygenation and hemodynamic parameters. Application of selective PEEP or higher PEEP levels to the transplanted lung may protect the native lung from overinflation and recruit alveoli.

7.2.3 Bronchopleural Fistula

Management of BPF should focus on relieving tension pneumothorax if present, healing of the BPF, and maintaining an adequate gas exchange. Treatment options include surgical and medical procedures to reduce or seal air leak including manipulation of chest tube suction, ILV, HFOV, and application of glues, coils, or sealants.

Maintaining adequate oxygenation while decreasing fistula air leak is conflicting. Chest tube suction devices are needed to prevent the development of tension pneumothorax. Positive pressure from ventilation summed to the negative pressure from chest suction increases the leakage through the fistula, delaying its healing [2]. When conventional ventilation fails, ILV with DLT is an alternative [2, 7, 30].

ILV allows optimal ventilation of the noninvolved lung while minimizing airway pressures and, therefore, pressure gradient across the BPF. The noninvolved lung can be managed with conventional ventilation, while in the fistula side, management is directed at decreasing airway pressure and minimizing pleural suctioning pressure. In order to achieve this, tidal volume, respiratory rate, PEEP, and inspiratory time are set to the lowest possible [30].

7.2.4 Unilateral Airway Obstruction

The involved side is supported with ILV with a low respiratory rate, low tidal volume, and prolonged expiratory time, to prevent auto-PEEP, while the noninvolved side is managed with conventional ventilation [87].

8 Weaning of ILV

Continuous evaluation of lung mechanics of each lung should be performed. Ventilator parameters of the involved lung can only be weaned when the patient shows significant resolution of the asymmetry of the disease process. With resolution of the unilateral process, lung mechanics will progressively converge.

The need for continuous use of ILV is determined by clinical, mechanical, and radiographic progress (Table 4). Continuation of ILV should be weighed against the

Table 4 Criteria for terminating independent lung ventilation

• Near-complete or complete resolution of the disease process (clinical or radiologically)
• Difference in PEEP in two circuits <5 cm H_2O with stable PaO_2
• Paw_{peak} difference < 5 cm H_2O on identical settings in both circuits
• Compliance difference between the two lungs <20%
• Tidal volume difference between the two lungs <100 cc
• Total minute ventilation <12 L/min (sum of the two systems)
• Ratio of ET_{CO2} or V_{CO2} ε0.88
• ET_{CO2} difference between the two lungs <20%

Abbreviations: Paw_{peak} peak airway pressure, *PEEP* positive end-expiratory pressure, PaO_2 partial pressure of oxygen, ET_{CO2} end-tidal carbon dioxide, V_{CO2} carbon dioxide production
Data from Thomas and Bryce [22], Berg et al. [88]
These parameters have been obtained from reported cases and have not been subject to scientific study; therefore, they serve as guidelines to be considered in the context of the patient

risk associated to the duration of ILV. Sedation minimizes patients' ventilatory effort and prevents participation in physical therapy, resulting in muscle atrophy. In addition, prolonged duration of ILV may increase the risk of bronchial injury from DLT.

9 Complications

Complications are related to both the technique of lung separation used (see Sect. 6) and mechanical ventilation. Mechanical ventilation can lead to ventilator-induced lung injury (VILI), which includes barotrauma, volutrauma, atelectrauma, and biotrauma. Therefore, frequent assessments of lung mechanics are necessary to decrease the risk of these complications. In addition, correct positioning of the tube is vital, as an incorrect position of the tube could not only be ineffective but also compromise the patient's life.

10 Conclusion

ULDs can cause changes in the mechanical properties of each lung. If the involved lung has a reduced compliance, most of the volume and pressure are diverted to the nonaffected lung, while if the involved lung has an increased compliance, ventilation is mostly diverted to the affected lung. Conventional ventilatory support maintains adequate gas exchange and hemodynamic stability in most patients. ILV is usually instituted as a rescue strategy when conventional ventilation fails to maintain adequate ventilation and oxygenation.

Data supporting the use of ILV in a critical care setting is limited to case reports and series; therefore, indications are poorly defined. Decision to attempt ILV should take into account the technical difficulties associated with the procedure. ILV is a technically demanding procedure that requires skilled nursing care, specialized monitoring devices, and readily available FOB.

References

1. Tuxen D. Independent lung ventilation. In: Tobin MJ, editor. Principles and practice of mechanical ventilation. New York: McGraw-Hill; 1994. p. 571–88.
2. Ost D, Corbridge T. Independent lung ventilation. Clin Chest Med. 1996;17:591–601.
3. Skjeflo GW, Dybwik K. A new method of securing the airway for differential lung ventilation in intensive care. Acta Anaesthesiol Scand. 2014;58:463–7.
4. Stow PJ, Grant I. Asynchronous independent lung ventilation. Its use in the treatment of acute unilateral lung disease. Anaesthesia. 1985;40:163–6.
5. Shivaram U, Finch P, Nowak P. Plastic endobronchial tubes in the management of life-threatening hemoptysis. Chest. 1987;92:1108.
6. Badesch DB, Zamora MR, Jones S, Campbell DW, Fullerton DA. Independent ventilation and ECMO for severe unilateral pulmonary edema after SLT for primary pulmonary hypertension. Chest. 1995;107:1766–70.
7. Carvalho P, Thompson WH, Riggs R, Carvalho C, Charan N. Management of bronchopleural fistula with a variable resistance valve and a single ventilator. Chest. 1997;111:1452–4.
8. Cinnella G, Dambrosio M, Brienza N, Bruno F, Brienza A. Compliance and capnography monitoring during independent lung ventilation: report of two cases. Anesthesiology. 2000;93:275–8.
9. Graciano AL, Barton P, Luckett PM, Morriss F, Sommerauer JF, Toro-Figueroa LO. Feasibility of asynchronous independent lung high-frequency oscillatory ventilation in the management of acute hypoxemic respiratory failure: a case report. Crit Care Med. 2000;28:3075–7.
10. Cinnella G, Dambrosio M, Brienza N, Giuliani R, Bruno F, Fiore T, Brienza A. Independent lung ventilation in patients with unilateral pulmonary contusion. Monitoring with compliance and EtCO(2). Intensive Care Med. 2001;27:1860–7.
11. Pilcher DV, Auzinger GM, Mitra B, Tuxen DV, Salamonsen RF, Davies AR, Williams TJ, Snell GI. Predictors of independent lung ventilation: an analysis of 170 single-lung transplantations. J Thorac Cardiovasc Surg. 2007;133:1071–7.
12. Rico FR, Cheng JD, Gestring ML, Piotrowski ES. Mechanical ventilation strategies in massive chest trauma. Crit Care Clin. 2007;23:299–315.
13. Shekar K, Foot CL, Fraser JF. Independent lung ventilation in the intensive care unit: desperate measure or viable treatment option? Crit Care Resusc. 2008;10:144–8.
14. Fujita M, Tsuruta R, Oda Y, Kaneda K, Miyauchi T, Kasaoka S, Maekawa T. Severe legionella pneumonia successfully treated by independent lung ventilation with intrapulmonary percussive ventilation. Respirology. 2008;13:475–7.
15. Yamakawa K, Nakamori Y, Fujimi S, Ogura H, Kuwagata Y, Shimazu T. A novel technique of differential lung ventilation in the critical care setting. BMC Res Notes. 2011;4:134.
16. Achar SK, Chaudhuri S, Krishna H, Sagar M. Re-expansion pulmonary edema - differential lung ventilation comes to the rescue. Indian J Anaesth. 2014;58:330–3.
17. Sarnaik A. The use of independent lung ventilation for unilateral pulmonary hemorrhage. Int J Respir Pulm Med. 2015;2:13.
18. Minhas JS, Halligan K, Dargin JM. Independent lung ventilation in the management of ARDS and bronchopleural fistula. Heart Lung. 2016;45:258–60.
19. Glass DD, Tonnesen AS, Gabel JC, Arens JF. Therapy of unilateral pulmonary insufficiency with a double lumen endotracheal tube. Crit Care Med. 1976;4:323–6.

20. Powner D, Eross B, Grenvik A. Differential lung ventilation with PEEP in treatment of unilateral pneumonia. Crit Care Med. 1977;5:170–2.
21. Anatham D, Jagadesan R, Tiew PEC. Clinical review: independent lung ventilation in critical care. Crit Care. 2005;9:594–600.
22. Thomas A, Bryce T. Ventilation in the patient with unilateral lung disease. Crit Care Clin. 1998;14(4):743–73.
23. Siegel JH, Stoklosa JC, Borg U, Wiles CE, Sganga G, Geisler FH, Belzberg H, Wedel S, Blevins S, Goh KC. Quantification of asymmetric lung pathophysiology as a guide to the use of simultaneous independent lung ventilation in posttraumatic and septic adult respiratory distress syndrome. Ann Surg. 1985;202:425–39.
24. Carlon GC, Kahn R, Howland WS, et al. A case of life-threatening ventilation-perfusion inequality: an indication for independent lung ventilation. Crit Care Med. 1978a;6:380–3.
25. Carlon GC, Ray C, Klein R, et al. Criteria for selective positive end-expiratory pressure and independent lung ventilation of each lung. Chest. 1978b;74:501–7.
26. Hurst JM, DeHaven CB Jr, Branson RD. Comparison of conventional mechanical ventilation and synchronous independent lung ventilation (SILV) in the treatment of unilateral lung injury. J Trauma. 1985;25:766–70.
27. Parish JM, Gracey DR, Southorn PA, Pairolero PA, Wheeler JT. Differential mechanical ventilation in respiratory failure due to severe unilateral lung disease. Mayo Clin Proc. 1984;59:888–90.
28. Venus B, Pratap KS, Op'Tholt T. Treatment of unilateral pulmonary insufficiency by selective administration of continuous positive airway pressure through a double-lumen tube. Anesthesiology. 1980;53:74–7.
29. Zandstra DF, Stoutenbeek CP, Bams JL. Monitoring lung mechanics and airway pressures during differential lung ventilation (DLV) with emphasis on weaning from DLV. Intensive Care Med. 1989;15:458–63.
30. Baumann MH, Sahn SA. Medical management and therapy of bronchopleural fistulas in the mechanically ventilated patient. Chest. 1990;97:721–8.
31. Pierson D. Management of bronchopleural fistula in the adult respiratory distress syndrome. New Horiz. 1993;1:512–21.
32. Kaiser L, Cooper JD, Trulock E, et al. The evolution of single lung transplant for emphysema. J Thorac Cardiovasc Surg. 1991;102:333–41.
33. Adoumie R, et al. Differential lung ventilation: applications beyond the operating room. J Thorac Cardiovasc Surg. 1993;105:229–33.
34. Kollef MH. Recurrent unilateral lung hyperinflation as a manifestation of "auto-PEEP". Heart Lung. 1993;22:84–8.
35. Kollef MH, Turner JF. Intrinsic PEEP and unilateral lung hyperinflation. Pathophysiology and clinical significance. Chest. 1992;102:1220–4.
36. Everloff SE, Rounds S, Braman SS. Unilateral lung hyperinflation and herniation as a manifestation of intrinsic PEEP. Chest. 1990;98:228–9.
37. Hillman KM, Barber JD. Asynchronous independent lung ventilation (AILV). Crit Care Med. 1980;8:390–5.
38. Marraro G, Marinari M, Rataggi M. The clinical application of synchronized independent lung ventilation (S.I.L.V.) in pulmonary disease with unilateral prevalence in pediatrics. Int J Clin Monit Comput. 1987;4:123–9.
39. Charan NB, Cg C, Hawk P, Crowley JJ, Carvalho P. Independent lung ventilation with a single ventilator using a variable resistance valve. Chest. 1995;107:256–60.
40. Roupie E, Dambrosio M, Servillo G, et al. Titration of tidal volume and induced hypercapnia in acute respiratory distress syndrome. Am J Respir Crit Care Med. 1995;152(1):121–8.
41. Amato MB, Meade MO, Slutsky AS, Brochard L, Costa EL, Schoenfeld DA, Stewart TE, Briel M, Talmor D, Mercat A, Richard JC, Carvalho CR, Brower RG. Driving pressure and survival in the acute respiratory distress syndrome. N Engl J Med. 2015;372:747–55.

42. Katsaragakis S, Stamou K, Androulakis A. Independent lung ventilation for asymmetrical chest trauma: effect on ventilatory and haemodynamic parameters. Int J Care Injured. 2005;36:501–4.
43. Di Nardo M, Perrotta D, Stoppa F, Cecchetti C, et al. Independent lung ventilation in a newborn with asymmetric acute lung injury due to respiratory syncytial virus: a case report. J Med Case Rep. 2008;2:212.
44. Konstantinov I, Saxena P. Independent lung ventilation in the postoperative management of large bronchopleural fistula. J Thorac Cardiovasc Surg. 2010;139:e21–2.
45. Papadakos P, Karcz M, Lachmann B. Mechanical ventilation in trauma. Curr Opin Anaesthesiol. 2010;23:228–32.
46. Campos JH. An update on bronchial blockers during lung separation techniques in adults. Anesth Analg. 2003;97:1266–74.
47. Cohen E. Methods of lung separation. Minerva Anestesiol. 2004;70:313–8.
48. Chen KP, Chan HC, Huang SJ. Foley catheter used as bronchial blocker for one lung ventilation in a patient with tracheostomy: a case report. Acta Anaesthesiol Sin. 1995;33:41–4.
49. Park HP, Bahk JH, Park JH, Oh YS. Use of a Fogarty catheter as a bronchial blocker through a single-lumen endotracheal tube in patients with subglottic stenosis. Anaesth Intensive Care. 2003;31:214–6.
50. Campos JH, Kernstine KH. A comparison of a left-sided Broncho-Cath with the torque control blocker Univent and the wire-guided blocker. Anesth Analg. 2003;96:283–9.
51. Bauer C, Winter C, Hentz JG, Duerocq X, Steib A, Dupeyron JP. Bronchial blocker compared to double-lumen tube for one-lung ventilation during thoracoscopy. Acta Anaesthesiol Scand. 2001;45:250–4.
52. Tsai KM. Lung isolation update. Sem anesthesia, perioperative. Med Pain. 2003;22:88–105.
53. Inoue H, Shotsu A, Ogawa J, et al. New device for one-lung anesthesia: endotracheal tube with moveable blocker. Thorac Cardiovasc Surg. 1982;83:940–1.
54. Gayes JM. Pro: one-lung ventilation is best accomplished with the Univent endotracheal tube. J Cardiothor Vasc Anesth. 1993;7:103–7.
55. Kelley JG, Gaba DM, Brodsky JB. Bronchial cuff pressures of two tubes used in thoracic surgery. J Cardiothor Vasc Anesth. 1992;6:190–2.
56. Campos JH. Lung isolation. In: Slinger P, editor. Principles and practice of anesthesia for thoracic surgery. New York: Springer; 2011. p. 227–46.
57. Burton NA, Watson DC, Brodsky JB, et al. Advantages of a new polyvinyl chloride double lumen tube in thoracic surgery. Ann Thorac Surg. 1983;36:78–84.
58. Brodsky JB, Mihm FG. Spit-lung ventilation. In: Hall JB, Schmidt GA, Wood LDH, editors. Principles of Critical Care. New York: McGraw-Hill; 1992. p. 160–4.
59. Benumof JL, Patridge BL, Salvatierra C, et al. Margin of safety in positioning modern double-lumen endotracheal tubes. Anesthesiology. 1987;67:729.
60. Strange C. Double-lumen endotracheal tubes. Clin Chest Med. 1991;12:12497–506.
61. Alfrey DD. Double-lumen endobronchial tube intubation using a retrograde wire technique. Anesth Analg. 1993;76:1374–5.
62. Benumof JL. Separation of the two lungs (double-lumen tube intubation). In: Anesthesia for thoracic surgery. 2nd ed. Philadelphia, PA: WB Saunders; 1995. p. 223–58.
63. Coe VL, Brodsky JB, Mark JBD. Double-lumen endobronchial tubes in patients with tracheostomies. Anesth Analg. 1984;63:882.
64. Taylor S, Walford A, McLellan I. A disposable double-lumen tracheostomy tube: a prototype. Anaesth Intensive Care. 1984;12:57.
65. Lieberman D, Littleford J, Horan T, Unruth H. Placement of left double-lumen endobronchial tubes with or without stylet. Can J Anaesth. 1996;43:238–42.
66. Smith GB, Hirsch NP, Ehrenwerth J. Placement of double-lumen endobronchial tubes. Br J Anaesth. 1986;58:1317–20.
67. McKenna MJ, Wilson RS, Botelho RJ. Right upper lobe obstruction with right-sided double-lumen endobronchial tubes: a comparison of two types. Cardiothorac Vasc Anesth. 1988;2:734–40.

68. Alliaume B, Coddens J, Deloof T. Reliability of auscultation in positioning double-lumen endotracheal tubes. Can J Anaesth. 1992;39:687–90.
69. Campos JH. Update on tracheobronchial anatomy and flexible fiberoptic bronchoscopy in thoracic anesthesia. Curr Opin Anaesthesiol. 2009;22:4–10.
70. Brodsky JB, Mark JB. Balloon method for detecting inadequate double-lumen tube cuff seal. Ann Thorac Surg. 1993;55:1584.
71. Spragg RG, Benumof JL, Alfery DD. New methods in the performance of unilateral lung lavage. Anesthesiology. 1982;57:535.
72. Inoue S, Nishimine N, Kitaguchi K, Furuya H, Taniguchi S. Double lumen tube location predicts tube malposition and hypoxaemia during one lung ventilation. Br J Anaesth. 2004;92:195–201.
73. Shankar KB, Moseley HSL, Kumar AY. Dual end-tidal CO, monitoring and double-lumen tubes. Can J Anaesth. 1991;39:100–1.
74. Bardoczky GI, Levarlet M, Engelman E, et al. Continuous spirometry for detection of double lumen endobronchial tube displacement. Br J Anaesth. 1993;70:499–502.
75. Iwasaka H, Itoh K, Miyakawa H, Taniguchi K, Honda N. Continuous monitoring of ventilatory mechanics during one-lung ventilation. J Clin Monit. 1996;12(161):164.
76. Szegedi LL, Bardoczky GI, Engelman EE, d'Hollander AA. Airway pressure changes during one-lung ventilation. Anesth Analg. 1997;84:1034–7.
77. Sivalingam P, Tio R. Tension pneumothorax, pneumomediastinum, pneumoperitoneum, and subcutaneous emphysema in a 15-year-old Chinese girl after a double-lumen tube intubation and one-lung ventilation. J Cardiothor Vasc Anesth. 1999;13:312–5.
78. Clapham MC, Vaughan RS. Bronchial intubation: a comparison between polyvinyl chloride and red rubber double-lumen tubes. Anaesthesia. 1985;40:1111.
79. Brodsky JB. Complications of double-lumen tracheal tubes. Probl Anesth. 1988;2:292.
80. Brodsky JB, Adkins MO, Gaba DM. Bronchial cuff pressures of double-lumen tubes. Anesth Analg. 1989;69:608–10.
81. Claypool WD, Rogers RM, Matuschak GM. Update on the clinical diagnosis, management, and pathogenesis of pulmonary alveolar proteinosis (phospholipidosis). Chest. 1984;85:550–8.
82. Rocke DA. Percutaneous lung biopsy. Anaesthesia. 1984;39:888–90.
83. Wendt M, et al. Differential ventilation with low-flow CPAP and CPPV in the treatment of unilateral chest trauma. Intensive Care Med. 1989;15:209–11.
84. Inoue H, et al. Selective exclusion of the injured lung. J Trauma. 1993;34:496–8.
85. Hedenstiema G, Baehrendtz S, Klingstedt C, et al. Ventilation and perfusion of each lung during differential ventilation with selective PEEP. Anesthesiology. 1984;61:369.
86. Gavazzeni V, Iapichino G, Mascheroni D, Langer M, Bordone G, Zannini P, Radrizzani D, Damia G. Prolonged independent lung respiratory treatment after single lung transplantation in pulmonary emphysema. Chest. 1993;103:96–100.
87. Narr BJ, Fromme GA, Peters SG. Unilateral bronchospasm during pleurodesis in an asthmatic patient. Chest. 1990;98:767–8.
88. Berg S, Bittner EA, Berra L, Kacmarek RM, Sonny A. Independent lung ventilation: implementation strategies and review of literature. World J Crit Care Med. 2019;8(4):49–58.

Mechanical Ventilation in Obstructive Lung Disease

Ivan Co and Robert C Hyzy

1 Chronic Obstructive Pulmonary Disease (COPD)

1.1 Objective of Ventilator Management

The goal of ventilator management of patients with COPD is to offload a patient's work of breathing and allow for better synchrony, optimize their exhalation time, and minimize secondary complication such as ventilator-associated pneumonia (VAP) and ventilator-induced lung injury (VILI).

1.2 Mode of Ventilation and Initial Setting

Using the above principle, the initial mode of ventilation should be assist-control (AC) over synchronized intermittent mandatory ventilation (SIMV). Choosing whether to use volume (VC) or pressure (PC) control can be left up to the bedside

I. Co (✉)
Emergency Medicine, Division of Emergency Critical Care, University of Michigan Health System, Ann Arbor, MI, USA

Internal Medicine, Division of Pulmonary and Critical Care, University of Michigan Health System, Ann Arbor, MI, USA
e-mail: coivan@med.umich.edu

R. C Hyzy
Internal Medicine, Division of Pulmonary and Critical Care, University of Michigan Health System, Ann Arbor, MI, USA

Division of Pulmonary and Critical Care Medicine, University of Michigan, Ann Arbor, MI, USA
e-mail: rhyzy@med.umich.edu

J. Hidalgo et al. (eds.), *Personalized Mechanical Ventilation*,
https://doi.org/10.1007/978-3-031-14138-6_23

clinician. This is because AC has been documented to offload work of breathing far better than patients on SIMV [1]. Preferentially, VC tends to be chosen over PC secondary to the ability to guarantee certain tidal volume (TV) and minute ventilation (V_E), ultimately helping to prevent volutrauma particularly in patients with superimposed parenchymal lung disease.

After selecting the mode of ventilation, the next step should be focused on setting the respiratory rate (RR) and tidal volume that optimizes exhalation in order to appropriately correct hypercapnic respiratory failure and respiratory acidosis. An initial RR between 8 and 12 per minute and a TV of 6 cc/kg of the patient's ideal body weight (IBW) with a flow rate of >60 L/min are reasonable initial settings. An initial positive end-expiratory pressure (PEEP) of 5 cm H_2O or less and a fraction of inspired oxygen (FiO_2) that targets a SpO_2 of 90% or PaO_2 of 55 mmHg are ideal. V_E should be titrated to an arterial partial pressure of carbon dioxide ($PaCO_2$) that results in a normal pH without the presence of $PEEP_i$ or more commonly auto-PEEP or air trapping. In patients with chronic hypercarbia at baseline who have acute-on-chronic hypercapnic respiratory failure from a COPD exacerbation, the above strategy is reasonable with the goal of normalizing pH to 7.4 *regardless* of what the corresponding $PaCO_2$ is. Improper correction of $PaCO_2$ to "normal" value of 40 in these groups of patients will result in loss of serum bicarbonate compensation and will result in the inability to wean and liberate from the ventilator.

Once the initial ventilator mode and settings are chosen, two ventilator maneuvers should be performed to obtain dynamic data to help with ventilator adjustment: plateau pressure ($P_{PLATEAU}$) and auto-PEEP. $P_{PLATEAU}$ can be measured using an inspiratory hold maneuver, which measures the alveolar pressure at end inspiration without any dynamic airflow. A goal of less than 30 cm H_2O is crucial to avoid alveolar overdistention and lung injury (Fig. 1).

After $P_{PLATEAU}$ is measured and adjustments are made, the next ventilator maneuver to perform is expiratory hold to evaluate for auto-PEEP or $PEEP_i$. $PEEP_i$ is the notion that there is trapped volume of air in a closed-loop circuit that has not been fully exhaled prior to the next breath being initiated (Fig. 2). Failure to recognize the

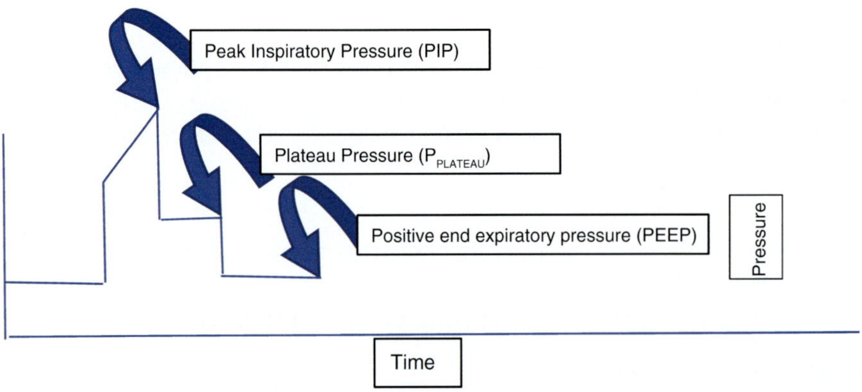

Fig. 1 Pressure over time graph of patients in assist-control, volume-control (ACVC) mode

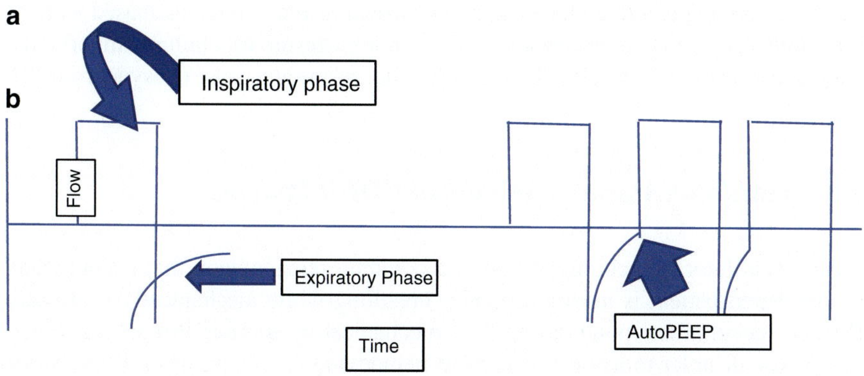

Fig. 2 Flow over time graph of patients in assist-control, volume-control (ACVC) mode. B. Auto-PEEP expiratory phase in flow over time graph does not return to baseline prior to the next inspiratory cycle

presence of auto-PEEP will result in additive increase in intrathoracic pressure resulting in hemodynamic decompensation secondary to lack of venous return as well as worsening hypercarbic respiratory failure and acidosis, which will ultimately precipitate in right ventricular (RV) dysfunction.

Correction of auto-PEEP entails maximizing exhalation time for patients with acute obstructive lung disease being supported on the ventilator. There are multiple interventions that allows for prolonged exhalation in a ventilated patient, i.e., increasing expiratory time (Te). These includes decreasing inspiratory time (T_i), reducing RR, or decreasing TV. The most effective strategy to allow for prolonged exhalation in patients with auto-PEEP is to reduce RR. This completely eliminates respiratory cycle allowing for natural prolongation of exhalation time. Reduce RR by 1–2 breaths/minute and perform expiratory hold to ensure resolution of auto-PEEP. Increased sedation to blunt intrinsic respiratory drive may be required once paralytic agents used to perform endotracheal intubation are metabolized. Episodically disconnecting the patient from the ventilator may additionally be useful to exhale trapped gas causing intrinsic PEEP until adequate elimination of auto-PEEP.

If there is no auto-PEEP present, a gradual increase in RR is warranted to allow for adequate V_E and correction of the acute component of the patient's respiratory acidosis. This allows for an appropriate balance between minimizing dynamic hyperinflation with adequate V_E that results in adequate gas exchange to target the ventilated patient back to his/her baseline $PaCO_2$ and pH.

Once paralytics used during rapid sequence intubation (RSI) wear off, it is important to ensure that the patient receives adequate sedation during the acute phase of critical disease to allow for appropriate patient-ventilator synchrony, thereby permitting initiation of appropriate ventilator strategies for obstructive lung disease patients on the ventilator. Additionally, this allows sufficient time for therapeutics such as antibiotics, corticosteroids, and bronchodilators to take effect, which serves to correct the altered lung mechanics which resulted in the increased work of breathing responsible for the presence of hypercarbic respiratory failure. Importantly, undersedation can result in ineffective triggering, a common cause of asynchrony [2].

1.3 Ventilator Alarm in Ventilated COPD Patients

Patient-ventilator asynchrony (PVA) is a common phenomenon that occurs when the intubated patient is having difficulty breathing while mechanically ventilated. PVA can occur at any point during their mechanical ventilation. Prompt identification is key in order to avoid and prevent hemodynamic compromise. PVA can be broken down into two broad categories: patient related and ventilator related (Table 1). Once PVA has been identified in a mechanically ventilated patient, the first thing to consider is to disconnect the patient from the ventilator and perform bag-valve mask (BVM) ventilation being cognizant of excessive volume and rate of breath administered. If distress resolves once BVM is initiated, the cause of PVA is likely to be ventilator related. If patient distress does not resolve once BVM is initiated, the cause of PVA is likely secondary to patient-related issues. Once a patient-related issue is identified, the next step would be to pass a suction catheter down the endotracheal tube (ETT) to evaluate for airway patency. Chest auscultation, evaluation of airway pressure, bedside thoracic ultrasound, and portable chest X-ray should be sequentially performed to further delineate the etiology of patient-related cause of PVA [3].

1.4 High-Pressure Alarm in Ventilated COPD Patients

One of the common but concerning ventilator alarms in ventilated COPD patients is the high-pressure alarm. The high-pressure alarm is usually set to be around 10 cm H_2O above PIP. When this is reached, this results in termination of inspiration to prevent further increase and rise in intrathoracic pressure. Common scenarios that

Table 1 Common patient- and ventilator-related problems causing patient-ventilator asynchrony in patients with acute COPD on mechanical ventilation [3]

Common causes of patient-ventilator asynchrony in COPD	
Patient related	Ventilator related
Bronchospasm	Circuit leak or disconnection
Secretion and mucous plugging	Ventilator malfunction
Anxiety/pain	Inappropriate trigger sensitivity
Pneumothorax	Inappropriate PEEP setting
Hyperinflation	Inappropriate flow setting
Acute airway problem (tube migration, kinking)	Inadequate ventilator support setting

Table 2 Common high airway pressure alarm in ventilated COPD patients [11]

Common high-pressure alarm in ventilated COPD patients		
Airway	Lung parenchyma	Ventilator
Secretion	Pneumothorax	Circuit obstruction
ETT obstruction (biting, kinking)	Bronchospasm	Ventilator malfunction
ETT migration	Interstitial edema	Water accumulation in circuit
	Patient-ventilator asynchrony	Valve malfunction

Table 3 Common low airway pressure alarm in ventilated COPD patients [11]

Common low-pressure alarm in ventilated COPD patients	
Airway	Ventilator
ETT-ventilator disconnect	Circuit leak
Pilot balloon malfunction	Ventilator malfunction
ETT balloon malfunction	Inspiratory circuit leak
ETT balloon malposition	Expiratory circuit leak
Bronchopleural fistula	Ventilator valve leak

trigger high-pressure alarm are briefly summarized in Table 2. Given that high-pressure alarm ends inspiration cycle prematurely, proper identification is crucial to differentiate pathologic vs. physiologic. Clinicians must work through the pathologic causes of high pressure alarm (Table 2). Once all pathologic causes are ruled out, physiologic causes of high pressure alarm can then be addressed, temporarily by increasing high pressure threshold alarm and decreasing flow rate while therapeutics takes effect, which will require time. Failure to recognize pathologic causes of high pressure alarm with subsequent increase in threshold alarm will result in iatrogenesis such as pneumothoraces. On the flip side, inaction when it comes to high pressure alarm will results in inadequate V_E resulting in worsening respiratory acidosis.

1.5 Low-Pressure Alarm in Ventilated COPD Patients

Low-pressure alarm is almost always a consequence of a circuit leak somewhere. If there is inadequate V_E, the patient should be disconnected from the ventilator and BVM should be initiated. Common causes of low-pressure alarm are summarized in Table 3.

1.6 Liberation from Mechanical Ventilation

Once the acute disease process requiring mechanical ventilation has been reversed, the patient should be evaluated for the possibility of liberation from mechanical ventilation. This process involves the implementation of a spontaneous breathing

Table 4 Criteria for initiation of SBT and ventilator liberation [12, 13]

Criteria for spontaneous breathing trial	Criteria for ventilator liberation
Reversal of underlying process	Ability to maintain airway patency
Can generate spontaneous breath	Intact cough and gag
Correction of acidosis	Management of secretion
$FiO_2 < 50\%$	Following complex command
PEEP < or equal to 8	

trial (SBT), which has proven in clinical trials to represent the most expeditious transition of patients to successful extubation. Many approaches to an SBT have been advocated, often utilizing some form of partial ventilatory support through the ventilator with pressure-support ventilation, with or without continuous positive airway pressure (CPAP), although breathing spontaneously without the ventilator via a t-piece adapter also has its proponents. A recent trial demonstrated the superiority of a 30-minute SBT using a PSV of 8 cm H_2O when compared to a 2-h T-piece trial in the percentage of patients successfully extubated [4]. Criteria prior to initiating patients on PS SBT are outlined in Table 4. Setting the level of pressure support for SBT should not exceed the airway resistance of the ETT and the circuit. This results in allowing the patient to breathe spontaneously as close to "physiologic" as possible in order to have a true evaluation if failure during SBT occurs.

Once a patient successfully passes an SBT, Table 4 outlines some criteria separate from the criteria for SBT in order to be able to safely remove the ETT. No one particular criterion is absolute prior to extubation. A holistic approach evaluating a patient's ability to maintain a patent airway, minute ventilation, and hemodynamics should take place that is guided by the criteria listed in Table 4.

1.7 Postextubation Management

There is good evidence for the transition from mechanical ventilation to noninvasive ventilation (NIV) for patients with chronic hypercarbia postextubation [5, 6]. It has been found to decrease the work of breathing in a "stepwise" fashion, decrease the likelihood of reintubation, decrease the incidence of ventilator-associated pneumonia (VAP), improve mortality, and shorten the ICU length of stay. Initiation of NIV requires the ability of the patient to maintain his/her own airway, awake following commands, as well as the ability to generate V_E spontaneously. Heated high-flow nasal cannula provides a low level of CPAP, which can partially unload hyperinflation in COPD patients and thereby decrease work of breathing can be considered as an alternative or additive to NIV in the chronic hypercapnic COPD patient after extubation, particularly if NIV is not tolerated [7]. Therapeutics such as antibiotics, steroids, bronchodilators, and diuretics should be continued, and the patient should continue to have optimization of their nutritional status as well as exercise to prevent critical illness weakness.

2 Status Asthmaticus

2.1 *Objective of Ventilator Management*

Ventilator management for patients with status asthmaticus is one of the *most* challenging situations in critical care. It comes with increased risk of complications as well as morbidity. This is because of increased R_{AW} as a result of bronchospasm, increased secretions that lead to increased work of breathing which leads to increased air trapping, dynamic hyperinflation, and lung injury. Intubation in status asthmaticus should be avoided whenever clinically feasible. Some clinical triggers to intubate status asthmaticus are listed in Table 5. The goal of ventilator management for status asthmaticus is not only to oxygenate the patient but, importantly, to promote exhalation time in order to avoid hypotension and barotrauma, in order to allow for sufficient time to reverse the increased R_{AW} with therapeutics while preventing barotrauma. This requires a fine balance between effective V_E and adequate exhalation to prevent air trapping and barotrauma [8].

2.2 *Mode of Ventilation and Initial Setting*

Similar to COPD, patients with status asthmaticus should be ventilated initially with AC-VC to ensure adequate tidal volume and minute ventilation. Most patients with status asthmaticus will require heavy sedation, often with neuromuscular blockade, during the acute phase of their critical illness to prevent patient-ventilator asynchrony and air trapping. Minute ventilation should be set low to start with the focus on maximum exhalation time to prevent air trapping or auto-PEEP. This is counter-intuitive particularly if the patient has acute hypercarbic respiratory failure or the clinician is intent on "matching" pre- and post-intubation minute ventilation. Patients with status asthmaticus have increased R_{AW} secondary to edema, bronchospasm, and secretion. This leads to dynamic hyperinflation as a consequence of increased R_{AW}. Dynamic hyperinflation in status asthmaticus has been proven to be detrimental and a major determinant of barotrauma and cardiovascular collapse [9]. This is a result of additive end-inspiratory volume (V_{EI}), essentially "trapped gas," that is unable to be exhaled as a consequence of severe airway obstruction in status asthmaticus (Fig. 3). Factors such as VE greater than 13 L/min as well as V_{EI} greater

Table 5 Some clinical indications to intubate status asthmaticus [14]

Clinical indication to mechanically ventilate status asthmaticus	
Respiratory arrest	Bradypnea
Respiratory fatigue with pseudo-normalization of respiratory alkalosis	Altered mental status
Acute hypercapnic respiratory failure	Ongoing respiratory distress despite maximum medical therapy

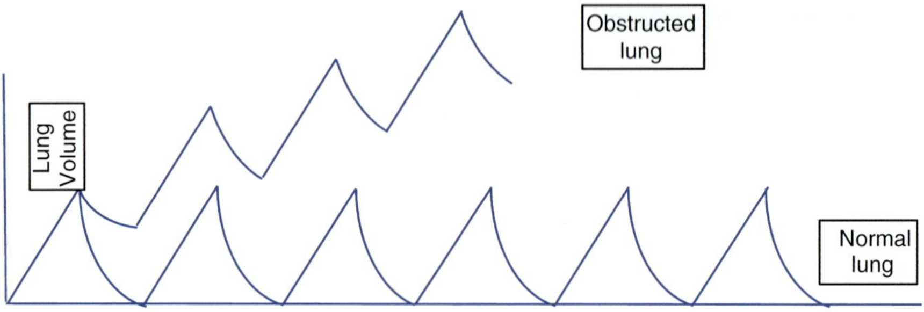

Fig. 3 Volume over time graph demonstrating dynamic hyperinflation with additive volume at end inspiration (Vei) in patients with status asthmaticus

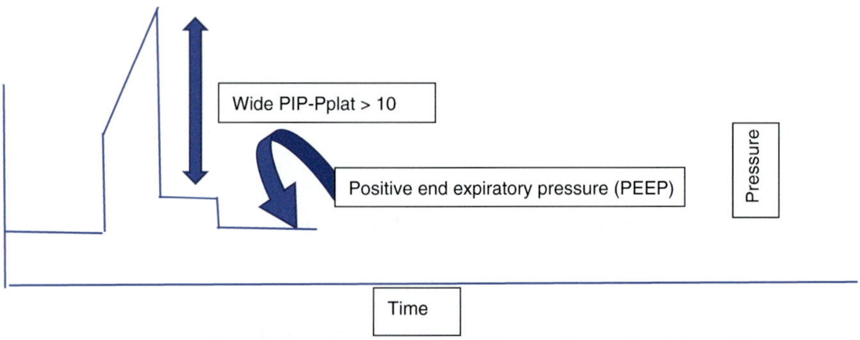

Fig. 4 Pressure over time graph of patients in assist-control, volume-control (ACVC) mode with status asthmaticus. Wide PIP-Pplat suggestive of high R_{AW} with a normal lung compliance

than 1.4 L have been demonstrated to be predictive of barotrauma in patients with status asthmaticus on mechanical ventilation [9].

To start, set the initial RR at 8 with a tidal volume of 6 cc/kg of the patient's ideal body weight (IBW) and a fast inspiratory time (<1 s) and flow (80–100 L/min). This strategy goes with "get the volume in as fast as possible so the rest of the time is spent on exhalation" with an average inspiratory:expiratory ratio of ~1:5. This will result in an elevated PIP as a consequence of both the pathologies of increased R_{AW} and ventilator setting. This is *ok* since in most scenarios, alveolar, $P_{PLATEAU}$, pressure will be low, <30 cm H_2O, suggesting the absence of a significant risk of barotrauma (Fig. 4).

An end-expiratory hold should be performed to evaluate for air trapping or auto-PEEP. Adjustment to eliminate auto-PEEP by further decreasing RR and/or tidal volume from the initial setting is similar to above and is *crucial* given the additive effect this have on the patient's hemodynamic coupled with the severe degree of bronchospasm and the elevated R_{AW}. The goal of mechanical ventilation in asthma is to oxygenate the patient and to avoid barotrauma due to trapped gas, which historically had resulted in a significant mortality in these patients. Avoiding a Pplat >30 cm H_2O by maximizing exhalation via sedation, a low tidal volume, and a high-flow delivery of ventilator gas are helpful in achieving this goal. Additionally, neuromuscular blockade with permissive hypercapnia, sometimes for several days, may be required. Hypercapnia should be permitted in the acute phase with slow normalization over days as disese process is improving with therapy. Be aware of hypercarbia in pregnant patients, patients with elevated intracranial pressure and patients with underlying right ventricular dysfunction. Sodium bicarbonate administration may be required to achieve a satisfactory pH (7.20) in this setting.

It is important to keep the amount of applied PEEP minimal in these patients (perhaps no greater than a PEEP of 5 cm H_2O), as titration of PEEP in status asthmaticus patients can precipitate worsening alveolar pressure, causing overdistention, iatrogenic hypoxia, and barotrauma [10]. If an intubated patient with status asthmaticus is spontaneously breathing on the ventilator with auto-PEEP and cannot trigger each attempted breath as a result (i.e., "locked out"), increasing the PEEP to ~80% of auto-PEEP can help a patient trigger the ventilator with each attempted inhalation. However, if this strategy results in a significant increase in PIP, additional sedation and paralytics might be warranted.

FiO_2 should be titrated to a goal of SpO_2 of ~90% or a PaO_2 of ~55 mmHg. Ensure ongoing dynamic assessment of hemodynamic and cardiac function. One should be cautious with aggressive fluid resuscitation in these group of patients as parenchymal edema can compound the clinical picture if a patient subsequently becomes acutely hypoxic (barotrauma vs. lung water vs. pulmonary embolism).

2.3 Ventilator Alarm in Ventilated Status Asthmaticus

Common ventilator alarms between patients with COPD and status asthmaticus are similar and are reviewed in Table 2. Close attention should be paid in status asthmaticus to the high airway pressure alarm given that they are at increased risk for barotrauma and pneumothorax. However, plateau pressure is more closely associated with barotrauma in this setting as peak pressure may be less indicative of transalveolar pressure, the actual source of barotrauma. Hence, this needs to be ruled out from the disease course of status asthmaticus in which increased airway resistance yields the activation of the high airway pressure alarm resultant from the rapid flow of ventilator gas in an attempt to shorten inhalation time and allow for maximum exhalation. Steps to evaluate high airway pressure alarm are highlighted above. The use of BVM, bedside ultrasound, and portable chest X-ray will help in delineating the etiology of high-pressure alarm.

2.4 High-Pressure Alarm in Ventilated Status Asthmaticus

High-pressure alarming is not uncommon in patients with status asthmaticus on the ventilator, owing to the considerations outlined in the above section. PIP threshold will be reached just from the initial ventilator setting compounded by increased R_{AW} from bronchospasm as well as secretions. The key is to be able to astutely distinguish when high-pressure alarm in status asthmaticus is pathologic and harmful to the patient. Ongoing, serial evaluation is important while therapeutics is employed. Slow liberation of initial ventilator settings can be employed once there is a notable improvement in PIP, which suggests improvement in bronchospasm and R_{AW}.

2.5 Liberation from Mechanical Ventilation

Liberation from mechanical ventilation in patients with status asthmaticus is no different than liberation from mechanical ventilation in COPD patients. Daily SBT should be employed once the criteria for SBT are met (Table 4). CPAP/PS should be the mainstay of SBT mode, setting the level of support no more than to overcome airway resistance of ETT and ventilator circuit to allow spontaneous respiration as close to "physiologic" as possible. In certain group of patients who still have some degree of air trapping and auto-PEEP, ensuring that their set PEEP matches ~80% of their intrinsic PEEP is helpful to ensure that the patient is able to trigger the ventilator on a spontaneous mode. This particular scenario should be rare since the majority of patients at this point will have resolution of their bronchospasm.

2.6 Postextubation Management

There is no data supporting the use of NIV to transition patients from mechanical ventilation who have recovered from status asthmaticus. Therapeutics such as antibiotics, steroids, bronchodilators, and diuretics should be continued, and postextubation patients should continue to have their nutrition and strength optimized as they transition from critical care recovery.

2.7 Summary

Mechanical ventilation is required for obstructive lung disease patients who do not respond to medical management (asthma) or medical management plus NIV (COPD). The overarching goal is to correct and further minimize dynamic hyperinflation through reduction in minute ventilation, shortening inspiratory time, and increasing inspiratory flow rate and lung-protective tidal volume. This will ultimately result in some degree of permissive hypercapnia particularly in patients with status asthmaticus, which will correct over time with medical therapy. A brief summary of initial ventilator setting is outlined in Table 6. It is important to remember to individualize ventilator settings and adjust accordingly depending on the severity of obstructive lung disease process.

Table 6 Summary of initial ventilator setting for patients with obstructive lung pathology

Generic outline for initial ventilator settings		
	COPD	Status asthmaticus
Mode	VC	VC
Respiratory rate	8–10	8
Tidal volume	6 cc/kg of IBW to start	6 cc/kg of IBW to start
FiO_2	Target SpO_2 of 90%	Target SpO_2 of 90%
PEEP	5	5
Flow rate	80–100 L/min	80–100 L/min

References

1. Sethi JM, Siegel MD. Mechanical ventilation in chronic obstructive lung disease. Clin Chest Med. 2000;21:799.
2. Wit M, Pedram S, Best AM, Epstein S. Observational study of patient-ventilator asynchrony and relationship to sedation level. J Crit Care. 2009;24(1):74–80.
3. Tobin MJ. What should a clinician do when a patient 'fights the ventilator? Respir Care. 1991;36:395–406.
4. Subria C, Hernandez G, Vazquez A, et al. Effect of pressure support vs T-piece ventilation strategies during spontaneous breathing trials on successful extubation among patients receiving mechanical ventilation. JAMA. 2019;321(22):2175–82.
5. Hernandez G, Vaquero C, Colinas L, et al. Effect of postextubation high-flow nasal cannula vs noninvasive ventilation on reintubation and postextubation respiratory failure in high-risk patients. JAMA. 2016;316(15):1565–74.
6. Glossop AJ, Shephard N, Bryden DC, Mills GH. Non-invasive ventilation for weaning, avoiding reintubation after extubation and in the postoperative period: a meta-analysis. Br J Anaesth. 2012;109(3):305–14.
7. Hernandez G, Vaquero C, Colinas L, et al. Effect of postextubation high-flow nasal cannula vs noninvasive ventilation on reintubation and postextubation respiratory failure in high-risk patients: a randomized clinical trial. JAMA. 2016;316(15):1565–74.
8. Hallstrand TS, Fahy JV. Practical management of acute asthma in adults. Respir Care. 2002;47:171.
9. Williams TJ, Tuxen DV, Scheinkestel CD, et al. Risk factors for morbidity in mechanically ventilated patients with acute severe asthma. Am Rev Respir Dis. 1992;146(3):607–15.
10. Georgopoulos D, Kondili E, Prinianakis G. How to set the ventilator in asthma. Monaldi Arch Chest Dis. 2000;55:74.
11. Cairo JM, Pilbeam SP: Mosby's respiratory care equipment, 7, St. Louis, MI, Mosby; 2004
12. Mcintyre NR, Cook DJ, et al. ACCP/AARC/SCCM task force: evidence-based guidelines for weaning and discontinuing mechanical ventilator support. Chest. 2001;120(6):375S.
13. AARC Clinical Practice Guideline: Removal of the endotracheal tube. Respir Care. 2007;52:81.
14. Demoule A, Brochard L, Dres M, et al. How to ventilate obstructive and asthmatic patients. Intensive Care Med. 2020;46:2436.

Mechanical Ventilation Strategies for Patients on Extracorporeal Membrane Oxygenation Support

Alexis K. Nickols and Pauline K. Park

1 Introduction

Mortality in acute respiratory distress syndrome (ARDS) remains disappointingly high. In recent international series, crude mortality for severe ARDS (PaO_2/FiO_2 ratio < 100) [1] remained 37–48.6% [2–4]. In this subset of patients, oxygenation and ventilation requirements can exceed the limits of conventional mechanical ventilation, risking further complications from ventilator-induced lung injury (VILI).

Extracorporeal membrane oxygenation (ECMO) can provide additional respiratory support via an extracorporeal circuit with a centrifugal pump propelling blood flow over an external membrane oxygenator. ECMO is primarily employed in three scenarios: (1) refractory hypoxia, (2) refractory hypercarbia with respiratory acidosis, and (3) severely diminished compliance, with concern for worsening VILI. Oxygen delivery by the ECMO circuit varies with the oxygen-carrying capacity of the blood and the volume of blood flow across the membrane. Carbon dioxide clearance varies with the sweep gas flow rate as well as the volume of blood flow past the sweep gas. By adjusting these parameters, respiratory gas exchange can be managed via the ECMO circuit, thereby reducing reliance on toxic mechanical ventilator support.

A. K. Nickols
Department of Surgery, Division of Trauma, Surgical Critical Care, University of Kentucky, Lexington, KY, USA
e-mail: alexis.nickols@uky.edu

P. K. Park (✉)
Department of Surgery, Division of Acute Care Surgery, University of Michigan, Ann Arbor, MI, USA
e-mail: parkpk@med.umich.edu

J. Hidalgo et al. (eds.), *Personalized Mechanical Ventilation*,
https://doi.org/10.1007/978-3-031-14138-6_24

Use of venovenous ECMO has increased substantially since the first report of ECMO support of adult respiratory failure in 1972 [5]. Clinical adoption has been accelerated by device improvements, two randomized controlled clinical trials suggesting the benefit in severe ARDS (CESAR [6] and EOLIA [7]), and early clinical success during the H1N1 and COVID pandemics. During the last decade, 4.4–6.6% of adult severe ARDS patients received ECMO support [3, 4]. As of 2021, the Extracorporeal Life Support Organization (ELSO) registry reported 43,072 adult respiratory support cases in over 500 centers, with an overall survival rate of 58% [8].

As ECMO has become an accepted rescue strategy for severe ARDS, attention has turned towards optimizing mechanical ventilation during extracorporeal support. The ideal targets and modes remain incompletely understood, and ventilator management has been identified as one of the ten top priorities for ongoing ECMO research [9]. This chapter summarizes recommendations based on the available evidence.

2 Ventilator Management Prior to ECMO Initiation

Consensus recommendations place ECMO as a rescue therapy in severe ARDS, to be considered after conventional critical care measures have been exhausted. As ECMO does not treat underlying lung injury, the decision for cannulation balances the potential benefits of reducing toxic ventilator support against the risks of complications from sustained extracorporeal bypass.

In severe ARDS, prompt identification of the underlying cause should be sought. Lung-protective ventilation [10], with tidal volumes (V_T) of 6 mL/kg predicted body weight (PBW) and controlled plateau pressures (P_{plat}) <30 mm H_2O, remains the mainstay of ARDS ventilator management. Other adjuvants should be considered in a stepwise fashion. Higher levels of positive end-expiratory pressure (PEEP) are associated with lower mortality in moderate-severe ARDS [11]. Evidence also supports the use of early prone positioning in moderate-severe ARDS [12], and a recent meta-analysis suggested the benefit in continuing prone positioning after ECMO has been initiated [13]. Early neuromuscular blockade, aimed at reducing ventilator dyssynchrony and minimizing work of breathing, is frequently used in this setting, although no mortality advantage was seen in a recent large, randomized trial [14]. Inhaled pulmonary vasodilators and judicious fluid management strategies are additional strategies that can be considered. Once a patient fails conventional measures, evaluation of candidacy for ECMO is reasonable.

ELSO guidelines for initiating support for ARDS include (1) severe hypoxemic respiratory failure with sustained PaO_2/FiO_2 ratio < 80, following, in the absence of contraindications, a trial of prone positioning, and (2) severe hypercapnic respiratory failure with a pH < 7.25 with $PaCO_2 \geq 60$ mm Hg after optimal conventional management, including a respiratory rate of 35 breaths per minute and plateau pressure ≤ 30 mm Hg [15]. The only absolute contraindication to extracorporeal support is the presence of an irreversible medical condition; relative contraindications include neurologic and anticoagulation risks, older age, immunosuppression, and mechanical ventilation for more than 7 days with P_{plat} > 30 mm H_2O and $FiO_2 > 90\%$.

3 Ventilator Management on ECMO

Once ECMO is initiated to support oxygenation and CO_2 clearance effectively, ventilator support can be reduced. Prospective randomized trials of the optimal "dose" of mechanical ventilation while on ECMO are difficult to conduct and, to date, are limited. It is not clear that evidence in less severe cases can be generalized to cases of previously unsurvivable lung injury or even if specific variables can be targeted by a precision medicine approach. Additional complexity is present as short-term surrogate outcomes are not clearly correlated with longer term outcomes of morbidity and mortality. "Best practice" mechanical ventilator strategies on ECMO thus are generally consensus based, and research priorities extend from our knowledge of ventilation in less severe cases.

3.1 Historical Management, Observational Studies

Ventilator management on ECMO historically has focused on the reduction of ventilator-delivered airway pressures and FiO_2. For many years, ELSO advocated a set "lung rest" strategy of pressure-controlled ventilation with FiO_2 0.30, P_{plat} 20 cm H_2O, PEEP 10 cm H_2O, respiratory rate 10 breaths per minute, and inspiratory:expiratory ratio at 1:1 [15]. Oxygenation goals may be titrated to SvO_2 as a more meaningful reflection of adequate oxygenation than PaO_2. Nevertheless, in a 2014 international survey, only 27% of ECMO centers maintained explicit ventilation protocols for patients on ECMO, with 77% reporting "lung rest" as the goal and 9% stressing "lung recruitment" [16].

Observational studies recording ventilator settings before and after ECMO initiation predictably demonstrate reductions in ventilator settings following cannulation (Table 1) [17–19]. Notably, on average, V_T and minute ventilation (V_E) were cut by one-third to one-half, P_{plat} kept below 25 cm H_2O, and driving pressure (ΔP) reduced from around 20 cm H_2O to 15 cm H_2O. One retrospective study suggested that higher PEEP levels during the first 3 days of ECMO support were independently associated with lower mortality; however, in a follow-up multicenter prospective observational study (LIFEGARDS [18]), mechanical ventilation settings during ECMO did not impact prognosis. In this series, the cohort included medium- to high-volume centers that had already largely adopted a strategy of

Table 1 Change in mechanical ventilator settings following ECMO initiation: Ventilator management variables pre- and post-initiation of VV-ECMO from three large multi-institutional observational studies. All variables are reduced towards lung-protective ventilation following cannulation

	Pre-cannulation			Post-cannulation		
	Schmidt et al. [17]	LIFEGARDS [18]	Serpa Neto et al. [19]	Schmidt et al. [17]	LIFEGARDS [18]	Serpa Neto et al. [19]
FiO_2 (%)	N/A	100	90	N/A	50	70
V_T (ml/kg PBW)	6.3	6.4	6.0	3.9	3.7	4.0
P_{plat} (cm H_2O)	32.2	32	31.1	26.4	24	26.2
ΔP (cm H_2O)	19.0	20	17.7	13.7	14	13.7
PEEP (cm H_2O)	13	12	13.7	12	11	12.9
RR (breaths/min)	N/A	26	21.9	N/A	14	17.8
V_E (L/min)	8.8	N/A	9.1	3.6	N/A	5.0

Abbreviations: FiO_2 fraction of inspired oxygen, V_T tidal volume, *PBW* predicted body weight, P_{plat} plateau pressure, *cm* H_2O centimeters of water, ΔP driving pressure, *PEEP* positive end-expiratory pressure, *RR* respiratory rate, V_E minute ventilation, *L/min* liters per minute

ultraprotective lung ventilation (<4 cc/kg PBW). In a patient-level meta-analysis using a time-dependent model of ventilator settings during the first 3 days of ECMO support for refractory hypoxemia, ΔP, rather than P_{plat} or PEEP, was identified as the only ventilator setting showing an independent association with in-hospital mortality [19].

3.2 *Lung-Protective Ventilation Remains the Standard*

In the face of limited evidence, reducing ventilator settings to maintain lung-protective ventilation by controlling V_T to 6 ml/kg PBW and $P_{plat} < 30$ cm H_2O should be considered as a minimum goal once ECMO support is initiated. Suggested ventilator settings and targets are detailed in Fig. 1. In cases where pre-ECMO mechanical ventilation is at extremely high levels, titration to lower settings may be spaced over 24 h, based on patient status. Primary management of oxygen delivery and respiratory acidosis should be titrated through the ECMO circuit to give priority to achieving lung-protective ventilator settings. As the underlying lung compliance remains unchanged by the circuit, decreased ventilator support may lead to complete lung atelectasis or "white out" on chest X-ray. This is managed expectantly, with the anticipation that aeration will return once lung compliance improves. Tidal

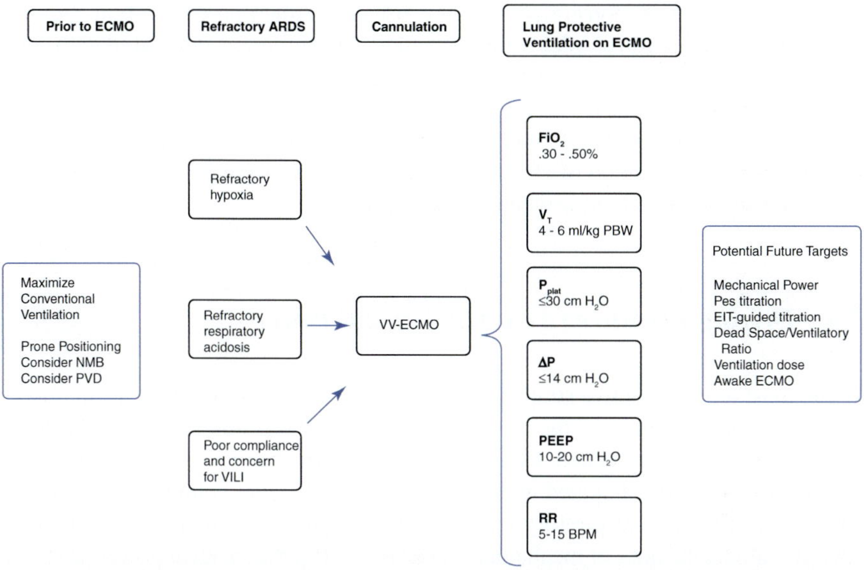

Fig. 1 Mechanical ventilation on ECMO: Flow diagram illustrating the current approach to and targets for mechanical ventilation on ECMO. Abbreviations: *ECMO* extracorporeal membrane oxygenation, *ARDS* acute respiratory distress syndrome, *NMB* neuromuscular blockade, *PVR* pulmonary vasodilators, *VILI* ventilator-induced lung injury, *VV-ECMO* venovenous extracorporeal membrane oxygenation, FiO_2 fraction of inspired oxygen, V_T tidal volume, *PBW* predicted body weight, P_{plat} plateau pressure, *cm* H_2O centimeters of water, ΔP driving pressure, *PEEP* positive end-expiratory pressure, *RR* respiratory rate, P_{es} esophageal pressure, *EIT* electrical impedance tomography

volumes may remain well below 6 mL/kg PBW during ECMO; native lung recovery may be more easily identified on pressure control ventilator modes, by observing for steady increases in tidal volumes on stable pressure settings. Forced recruitment maneuvers are discouraged, as without increasing the primary ventilator setting, reinflation will only be transient.

3.3 Ultraprotective Lung Ventilation, Promise Unrealized

Given that the overarching goal of protective lung ventilation is avoidance of VILI rather than gas exchange, intentional ventilation with tidal volumes less than 4 ml/kg and Pplat ≤25 cm H_2O ("ultraprotective" lung ventilation) has been explored as a strategy on ECMO. Initial preclinical and pilot human studies demonstrated reduced injury biomarkers with apneic ventilation [20, 21], and the SUPERNOVA trial demonstrated the feasibility of using lower flow extracorporeal devices to remove excess CO_2 and facilitate ultralow tidal volume ventilation [22]. Nevertheless, the recent multicenter randomized, prospective REST trial [23] in acute hypoxemic respiratory failure demonstrated that the use of extracorporeal carbon dioxide removal to facilitate lower tidal volume mechanical ventilation, compared with conventional lung-protective ventilation, did not significantly reduce 90-day mortality. The study was terminated early for suggestion of increased adverse events with extracorporeal support. While early termination resulted in the trial being underpowered for determination of efficacy, an ultraprotective strategy cannot be recommended over standard lung-protective ventilation.

3.4 Driving Pressure (ΔP), Mechanical Power

While most lung-protective strategies have focused on setting V_T and P_{plat}, in observational mediation analysis, the driving pressure or ΔP was observed to be the pressure variable most associated with mortality [24]. Mechanical power, a summary variable that can be calculated at the bedside based on tidal volume, driving pressure, flow, PEEP, and respiratory rate, has been proposed as a more complete measure to evaluate the dose of mechanical ventilation [25]. Mechanical power has been associated with mortality during controlled mechanical ventilation in ARDS, but a simpler model, using only the ΔP and RR, was an equivalent predictor of mortality, with the ΔP accounting for the majority of the effect [26]. Clinical trials testing the efficacy of manipulating drive pressure as a therapeutic maneuver are in progress; in the meantime, maintaining a ΔP goal of ≤14 mm H_2O is reasonable.

3.5 Future Directions in Mechanical Ventilation

Hypotheses considering optimal ventilation on ECMO parallel ongoing research on improving mechanical ventilation in general. In particular, the role of spontaneous ventilation and its impact on lung recruitment and contribution to lung injury remain a critical area for study, particularly in the setting of decreased sedation. Transpulmonary pressure measurement may allow individualized titration of PEEP [27] to minimize atelectrauma, particularly in high-BMI patients. Electrical impedance tomography has been proposed as a means to visualize heterogeneously collapsed lung regions to titrate ventilator recruitment on ECMO [28]. The impact of other ventilatory variables, particularly in long-term ECMO support, remains incompletely studied. Proposed targets include inverse ratio ventilation and inspiratory flows, dead space and ventilatory ratio, dose of ventilation over time, impact on right ventricular function, and short-term surrogate outcomes.

3.6 Awake ECMO/Early Extubation

The concept of reducing ventilator support can be logically extended to removing the ventilator entirely prior to discontinuing ECMO. With the advent of single-site cannulation (either bicaval or pulmonary arterial), aggressive reduction of sedation, early mobilization, and even early extubation with sole reliance on extracorporeal support are feasible. A single-center series demonstrated excellent results using this strategy, with intentionally lower sedation, low tracheostomy rate, and high survival to hospital discharge [29]. Propensity-matched analysis suggested benefits to this in both COVID and non-COVID cohorts [30]. As a cautionary note, an even more forward strategy of initiating ECMO *instead* of intubation for mechanical ventilation led to an increase in adverse events in the ECMO-only arm [31]. The contrasting results highlight the need for ongoing meticulous research to identify the patients most likely to benefit.

3.7 Ventilation Strategy During Lung Recovery and ECMO Weaning

As native lung recovery proceeds, systemic oxygenation and $PaCO_2$ will spontaneously improve without increases in ECMO blood flow, sweep gas flow rate, or hemoglobin. With improvement in pulmonary compliance, V_T will begin to increase spontaneously on stable pressure control settings. The development of higher V_T and lower driving pressures over time is, not surprisingly, associated with better outcomes [18]. Extracorporeal support can then be weaned in a stepwise fashion, by

Table 2 Ventilator weaning on ECMO: Goal ventilator settings and physiologic evaluation prior to decannulation

	Trial settings	Physiologic goals
Oxygenation	$FiO_2 < 60\%$ $V_T < 6$ ml/kg PBW $P_{Plat} < 28$ cm H_2O PEEP <10 cm H_2O For non-intubated patients: $PaO_2 > 70$ on no more than moderate supplemental O_2 (6 LPM NC or face mask, <40 L/min, FiO_2 30% HHFNC)	$PaO_2 > 70$ mm Hg
Ventilation	Comfortable and able to meet ventilatory demand without excessive work of breathing	$PaCO_2 \leq 60$ pH ≥7.25 RR ≤35 BPM V_E 8–12 L/min
Imaging		Improved CXR appearance

Abbreviations: *FiO_2* fraction of inspired oxygen, *V_T* tidal volume, *PBW* predicted body weight, *P_{plat}* plateau pressure, *cm H_2O* centimeters of water, *PEEP* positive end-expiratory pressure, *PaO_2* partial pressure of oxygen, *O_2* oxygen, *L/min* liters per minute, *NC* nasal cannula, *HHFNC* heated high-flow nasal cannula, *$PaCO_2$* partial pressure of carbon dioxide, *RR* respiratory rate, *V_E* minute ventilation decreasing circuit flow and sweep gas to maintain a goal $SpO_2 > 92\%$ or $PaO_2 > 70$ mm Hg. During ECMO weaning, the ventilator should continue on lung-protective settings. Sweep gas can be titrated down in increments of 0.5–1 L, checking arterial blood gases at each reduction to maintain acceptable pH and work of breathing. It is important not to allow the pCO_2 to fall quickly, as rapid decreases are associated with increased adverse neurologic events [21]. A final trial of sweep gas for 2–3 h minimum is mandatory prior to decannulation [15, 32] (Table 2). Patients with larger tidal volume, heart rate, ventilatory ratio, and esophageal pressure variations during trial are less likely to achieve safe liberation from VV-ECMO [33]. If the trial is not tolerated, ECMO support can be reinstituted by resuming sweep gas flow, and a search for cause of failure can be conducted. Once sufficient native lung function has returned, decannulation can proceed.

4 Summary and Recommendations

"Lung rest" during ECMO in severe ARDS patients aims to prevent further VILI secondary to excessively high ventilator settings required to maintain oxygenation and ventilation through a noncompliant, diseased lung. By conducting all gas exchange extracorporeally and targeting lung-protective ventilator settings, venovenous ECMO permits support beyond conventional mechanical ventilation in severe ARDS patients with refractory hypoxemia and hypercarbia.

With the evidence currently available, once ECMO is initiated, a lung-protective strategy is favored, with intentional reduction of plateau pressures and drive pressures. It remains unclear if allowing complete lung collapse or maintaining aeration with higher PEEP offers advantages. Evidence from trials of ultraprotective ventilation during ECMO suggests that any additional benefit from further reduction in tidal volumes may not be sufficient to offset the risks of extracorporeal support. Similarly, awake extubation on ECMO presents an exciting new paradigm, permitting early ambulation and mobilization; however, multicenter follow-up is needed to ensure that adverse effects do not limit application. Further research on mechanical ventilation during ECMO will focus on clarifying the heterogeneity in patient selection and response to ventilation, identifying the most relevant targets for precision ventilator management and the short-term goals that correlate with long-term morbidity and mortality in these most critically ill patients.

References

1. Ranieri VM, Rubenfeld GD, Thompson BT, et al. Acute respiratory distress syndrome: the Berlin definition. JAMA. 2012;307(23):2526–33. https://doi.org/10.1001/jama.2012.5669.
2. Duan EH, Adhikari NKJ, D'Aragon F, et al. Management of acute respiratory distress syndrome and refractory hypoxemia. A multicenter observational study. Ann Am Thorac Soc. 2017;14(12):1818–26. https://doi.org/10.1513/AnnalsATS.201612-1042OC.

3. Bellani G, Laffey JG, Pham T, et al. Epidemiology, patterns of care, and mortality for patients with acute respiratory distress syndrome in intensive care units in 50 countries. JAMA. 2016;315(8):788–800. https://doi.org/10.1001/jama.2016.0291.
4. Qadir N, Bartz RR, Cooter ML, et al. Variation in early management practices in moderate-to-severe ARDS in the United States: the severe ARDS: generating evidence study. Chest. 2021;160(4):1304–15. https://doi.org/10.1016/j.chest.2021.05.047.
5. Hill JD, O'Brien TG, Murray JJ, et al. Prolonged extracorporeal oxygenation for acute post-traumatic respiratory failure (shock-lung syndrome). Use of the Bramson membrane lung. N Engl J Med. 1972;286(12):629–34. https://doi.org/10.1056/NEJM197203232861204.
6. Peek GJ, Mugford M, Tiruvoipati R, et al. Efficacy and economic assessment of conventional ventilatory support versus extracorporeal membrane oxygenation for severe adult respiratory failure (CESAR): a multicentre randomised controlled trial. Lancet. 2009;374(9698):1351–63. https://doi.org/10.1016/S0140-6736(09)61069-2.
7. Combes A, Hajage D, Capellier G, et al. Extracorporeal membrane oxygenation for severe acute respiratory distress syndrome. N Engl J Med24. 2018;378(21):1965–75. https://doi.org/10.1056/NEJMoa1800385.
8. Organization TELS. ELSO registry, International Summary; October, 2021. https://www.elso.org/Registry/InternationalSummaryandReports/InternationalSummary.aspx. Accessed 31 Mar 2022.
9. Combes A, Brodie D, Chen YS, et al. The ICM research agenda on extracorporeal life support. Intensive Care Med. 2017;43(9):1306–18. https://doi.org/10.1007/s00134-017-4803-3.
10. Brower RG, Matthay MA, Morris A, et al. Ventilation with lower tidal volumes as compared with traditional tidal volumes for acute lung injury and the acute respiratory distress syndrome. N Engl J Med. 2000;342(18):1301–8. https://doi.org/10.1056/NEJM200005043421801.
11. Briel M, Meade M, Mercat A, et al. Higher vs lower positive end-expiratory pressure in patients with acute lung injury and acute respiratory distress syndrome: systematic review and meta-analysis. JAMA. 2010;303(9):865–73. https://doi.org/10.1001/jama.2010.218.
12. Guérin C, Reignier J, Richard JC, et al. Prone positioning in severe acute respiratory distress syndrome. N Engl J Med. 2013;368(23):2159–68. https://doi.org/10.1056/NEJMoa1214103.
13. Papazian L, Schmidt M, Hajage D, et al. Effect of prone positioning on survival in adult patients receiving venovenous extracorporeal membrane oxygenation for acute respiratory distress syndrome: a systematic review and meta-analysis. Intensive Care Med. 2022;48(3):270–80. https://doi.org/10.1007/s00134-021-06604-x.
14. Moss M, Huang DT, Brower RG, et al. Early neuromuscular blockade in the acute respiratory distress syndrome. N Engl J Med. 2019;380(21):1997–2008. https://doi.org/10.1056/NEJMoa1901686.
15. Tonna JE, Abrams D, Brodie D, et al. Management of adult patients supported with venovenous extracorporeal membrane oxygenation (VV ECMO): guideline from the extracorporeal life support organization (ELSO). ASAIO J. 2021;67(6):601–10. https://doi.org/10.1097/MAT.0000000000001432.
16. Marhong JD, Telesnicki T, Munshi L, Del Sorbo L, Detsky M, Fan E. Mechanical ventilation during extracorporeal membrane oxygenation. An international survey. Ann Am Thorac Soc. 2014;11(6):956–61. https://doi.org/10.1513/AnnalsATS.201403-100BC.
17. Schmidt M, Stewart C, Bailey M, et al. Mechanical ventilation management during extracorporeal membrane oxygenation for acute respiratory distress syndrome: a retrospective international multicenter study. Crit Care Med. 2015;43(3):654–64. https://doi.org/10.1097/CCM.0000000000000753.
18. Schmidt M, Pham T, Arcadipane A, et al. Mechanical ventilation management during extracorporeal membrane oxygenation for acute respiratory distress syndrome. an international multicenter prospective cohort. Am J Respir Crit Care Med. 2019;200(8):1002–12. https://doi.org/10.1164/rccm.201806-1094OC.
19. Serpa Neto A, Schmidt M, Azevedo LC, et al. Associations between ventilator settings during extracorporeal membrane oxygenation for refractory hypoxemia and outcome in patients with acute respiratory distress syndrome: a pooled individual patient data analysis: mechanical ventilation during ECMO. Intensive Care Med. 2016;42(11):1672–84. https://doi.org/10.1007/s00134-016-4507-0.

20. Araos J, Alegria L, Garcia P, et al. Near-apneic ventilation decreases lung injury and fibroproliferation in an acute respiratory distress syndrome model with extracorporeal membrane oxygenation. Am J Respir Crit Care Med. 2019;199(5):603–12. https://doi.org/10.1164/rccm.201805-0869OC.
21. Cavayas YA, Munshi L, Del Sorbo L, Fan E. The early change in Pa. Am J Respir Crit Care Med. 2020;201(12):1525–35. https://doi.org/10.1164/rccm.202001-0023OC.
22. Combes A, Fanelli V, Pham T, Ranieri VM, investigators ESoICMTGatSoU-PlvwECRfN-OmtsAS. Feasibility and safety of extracorporeal CO. Intensive Care Med. 2019;45(5):592–600. https://doi.org/10.1007/s00134-019-05567-4.
23. McNamee JJ, Gillies MA, Barrett NA, et al. Effect of lower tidal volume ventilation facilitated by extracorporeal carbon dioxide removal vs standard care ventilation on 90-day mortality in patients with acute hypoxemic respiratory failure: the rest randomized clinical trial. JAMA. 2021;326(11):1013–23. https://doi.org/10.1001/jama.2021.13374.
24. Amato MB, Meade MO, Slutsky AS, et al. Driving pressure and survival in the acute respiratory distress syndrome. N Engl J Med. 2015;372(8):747–55. https://doi.org/10.1056/NEJMsa1410639.
25. Gattinoni L, Tonetti T, Cressoni M, et al. Ventilator-related causes of lung injury: the mechanical power. Intensive Care Med. 2016;42(10):1567–75. https://doi.org/10.1007/s00134-016-4505-2.
26. Costa ELV, Slutsky AS, Brochard LJ, et al. Ventilatory variables and mechanical power in patients with acute respiratory distress syndrome. Am J Respir Crit Care Med. 2021;204(3):303–11. https://doi.org/10.1164/rccm.202009-3467OC.
27. Beitler JR, Sarge T, Banner-Goodspeed VM, et al. Effect of titrating positive end-expiratory pressure (PEEP) with an esophageal pressure-guided strategy vs an empirical high PEEP-Fio2 strategy on death and days free from mechanical ventilation among patients with acute respiratory distress syndrome: a randomized clinical trial. JAMA. 2019;321(9):846–57. https://doi.org/10.1001/jama.2019.0555.
28. Franchineau G, Bréchot N, Lebreton G, et al. Bedside contribution of electrical impedance tomography to setting positive end-expiratory pressure for extracorporeal membrane oxygenation-treated patients with severe acute respiratory distress syndrome. Am J Respir Crit Care Med. 2017;196(4):447–57. https://doi.org/10.1164/rccm.201605-1055OC.
29. Gurnani PK, Michalak LA, Tabachnick D, Kotwas M, Tatooles AJ. Outcomes of extubated COVID and non-COVID patients receiving awake venovenous extracorporeal membrane oxygenation. ASAIO J. 2022;68(4):478–85. https://doi.org/10.1097/MAT.0000000000001632.
30. Mustafa AK, Joshi DJ, Alexander PJ, et al. Comparative propensity matched outcomes in severe COVID-19 respiratory failure-extracorporeal membrane oxygenation or maximum ventilation alone. Ann Surg. 2021;274(5):e388–94. https://doi.org/10.1097/SLA.0000000000005187.
31. Mang S, Reyher C, Mutlak H, et al. Awake extracorporeal membrane oxygenation for COVID-19-induced acute respiratory distress syndrome. Am J Respir Crit Care Med. 2022;205(7):847–51. https://doi.org/10.1164/rccm.202105-1189LE.
32. Bartlett RH. Physiology of gas exchange during ECMO for respiratory failure. J Intensive Care Med. 2017;32(4):243–8. https://doi.org/10.1177/0885066616641383.
33. Al-Fares AA, Ferguson ND, Ma J, et al. Achieving safe liberation during weaning from VV-ECMO in patients with severe ARDS: the role of tidal volume and inspiratory effort. Chest. 2021;160(5):1704–13. https://doi.org/10.1016/j.chest.2021.05.068.

Mechanical Ventilation in Neurocritical Care Patient

Jamil R. Dibu

1 Introduction

Patients with severe acute brain injury often require intubation to protect their airways, and mechanical ventilation due to respiratory failure secondary to numerous etiologies such as lung contusions, aspiration pneumonia, and acute respiratory distress syndrome [1, 2].

Patients admitted to the neurologic critical care units are prone to numerous pulmonary complications secondary to their primary etiology of brain injury, including their inability to protect the airway with secondary aspiration pneumonia resulting in hypoxic respiratory failure, neurogenic pulmonary edema such as in severe subarachnoid hemorrhage cases, and pulmonary embolism in hemiplegic and comatose patients. Hospital-acquired pneumonia, more specifically ventilator-associated pneumonia, can occur in up to 36% of traumatic brain injury patients [3] and up to 56.6% of acute ischemic stroke patients [4]. Common risk factors for ventilator-associated pneumonia include decreased level of consciousness and inability to cough and swallow [5]. These respiratory complications contribute to longer duration of mechanical ventilation, increased intensive care unit length of stay [3], and worse outcomes and lead to higher mortality in patients with acute brain injury [6].

Managing respiratory failure in a brain-injured patient is challenging as it requires deep understanding of the brain-lung pathophysiological interplay with the goal of mitigating secondary brain injury and treating concomitant respiratory failure (Fig. 1). Furthermore, these patients like any other critically ill patients will require

J. R. Dibu (✉)
Neurologic Critical Care Unit, Critical Care Institute, Cleveland Clinic Abu Dhabi, Abu Dhabi, UAE
e-mail: dibuj@clevelandclinicabudhabi.ae

J. Hidalgo et al. (eds.), *Personalized Mechanical Ventilation*,
https://doi.org/10.1007/978-3-031-14138-6_25

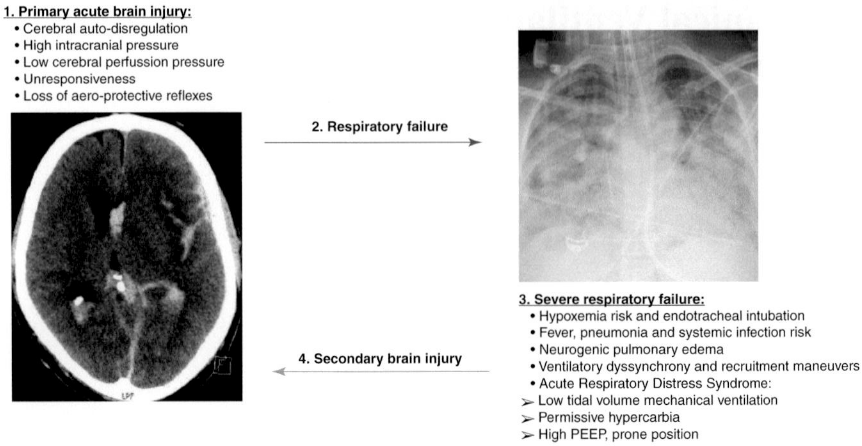

Fig. 1 Brain and lungs interplay with severe acute brain injury (1) leading to respiratory failure (2), treatment of severe respiratory failure with its strategies that could lead to secondary brain injury (4)

liberation from mechanical ventilation, which can be challenging while trying to understand the extent of the central or peripheral nervous system damage that may ultimately result in mechanical ventilation weaning and extubation success, or failure.

Throughout this chapter, we will be discussing steps involving airway protection, ventilation, and liberation from mechanical ventilation for neurocritical care patients with special considerations dedicated to each step.

2 Airway Management of a Patient with Intracranial Pathology

Securing the airway of a patient presenting with a neurological emergency can be lifesaving as failure to protect the lungs will lead to a myriad of complications such as hypoxia, acute respiratory distress syndrome, secondary brain injury including worsening cerebral edema, all of which will increase the morbidity and mortality chance of these patients. Following intubation of critically ill patients, up to 25% may develop severe hypotension or severe hypoxia and about 2% can suffer cardiac arrest [7, 8], and these will trigger secondary brain injury in neurocritical care patients. Understanding the location of the brain damage will help intensivists manage the neurocritically ill patient's airway and determine the correct indications to intubate the patients. Ischemic strokes affecting the patients' medullary respiratory rhythm generator can cause central apnea and possibly respiratory arrest, while damage to specific pontine nuclei and subcortical and cortical brain areas that modulate the respiratory pattern such as the depth, rise, and rate, could lead to unstable ventilatory patterns such as "ataxic" and "cluster" patterns [9, 10]. Conversely,

Table 1 Special considerations of intubating a neurocritically ill patient

Pre-intubation	Intubation	Post-intubation
Premedication choice to consider: Lidocaine, ketamine, and fentanyl	Adequate sedation	Adequate sedation
Keep the head of the bed at 30–45° till intubation and then back upright after securing airway	Adequate analgesia	Adequate analgesia
Anticipation of low blood pressure: Vasopressor availability and volume repletion	Adequate post-sedation paralytics	Minimize cough/gag
Anticipation for difficult airway: Equipment and right personnel	Minimize sympathetic and laryngeal reflexes	Adequate ventilation settings: PEEP, PaO_2, $PaCO_2$
ICP-lowering agent's peri-intubation: hypertonic saline or mannitol availability	Adequate positioning: Minimize flat position, in-line axial stability if indicated	Maintain target mean arterial pressure

certain abnormal respiratory patterns can be less problematic or potentially reversible indicating the presence of ongoing systemic disease processes such as "Cheyne-Stokes" pattern in heart failure, central hypoventilation secondary to oversedation or opioid overdose, and hyperventilation secondary to pulmonary embolism and sepsis. Summary of the special considerations for endotracheal intubation in neurocritical care patients can be found in Table 1.

2.1 Protecting the Airway Indications

Though strong level of evidence is lacking, a recent consensus recommends patients presenting with Glasgow Coma Scale (GCS) ≤8 to be considered as an indication for intubation [11] and particularly if admitted with neurological emergencies as they are unable to protect their airway. Intubating these patients helps secure their airways to prevent any aspiration episodes that could lead to pneumonia and subsequent respiratory failure [12, 13]. Impaired airway-protective reflexes in the form of dysphagia, lack of sensory input from the upper aerodigestive tracts, and weak or absent cough reflexes will increase the risk of aspiration, pneumonia, and respiratory failure as colonized oral secretions or regurgitated stomach content can enter the upper and lower airways; therefore, securing the airways to protect the lung of these patients is imperative. Neurocritical care patients who are unable to oxygenate or ventilate be it due to their primary brain injury or non-neurological systemic illness will also need to be intubated. Bedside examination of these patients reveals respiratory distress with labored breathing using accessory muscles to maintain a low oxygen saturation or rising end-tidal carbon dioxide level with deteriorating level of consciousness.

Other common indications to be considered when deciding if a patient with acute brain injury should be intubated include acute ischemic stroke patients with bulbar dysfunction, large middle cerebral artery infarct (more than 2/3 of the territory), seizures, high intracranial pressure signs and symptoms [14], combativeness, and severe agitation.

It is worthwhile re-emphasizing the negative impact on the outcome of brain-injured patients who deteriorate due to aspiration and respiratory failure, as patients may get hypoxic, hypercarbic, acidotic, and hemodynamically unstable leading up to mechanical ventilation, all of which would add insult to the primary brain injury.

2.2 *Planning Intubation and Difficult Airway Anticipation*

Similar to the approach for any procedure in the intensive care unit, planning for endotracheal intubation of a critically ill patient requires mental and physical checklists to avoid complications that could be life threatening. Endotracheal intubation is a process that starts with the preparation for the procedure itself by having the right equipment, personnel, and patient readiness followed by post-intubation critical care that needs early planning and anticipation in the pre-intubation phase. Often, all three phases can take place emergently over a few minutes' time span with rapid sequence induction in deteriorating patients, or non-emergently over a slightly longer period of time in slowly deteriorating patients with altered mental status requiring airway protection.

Preoxygenation for patients requiring rapid sequence intubation, if time allows, can help prevent possible peri-intubation desaturation episodes. Use of heated high-flow nasal cannula for preoxygenation during induction and throughout laryngoscopy known as apneic oxygenation at 60–70 L/min can increase the time to desaturation and first-pass success rate of intubation without hypoxemia [15]. Hypoxemic episodes in vulnerable brain injury will add insult to injury and worsen outcomes of these patients as will be discussed later in the chapter. It is important to emphasize the anticipation and planning for a difficult airway and bag-mask ventilation by following the LEMON and MOANS mnemonics for predicting difficult bag-and-mask ventilation and difficult tracheal intubation, respectively [16]. Failure to ventilate or oxygenate and hemodynamic instability that could ensue rapid sequence intubation will cause secondary brain injury in neurocritical care patients and can also increase the risk for cardiac arrest similar to all critically ill patients. Thus, planning for a difficult intubation if time allows can be lifesaving by having two providers present, one of which is experienced in airway management, a difficult airway cart with the right equipment such as adjunct airway devices, special blades, and bougie, with a readily available video laryngoscopy and fiber-optic bronchoscopy [17]. Maintaining the head of the bed at 30–45° and briefly bringing it down flat for intubation as well as avoiding CO_2 retention could prevent cerebral herniation in patients with suspected high intracranial pressure or cerebral edema.

Cervical spine instability should always be considered as a possibility in traumatic brain injury arriving to the emergency department especially after direct neck or head trauma with loss of consciousness. Caution must be taken in these cases by placing a stabilization device such as semirigid neck collar. Preparing for intubation includes removing the anterior part of the semirigid collar, appropriate difficult airway intubation equipment availability with the anticipation of difficult intubation in cases of mechanical upper airway obstruction, and presence of an assistant to help with manual in-line axial stability during intubation for uncleared cervical spine pending appropriate evaluation [18]. Standard intubation maneuvers for non-trauma patients such as head tilt and chin lift should be avoided, and use of video laryngoscopy is favored especially in cases of manual in-line axial stabilization [19]. Awake fiber-optic intubation should be considered in rare unstable cervical spine-injured awake patients. Reapplication of the anterior part of the semirigid collar post-intubation is important once the airway is secured.

2.3 *Preparing for Intubation Induction in a Patient with Acute Brain Injury*

Pre-intubation brief and focused neurological examination of the patient presenting with a neurological emergency, if circumstances and time allow, are crucial for the post-intubation therapeutic management of the patient, for example decision to insert an external ventricular drain or urgent need for electroencephalogram monitoring. Pre- and post-intubation sedation, analgesics, and paralytic medications will mask the neurological exam of the patient; therefore, obtaining pre-intubation baseline brief assessment is necessary.

The preferred method to intubate a patient with acute brain injury is with rapid sequence induction via simultaneous administration of fast-acting sedatives to induce immediate unresponsiveness followed by a paralytic agent for optimal intubation conditions and higher success rate. Rapid sequence intubation method is important for patients with cerebral edema or at risk of intracranial hypertension by limiting the potential risk that is associated with the physiologic responses accompanying laryngoscopy. When manipulating the airway, two responses are expected that could increase the intracranial pressure in brain-injured patients with autoregulation and exhausted intracranial compliance: first is the reflex sympathetic response whereby the patient's blood pressure and heart rate increase, and second is the direct laryngeal reflex that can increase the risk of high intracranial pressure independent of the reflex sympathetic response [16].

Alongside monitoring the standard vital signs of the patients getting intubated which include the blood pressure, heart rate, oxygen saturation, and end-tidal CO_2 (if available), monitoring the intracranial pressure and cerebral perfusion pressure if an intracranial pressure monitor device is in place can help mitigate secondary brain injury throughout the endotracheal intubation process. It is recommended to keep the intracranial pressure equal or less than 22 mmHg and cerebral perfusion pressure 60–70 mmHg bearing in mind the equation of CPP = MAP-ICP [20].

Using direct laryngoscopy for intubation can cause sympathetic stimulation with hypertension, tachycardia, and increased intracranial pressure [21]; therefore, two commonly used medications to prevent the direct laryngeal reflex and the reflex sympathetic response, respectively, include intravenous lidocaine and intravenous fentanyl, though supportive data is weak [22]. Lidocaine at 1.5 mg/kg can blunt the direct laryngeal reflex during direct laryngoscopy by reducing airway hyperactivity, tachycardia, and cerebral blood flow; however, it may decrease the mean arterial pressure. Fentanyl as a premedication analgesic at a dose of 2–3 mcg/kg can attenuate the reflex sympathetic response when administered 60 seconds prior to induction, to minimize the risk of hypoventilation or apnea [23]. Other measures to be considered when planning to intubate a patient with high intracranial pressure include reverse Trendelenburg position particularly in trauma patients requiring thoraco-lumbar spine immobilization, maintaining normal to elevated mean arterial pressure and cerebral perfusion pressure by use of vasopressors and volume repletion, treating pain and discomfort, and avoiding hypoventilation while maintaining normal oxygen saturation.

Induction medications that would cause hypotension in patients particularly with hypovolemia should be anticipated by volume repletion and vasopressor availability prior to, during, and after intubation. Avoiding hypotension during rapid sequence intubation and post-intubation in a pressure-dependent neurocritical care patient's clinical status can be lifesaving in certain scenarios, which is not uncommon when administering propofol or opioids. Patients admitted in the acute phase of ischemic stroke with flow-dependent extra or intracranial vessel-critical stenosis or with ischemic penumbra dependent on collaterals and compensatory physiological high blood pressure, might become symptomatic or complete their large stroke with the hypotensive episodes that could occur during or after rapid sequence intubation. Patients admitted with acute severe traumatic brain injury or high-grade subarachnoid hemorrhage and cerebral edema are at risk of high intracranial pressure and low cerebral perfusion pressure. Therefore, in such cases, induction medication such as etomidate is preferred, at a dose of 0.3 mg/kg. Etomidate is a GABA agonist drug that has sedative but no analgesic effects and does not lower the blood pressure with a tendency to reduce intracranial pressure. Side effects of etomidate to be aware of and consider avoiding its use include cases of seizures or status epilepticus as it may lower the seizure threshold, also in cases of sepsis and adrenal insufficiency with the concern of worsening shock and increased mortality rate [24]. Ketamine is another potential drug of choice in particular neurocritical care cases. Ketamine, a "dissociative" agent, provides analgesia, sedation, and amnesia at a dose of 2 mg/kg IV push without causing vasodilation nor lowering blood pressure, therefore not affecting the cerebral perfusion pressure. Though past reports showcase concern of increase in intracranial pressure with the use of ketamine in patients at risk [25, 26], it has been shown to be safe while co-administered with another sedative such as GABA agonist [27], but caution remains to be taken while using ketamine in neurocritical care patients as data remains weak.

When using neuromuscular blocking agents for intubation, special considerations must be taken regarding the drug of choice's duration of action; if the neurological exam of these patients is fluctuating or important to be closely monitored such as in patients at risk of hemicraniectomy, then shorter acting succinylcholine would be favored. Attention must be paid to the potential specific risk succinylcholine poses as a neuromuscular blockade agent such as hyperkalemia in patients with prolonged immobility, which applies to many of the severe brain injury patients, specifically in Guillain-Barre syndrome [28]. Another consideration for the choice of neuromuscular blocking agents is patients with myasthenia gravis: rocuronium is safe; however, it has a prolonged duration of action, and succinylcholine if used requires 2.5 times the normal dose to provide the same effect [29].

Finally, caution must be taken if the patient remains severely hypertensive in a setting of unsecured and ruptured aneurysm or arteriovenous malformation as it can cause rebleeding and deterioration of the patient's condition. Adequate sedation and pain control should be given prior to the administration of neuromuscular blocking agents to avoid hypertensive crisis during the intubation process and post-intubation by having readily available adequate intravenous sedation and analgesics medications. Ketamine in these circumstances will be avoided as it can cause sympathetic stimulation. Readily available blood pressure-lowering agents could play a role in certain rare cases of persistent hypertension despite adequate analgesia and sedation.

3 Mechanical Ventilation

Mechanical ventilation in patients with ischemic and hemorrhage strokes carries a mortality rate of up to 61% [30] with reported 20% of good functional outcome [31].

For neurocritical care patients with acute brain injury at risk of or with high intracranial pressure and concomitant respiratory failure mainly due to acute respiratory distress syndrome, concern arises when it comes to the right mode of mechanical ventilation, set positive end-expiratory pressure (PEEP), and alveolar recruitment maneuvers that could further increase the intracranial pressure, secondary to intracranial venous congestion from elevated intrathoracic pressures, and low cerebral perfusion due to low mean arterial pressure, while attempting to optimize oxygenation [32].

3.1 Is There a Right Setting for Neurocritical Care Patients?

One mechanical ventilation setting fits all neurocritical care patients is not established; rather, each patient's individual cerebral pathophysiology interplay with their underlying lung injury mechanism will dictate the ideal parameters for the ventilation strategy to mitigate secondary brain and lung damage [33]. The right balance of oxygen and carbon dioxide levels in brain-injured patients is vital to minimize the risk of worsening outcomes. Protective 6–8 ml/kg tidal volumes of predicted body weight (PBW) and plateau pressures <30 cm H_2O have been suggested to be protective in patients with brain injury [34]. A recent survey for the practice of mechanical ventilation for severe traumatic brain injury patient revealed a commonly adopted 6–8 ml/kg of PBW in patients with $PaO_2/FiO_2 > 150$ and 4–6 ml/Kg of PBW in half of the cases with $PaO_2/FiO_2 < 150$ [35]. A personalized approach should be adopted to choose the right ventilation strategy for patients with acute brain injury, depending on if the patient has clinically significant high intracranial pressure or acute respiratory distress syndrome and how severe it is. Generally, if a patient that is on mechanical ventilation has no significant high intracranial pressure with or without concurrent ARDS, lung-protective ventilation strategy should be used. If the patient has high intracranial pressure with or without concurrent ARDS, individualized approach should be considered if lung-protective mechanical ventilation is to be implemented taking into consideration the primary brain injury, its clinical status, the workup at hand including brain imaging, and importantly the presence or not of an intracranial monitor. Intracranial and cerebral perfusion pressure continuous monitoring would be valuable in vulnerable patients with exhausted intracranial compliance that could get worse with standard mechanical ventilation settings' change. Only two randomized controlled studies with very low quality of evidence have looked into different mechanical ventilation settings' approach, and both involved traumatic brain injury patients [36, 37]. Pressure-regulated volume control was shown to result in least fluctuations of intracranial pressure and $PaCO_2$ as compared to pressure-controlled modes in traumatic brain injury patients when compared to pressure-controlled ventilation [38], but that study had a small number of patients ($n = 11$) with high risk of bias and no blinding.

3.2 Positive End-Expiratory Pressure and Intracranial Pressure

Though higher level of PEEP carries a theoretical risk of higher intracranial pressure due to impaired venous return from the brain in the presence of higher intrathoracic pressure, study by Boone et al. showed that PEEP up to 15–20 cm H_2O can be safely used in patients with brain injury without an effect on intracranial pressure [39]; however, monitoring closely cerebral perfusion pressure is important as cardiac output may drop [40]. In a recent survey study, VENTILO (ventilatory strategies in patients with severe traumatic brain injury), PEEP ranging from 5 to 15 cm H_2O was used comfortably in patients with $PaO_2/FiO_2 < 300$ without intracranial hypertension, whereas PEEP limited to 10 cm H_2O was used in patients with high ICP under monitored conditions. Consensus recommendation is to keep PEEP at the same level for acute brain injury patients with clinically significant high intracranial pressure but without ARDS or need for high PEEP; however, if higher PEEP is needed to help with the respiratory failure clinical status of the patient, it would be important to titrate the PEEP level in the presence of an intracranial pressure monitor [11].

3.3 *Rescue Therapies for Patients with Severe Respiratory Failure and Acute Brain Injury*

Alveolar recruitment maneuvers are considered in critically ill patients admitted with respiratory failure, whereby hyperinflation can help improve hypoxemia particularly when clinically significant atelectasis is present. When faced with such a clinical scenario in a patient with acute brain injury, recruitment maneuvers can have a detrimental effect on the intracranial and cerebral perfusion pressures. In these cases, individualized approach is recommended to weigh the balance of the need of alveolar recruitment maneuvers versus the status of the intracranial compliance, pressure, and perfusion. Only one low level of evidence randomized controlled trial compared pressure control recruitment maneuver (CPAP 35/PEEP 15 mmHg) to continuous positive airway pressure recruitment maneuver (CPAP 15 mmHg) showing the latter group experiencing higher intracranial pressure and lower cerebral perfusion pressure values [41]. However, this study lacked blinding and intention to treat. Recruitment maneuvers are reserved in case of severe hypoxemia in patients with severe traumatic brain injury, under close and advanced neuromonitoring [42]. Along the same lines, neuromuscular blocking agents were favored over recruitment maneuvers in patients with combined brain and lung injury as a prior strategy step to improve oxygenation.

4 Carbon Dioxide Levels and the Brain: Effect of Hypercarbia and Hypocarbia

Respiratory care for patients with brain injury has some significant differences compared to medical intensive care unit patients, particularly when it comes to management of CO_2 levels. While permissive hypercarbia and respiratory acidosis are allowed in patients with acute respiratory distress syndrome as it would be of benefit [43], it can be harmful to neurocritical care patients with cerebral edema at risk of brain herniation.

Carbon dioxide levels play an important role in modifying the cerebral vasculature caliber and cerebral blood flow that would not generally impact healthy individuals with intact cerebral autoregulatory mechanism [44]. However, in brain-injured patients, cerebral autoregulation is disrupted; therefore, a rise in CO_2 level (hypercapnia) leads to vasodilatation of cerebral blood vessels, increasing cerebral blood flow which can contribute to rise in intracranial pressure, especially in patients with exhausted intracranial compliance such as in comatose severe traumatic brain injury patients or high-grade subarachnoid hemorrhage with diffuse cerebral edema. Conversely, hyperventilation will decrease CO_2 levels, leading to vasoconstriction of cerebral blood vessels and lowering of cerebral blood flow, which ultimately decreases intracranial pressure as a therapeutic measure in patients with intracranial hypertension at risk of cerebral herniation. However, hyperventilation can be detrimental in patients with acute ischemic stroke dependent on their collateral flow or flow-dependent critical intracranial or extracranial vessel stenosis for example, and hypocapnea ($PaCO_2 < 35$ mmHg) will increase the risk for delayed cerebral ischemia threefold in high-grade subarachnoid hemorrhage patients [45], worsen the 6-month functional outcome in severe traumatic brain injury [46] who in the acute setting are vulnerable to any reduction of cerebral blood flow.

Target CO_2 levels when hyperventilating patients with intracranial hypertension are 30–35 mmHg [47], which usually takes place over a few minutes' duration as it is considered a temporizing measure while providing longer lasting therapies (i.e., mannitol, 23.4%, sedation, or decompressive craniectomy), followed by slow normalization of CO_2 levels to 35–45 mmHg in the absence of cerebral herniation [20, 35]. Obtaining arterial blood gas if possible right before hyperventilation and monitoring quantitative CO_2 monitoring (end-tidal CO_2) during hyperventilation are suggested to avoid overshooting in target CO_2, acknowledging the possible discrepancy between the actual arterial PCO_2 and end-tidal values. Caution must be exerted in hyperventilating patients with high ICP and cerebral herniation, as prolonged hyperventilation with a $PaCO_2$ of <20–25 mmHg can cause cerebral ischemia and infarction, lower the blood pressure, and further impede venous return to the heart [48]. Monitoring cerebral oxygenation via a jugular venous oximetry or brain tissue oxygen monitor to detect cerebral ischemia could be of value in certain cases requiring prolonged mild hyperventilation.

When the patient exhibits hyperventilation, the questions that need to be asked are if this is physiologic (appropriate) or pathophysiologic (inappropriate) and is it a response to the initial brain insult or a compensatory mechanism to a systemic illness such as decompensated metabolic acidosis, whereby suppressing the respiratory drive is not recommended.

In summary, brief and effective hyperventilation is recommended only as a life-saving temporary measure in patients with cerebral herniation. Prolonged hyperventilation with lower than recommended levels in a patient with brain injury could be detrimental as it may cause secondary brain injury due to respiratory alkalosis and unwanted cerebral vasoconstriction [49].

5 Oxygen Levels: Impact of Hypoxia and Hyperoxia on Acute Brain Injury Patients

It is recommended to strictly monitor the peripheral oxygen saturation and keep the saturation level above 92–94% for acute ischemic and hemorrhagic strokes as well as for patients with severe traumatic brain injury [13, 47, 50]. Hyperoxia has been associated with worse outcomes in traumatic brain injury patients [51], after cardiac arrest [52], higher mortality at 6 months in a large multicenter study of 1100 patients ICH cohort across 21 sites [53], in acute ischemic stroke patients overall [54], and higher modified Rankin scores and mortality rates at 90 days in those who undergo mechanical thrombectomy for an anterior circulation occlusion with admission $PaO_2 > 120$ mmHg [55].

Supraphysiologic level of oxygen can stress the damaged and vulnerable brain tissue as reactive oxygen species will form that will overwhelm the antioxidants, therefore impairing mitochondrial function, leading to reperfusion injury and worse outcomes [52]. Hyperoxia can also cause direct injury to the lung by inducing inflammation and damage to the epithelium and alveoli and may cause reabsorption atelectasis. Similarly, the injured brain is vulnerable to low levels of oxygen or hypoxia, which would lead to secondary brain injury and worse outcomes for patients [56].

There is enough data to suggest the effect of hyperoxia and hypoxemia on patients with severe brain injury leading to unfavorable clinical outcomes. Following intubation, it is important to closely monitor the oxygenation saturation and decrease the FiO_2 support for the patient titrating it to normal oxygen saturation with a range of 95–100% [20] and PaO_2 80–120 mmHg [11], which is a slightly higher than the common target range of the general critical care patients [57].

6 Liberation from Mechanical Ventilation

Studies have shown the importance of early extubation of a critically ill mechanically ventilated patient as delays can have significant medical and economic implications [58, 59]. More mechanical ventilation days increase the chances of nosocomial pneumonia, muscle atrophy, intensive care unit-acquired weakness, and failure to extubate and increase the overall morbidity and mortality [58]. Moreover, patients on mechanical ventilation often require some type of analgo-sedation, which would make it challenging for a neurointensivist to get an accurate neurological examination, the latter which remains the cornerstone of evaluation and management of neurocritical care patients. Extubation failure rate has been reported to be up to 20% in critical care patients and up to 15% in neurocritical care patients [60].

Table 2 Contraindications to extubating a neurocritically ill patient

Neurological	Cardiorespiratory
Loss of airway-protective reflexes (cough, gag, swallowing)	Hemodynamic instability
GCS ≤ 8	$FiO_2 > 50\%$
Central apnea	PEEP > 8 cm H_2O
High intracranial pressure	RR > 35 breaths/min
Uncontrolled seizures/status epilepticus	Frequent suctioning and large amount of oro-tracheal secretions

Predictors of failure to extubate a critically ill patient include presence of pneumonia and atelectasis, duration of mechanical ventilation, lack of cough reflex, large secretion volume, female sex, and low Glasgow Coma Scale [61, 62].

Though extubation checklists and algorithms exist for medical intensive care unit patients [63], applying them to neurocritical care patients to predict extubation was shown to be unsuccessful [64]. There are additional weaning parameters and specific extubation considerations to be taken in the NCCU as compared to the rest of critically ill patients' population, particularly revolving around knowing where the lesion is in the neuroaxis of the neurocritically ill patient, and if the damage is reversible or not. For example, ischemic or hemorrhagic stroke to the cough center in the medulla or reticulating activating fiber locations along the brainstem structures will lead to impaired cough reflex and lack of consciousness, respectively, prohibiting the chance to extubate and committing to early tracheostomy in these patients. Contraindications to extubation in the neurologic critical care unit are found in Table 2. Alongside a successful spontaneous breathing trial, meeting all traditional weaning parameters and specific considerations for the neurocritical care patients, aggressive chest physiotherapy is often required for patients with brain injury to prevent reintubation as it has been shown to increase the odds of successful extubation, reduce the risk for respiratory complications, and decrease the length of stay [65].

7 Tracheostomy

Indications for tracheostomy in neurocritical care patients can vary. Irreversible ischemia to the central respiratory rhythm generator in the medulla, loss of aeroprotective reflex, and failed one or several extubation trials are straightforward indications for tracheostomy. Timing of tracheostomy is another important decision the neurointensivist has to take, early (within first few days of admission) versus late (after 10–14 days of endotracheal intubation), as this decision will help accelerate potential recovery after the severe brain injury. Early tracheostomy as compared to prolonged endotracheal intubation can lessen the number of mechanical ventilation days and pneumonia risk, leading to a shorter intensive care unit length of stay and improved mortality [66, 67]. More often, these patients, who originally were intubated for airway protection, can be weaned off mechanical ventilation rather quickly to oxygen mask and have a high chance to be decannulated should they recover their airway-protective reflexes and/or the level of consciousness. Tracheostomy can alleviate the oropharynx from the tube pressure and possible mouth or larynx lesions, improve orotracheal hygiene, and provide more patient comfort and early mobilization, all of which are key in neurologic critical care unit patients' recovery. Conversely, patients with active fluctuation of their mental status due to many reasons such as cerebral edema secondary to hemorrhagic stroke or toxic-metabolic encephalopathy can recover despite longer days on the mechanical ventilation as long as they have no irreversible brain damage in certain defining brain structures as evident on advanced brain imaging with a clinical bedside exam correlate. In these cases, it might be reasonable to avoid early tracheostomy as long as there is a treatable and reversible neurological condition without systemic critical illness such as multi-organ failure or intensive care unit-acquired severe weakness as indications for tracheostomy. The SET score is an internally validated scoring tool that was initially studied in random pilot trial, the Stroke-Related Early Tracheostomy Versus Prolonged Orotracheal Intubation in Neurocritical Care Trial (SETPOINT), to predict the feasibility and safety of early tracheostomy after severe stroke. The score comprises risk factors for prolonged (more than 14 days) period of mechanical ventilation, which were divided into three components: neurological function (maximum 10 points), neurological lesion (maximum 22 points), and general organ function or procedure (maximum 16 points). A SETscore >10 has a sensitivity of 64% and specificity of 86% in patients with severe stroke and respiratory failure to require tracheostomy with a suggested benefit in outcomes and mortality in favor of early tracheostomy in the small sample study size. This score currently is being further studied in SETPOINT 2 trial (NCT02377167) [68]. Other suggested scores include VISAGE score to predict extubation failure in subarachnoid hemorrhage patients [69] and TRACH score to identify intracerebral hemorrhage patients who may require tracheostomy [70].

8 Special Scenarios

8.1 Acute Respiratory Distress Syndrome in Patients with Brain Injury

Patients suffering from acute respiratory distress syndrome (ARDS) are treated with lung-protective mechanical ventilation strategies to prevent further injury to vulnerable inflamed lungs [43]. Lung-protective ventilation is a strategy of low tidal volumes and airway pressure with adequate positive end-expiratory pressure to prevent alveolar collapse and limit the utilization of high FiO_2. Low-tidal-volume mechanical ventilation leads to retention of CO_2 and acidosis, which is permitted in the management of ARDS patients. For moderate-to-severe ARDS cases, prone ventilation positioning for certain amount of hours instead of supine position has been shown to improve outcomes [71] as well as continuous neuromuscular blockage [72] as they minimize the risk of ventilator-induced lung injury. Neurointensivists managing neurocritical care patients with acute brain injury and concomitant ARDS are faced with a unique challenge of managing both brain and lungs to mitigate secondary injuries and worsening outcome. Up to a third of the patients with neurological injury can suffer from acute respiratory distress syndrome [42]. Brain-lung "cross talk" is critical to maintain the right treatment for the patient as a whole. While low tidal volume and permissive hypercapnia will help primary lung injury, caution must be taken in its implication on the cerebral blood flow and intracranial pressure. If the patient's brain injury is severe and cerebral autoregulation is disrupted with exhausted cerebral compliance, hypercapnia might worsen the patient's condition by causing high intracranial pressure and cerebral herniation. Similarly, proning a patient with exhausted intracranial compliance at risk of herniation will be a contraindication. However, in a patient without significant high intracranial pressure and concurrent severe ARDS with $PaO_2/FiO_2 < 150$, prone positioning should be considered particularly if an intracranial pressure monitor is in place, as improved oxygenation will improve both the ARDS and brain injury outcomes.

Small studies have shown that lung-protective ventilation strategies might be well tolerated despite the mild elevation of intracranial pressure due to hypercarbia [73], and proning benefits might offset the small increase in ICP with the significant oxygenation improvement [74], but further studies and solid data are required.

Managing a patient with moderate-to-severe ARDS and acute brain injury would be ideal with advanced multimodal monitoring of the intracranial pressure, compliance, intracerebral oxygenation, and metabolism to find the right balance between therapies of both the cerebral and pulmonary injuries, especially when allowing permissive hypercapnia and requiring prone ventilation [75].

8.2 *Neurogenic Pulmonary Edema*

Neurogenic pulmonary edema (NPE) is classified as a form of acute respiratory distress [76], triggered mainly by severe central nervous system insult, specifically the brain stem and hypothalamus [77]. While many acute brain and spinal cord injuries can precipitate neurogenic pulmonary edema, major etiologies are traumatic brain injury, epileptic seizures or status epilepticus, and intracranial hemorrhage such as subarachnoid or intracerebral hemorrhage. Among other reported etiologies include vertebral dissection [78], subdural hematomas [79], cryptococcal meningitis [80], multiple sclerosis [81], and ruptured spinal cord arteriovenous malformation [82]. Its pathogenesis is not fully understood but thought to be caused by a centrally triggered sympathetic overstimulation leading to systemic vasoconstriction, specifically involving the pulmonary vasculature, which increases hydrostatic pressure, permeability of the vessels that leak protein-rich fluid to the alveolar space, and interstitial pulmonary space [83].

Neurogenic pulmonary edema's onset is typically acute, occurring within 1–4 h of the acute brain injury, but can also occur at a relatively later onset within 12–72 h [84] and resolves within 48–72 h after onset [77]. Classic manifestations of NPE are shortness of breath, tachypnea, tachycardia with rales, crackles, and rhonchi on lung auscultation. Diagnosing a patient with NPE is challenging with the importance of excluding mimics such as aspiration pneumonia, ventilator-associated pneumonia, and cardiogenic pulmonary edema, which typically is evident in heart failure patients, with an enlarged heart on chest X-ray and depressed ejection fraction on echocardiography without fast resolution of the pulmonary edema as typical in cases of NPE. Supportive investigations for the diagnosis of NPE include bilateral alveolar infiltrates on chest X-ray and hypoxemia with low PaO_2/FiO_2 ratio < 200 correlating with a rapid clinical and radiographical resolution of abnormalities within 72 h of onset [77]. Treatment is generally supportive focused on addressing the main etiology behind the NPE and the patient's deterioration, which is generally a central nervous pathology. Diuretics can be used if the patient is not hypovolemic as well as oxygen supplementation ranging from mild support to high-flow nasal cannula, noninvasive positive-pressure ventilation, or invasive mechanical ventilation till it resolves.

8.3 *Pneumocephalus*

Pneumocephalus, or simply air inside the cranium, is seen most commonly after almost every neurosurgery, after head and facial trauma, and can occur spontaneously and less commonly following spinal surgeries [37]. Air usually can accumulate in every space inside the cranium and could be intracerebral or in the subarachnoid, subdural, epidural, and ventricular spaces. Pneumocephalus is usually a simple benign condition if the patient is asymptomatic, though patients can become symptomatic when it progresses to tension pneumocephalus. Symptomatic patients with tension pneumocephalus can exhibit a range of symptoms from persistent postoperative headaches to cerebrospinal fluid leak and seizures. The gold standard test to diagnose pneumocephalus is a plain head computed tomography with high sensitivity down to 0.55 ml of air that can be detected. Many signs have been described including the characteristic "Mount Fuji sign," whereby air accumulates mainly in the bifrontal region of the brain separating both frontal lobe tips [85] (Fig. 2). Treatment strategy is based on the type of pneumocephalus the patient has, as simple pneumocephalus cases are treated rather conservatively with bed rest, with head-of-the-bed elevation to 30° Fowler's position, avoiding Valsalva maneuvers such as sneezing or coughing, adequate pain control, and oxygen therapy. Oxygen therapy is most commonly delivered by non-rebreather mask at 100% FiO_2 with the aim of reducing the nitrogen concentration and absorption from the air collection inside or surrounding the brain tissue. Another suggested oxygen therapy

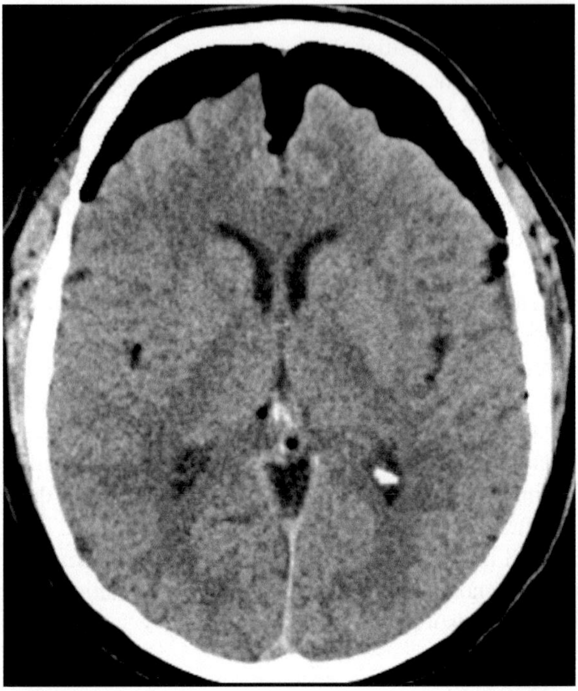

Fig. 2 "Mount Fuji Sign" pneumocephalus in routine postoperative CT brain without contrast after tumor resection

method is high-flow nasal cannula with heated and humidified high flow rate as it delivers consistent FiO_2 and higher flow rate that could expedite N_2 washout, provides more comfort to the patient, has been shown to increase tidal volumes, and provides some end-expiratory positive pressure which could be of help in certain postoperative patients [86]. The duration of oxygen therapy is unknown and can be limited to short or longer hours of duration, continuously or intermittently.

Key Notes

- Acute brain injury patients are at risk of respiratory failure due to namely loss of consciousness, therefore requiring endotracheal intubation and mechanical ventilation.
- Securing the airway of comatose neurocritical care patients is a delicate process including planning pre-intubation, intubation, and post-intubation with special considerations for intracranial and cerebral perfusion pressure preservation.
- There is not one setting or mode for mechanical ventilation strategies for neurocritical care patients; rather, it is a combined approach to the clinical status of both brain and lung injuries with special consideration for lung-protective ventilation in a setting of multimodal intracranial monitoring.
- Liberation from mechanical ventilation for acute brain injury patients requires understanding of the location and reversibility of the brain or spinal cord injury alongside traditional weaning and extubation parameters for critical care patients.

References

1. Asehnoune K, Roquilly A, Cinotti R. Respiratory management in patients with severe brain injury. Crit Care. 2018;22(1):76. https://doi.org/10.1186/s13054-018-1994-0.
2. Borsellino B, Schultz MJ, Gama de Abreu M, Robba C, Bilotta F. Mechanical ventilation in neurocritical care patients: a systematic literature review. Expert Rev Respir Med. 2016;10(10):1123–32. https://doi.org/10.1080/17476348.2017.1235976.
3. Li Y, Liu C, Xiao W, Song T, Wang S. Incidence, risk factors, and outcomes of ventilator-associated pneumonia in traumatic brain injury: a meta-analysis. Neurocrit Care. 2020;32(1):272–85. https://doi.org/10.1007/s12028-019-00773-w.
4. Hannawi Y, Hannawi B, Rao CP, Suarez JI, Bershad EM. Stroke-associated pneumonia: major advances and obstacles. Cerebrovasc Dis. 2013;35(5):430–43. https://doi.org/10.1159/000350199.
5. Smith CJ, Bray BD, Hoffman A, Meisel A, Heuschmann PU, Wolfe CD, et al. Can a novel clinical risk score improve pneumonia prediction in acute stroke care? A UK multicenter cohort study. J Am Heart Assoc. 2015;4(1):e001307. https://doi.org/10.1161/JAHA.114.001307.
6. Diringer MN, Bleck TP, Claude Hemphill J 3rd, Menon D, Shutter L, Vespa P, et al. Critical care management of patients following aneurysmal subarachnoid hemorrhage: recommendations from the Neurocritical Care Society's Multidisciplinary Consensus Conference. Neurocrit Care. 2011;15(2):211–40. https://doi.org/10.1007/s12028-011-9605-9.
7. Cook TM, Woodall N, Harper J, Benger J, Audit FN, P. Major complications of airway management in the UK: results of the Fourth National Audit Project of the Royal College of Anaesthetists and the Difficult Airway Society. Part 2: intensive care and emergency departments. Br J Anaesth. 2011;106(5):632–42. https://doi.org/10.1093/bja/aer059.
8. Simpson GD, Ross MJ, McKeown DW, Ray DC. Tracheal intubation in the critically ill: a multi-centre national study of practice and complications. Br J Anaesth. 2012;108(5):792–9. https://doi.org/10.1093/bja/aer504.
9. Feldman JL, Del Negro CA, Gray PA. Understanding the rhythm of breathing: so near, yet so far. Annu Rev Physiol. 2013;75:423–52. https://doi.org/10.1146/annurev-physiol-040510-130049.
10. Guyenet PG, Bayliss DA. Neural control of breathing and CO2 homeostasis. Neuron. 2015;87(5):946–61. https://doi.org/10.1016/j.neuron.2015.08.001.
11. Robba C, Poole D, McNett M, Asehnoune K, Bosel J, Bruder N, et al. Mechanical ventilation in patients with acute brain injury: recommendations of the European Society of Intensive Care Medicine consensus. Intensive Care Med. 2020;46(12):2397–410. https://doi.org/10.1007/s00134-020-06283-0.
12. von Elm E, Schoettker P, Henzi I, Osterwalder J, Walder B. Pre-hospital tracheal intubation in patients with traumatic brain injury: systematic review of current evidence. Br J Anaesth. 2009;103(3):371–86. https://doi.org/10.1093/bja/aep202.
13. Powers WJ, Rabinstein AA, Ackerson T, Adeoye OM, Bambakidis NC, Becker K, et al. Guidelines for the early management of patients with acute ischemic stroke: 2019 update to the 2018 guidelines for the early management of acute ischemic stroke: a guideline for healthcare professionals from the American Heart Association/American Stroke Association. Stroke. 2019;50(12):e344–418. https://doi.org/10.1161/STR.0000000000000211.
14. Seder DB, Jagoda A, Riggs B. Emergency neurological life support: airway, ventilation, and sedation. Neurocrit Care. 2015;23(Suppl 2):S5–22. https://doi.org/10.1007/s12028-015-0164-3.
15. Pavlov I, Medrano S, Weingart S. Apneic oxygenation reduces the incidence of hypoxemia during emergency intubation: a systematic review and meta-analysis. Am J Emerg Med. 2017;35(8):1184–9. https://doi.org/10.1016/j.ajem.2017.06.029.
16. Walls RMMM. Manual of emergency airway management. 3rd ed. Philadelphia: Lippincott Williams & Wilkins; 2008.
17. Higgs A, McGrath BA, Goddard C, Rangasami J, Suntharalingam G, Gale R, et al. Guidelines for the management of tracheal intubation in critically ill adults. Br J Anaesth. 2018;120(2):323–52. https://doi.org/10.1016/j.bja.2017.10.021.

18. Rajajee V, Riggs B, Seder DB. Emergency neurological life support: airway, ventilation, and sedation. Neurocrit Care. 2017;27(Suppl 1):4–28. https://doi.org/10.1007/s12028-017-0451-2.
19. Kill C, Risse J, Wallot P, Seidl P, Steinfeldt T, Wulf H. Videolaryngoscopy with glidescope reduces cervical spine movement in patients with unsecured cervical spine. J Emerg Med. 2013;44(4):750–6. https://doi.org/10.1016/j.jemermed.2012.07.080.
20. Carney N, Totten AM, O'Reilly C, Ullman JS, Hawryluk GW, Bell MJ, et al. Guidelines for the management of severe traumatic brain injury, Fourth Edition. Neurosurgery. 2017;80(1):6–15. https://doi.org/10.1227/NEU.0000000000001432.
21. Walls RM. Rapid-sequence intubation in head trauma. Ann Emerg Med. 1993;22(6):1008–13. https://doi.org/10.1016/s0196-0644(05)82743-x.
22. Salhi B, Stettner E. In defense of the use of lidocaine in rapid sequence intubation. Ann Emerg Med. 2007;49(1):84–6. https://doi.org/10.1016/j.annemergmed.2006.09.003.
23. Reynolds SF, Heffner J. Airway management of the critically ill patient: rapid-sequence intubation. Chest. 2005;127(4):1397–412. https://doi.org/10.1378/chest.127.4.1397.
24. Chan CM, Mitchell AL, Shorr AF. Etomidate is associated with mortality and adrenal insufficiency in sepsis: a meta-analysis. Crit Care Med. 2012;40(11):2945–53. https://doi.org/10.1097/CCM.0b013e31825fec26.
25. Wyte SR, Shapiro HM, Turner P, Harris AB. Ketamine-induced intracranial hypertension. Anesthesiology. 1972;36(2):174–6. https://doi.org/10.1097/00000542-197202000-00021.
26. Langsjo JW, Maksimow A, Salmi E, Kaisti K, Aalto S, Oikonen V, et al. S-ketamine anesthesia increases cerebral blood flow in excess of the metabolic needs in humans. Anesthesiology. 2005;103(2):258–68. https://doi.org/10.1097/00000542-200508000-00008.
27. Cohen L, Athaide V, Wickham ME, Doyle-Waters MM, Rose NG, Hohl CM. The effect of ketamine on intracranial and cerebral perfusion pressure and health outcomes: a systematic review. Ann Emerg Med. 2015;65(1):43–51 e2. https://doi.org/10.1016/j.annemergmed.2014.06.018.
28. Martyn JA, Richtsfeld M. Succinylcholine-induced hyperkalemia in acquired pathologic states: etiologic factors and molecular mechanisms. Anesthesiology. 2006;104(1):158–69. https://doi.org/10.1097/00000542-200601000-00022.
29. Abel M, Eisenkraft JB. Anesthetic implications of myasthenia gravis. Mt Sinai J Med. 2002;69(1-2):31–7.
30. Lahiri S, Mayer SA, Fink ME, Lord AS, Rosengart A, Mangat HS, et al. Mechanical ventilation for acute stroke: a multi-state population-based study. Neurocrit Care. 2015;23(1):28–32. https://doi.org/10.1007/s12028-014-0082-9.
31. Roch A, Michelet P, Jullien AC, Thirion X, Bregeon F, Papazian L, et al. Long-term outcome in intensive care unit survivors after mechanical ventilation for intracerebral hemorrhage. Crit Care Med. 2003;31(11):2651–6. https://doi.org/10.1097/01.CCM.0000094222.57803.B4.
32. Huynh T, Messer M, Sing RF, Miles W, Jacobs DG, Thomason MH. Positive end-expiratory pressure alters intracranial and cerebral perfusion pressure in severe traumatic brain injury. J Trauma. 2002;53(3):488–92; discussion 92–3. https://doi.org/10.1097/00005373-200209000-00016.
33. Pelosi P, Rocco PR. The lung and the brain: a dangerous cross-talk. Crit Care. 2011;15(3):168. https://doi.org/10.1186/cc10259.
34. Neto AS, Simonis FD, Barbas CS, Biehl M, Determann RM, Elmer J, et al. Lung-protective ventilation with low tidal volumes and the occurrence of pulmonary complications in patients without acute respiratory distress syndrome: a systematic review and individual patient data analysis. Crit Care Med. 2015;43(10):2155–63. https://doi.org/10.1097/CCM.0000000000001189.
35. Picetti E, Pelosi P, Taccone FS, Citerio G, Mancebo J, Robba C, et al. VENTILatOry strategies in patients with severe traumatic brain injury: the VENTILO Survey of the European Society of Intensive Care Medicine (ESICM). Crit Care. 2020;24(1):158. https://doi.org/10.1186/s13054-020-02875-w.
36. Aghadavoudi O, Alikiaii B, Sadeghi F. Comparison of respiratory and hemodynamic stability in patients with traumatic brain injury ventilated by two ventilator modes: Pressure regulated volume control versus synchronized intermittent mechanical ventilation. Adv Biomed Res. 2016;5:175. https://doi.org/10.4103/2277-9175.190991.

37. Schirmer CM, Heilman CB, Bhardwaj A. Pneumocephalus: case illustrations and review. Neurocrit Care. 2010;13(1):152–8. https://doi.org/10.1007/s12028-010-9363-0.
38. Schirmer-Mikalsen K, Vik A, Skogvoll E, Moen KG, Solheim O, Klepstad P. Intracranial pressure during pressure control and pressure-regulated volume control ventilation in patients with traumatic brain injury: a randomized crossover trial. Neurocrit Care. 2016;24(3):332–41. https://doi.org/10.1007/s12028-015-0208-8.
39. Boone MD, Jinadasa SP, Mueller A, Shaefi S, Kasper EM, Hanafy KA, et al. The effect of positive end-expiratory pressure on intracranial pressure and cerebral hemodynamics. Neurocrit Care. 2017;26(2):174–81. https://doi.org/10.1007/s12028-016-0328-9.
40. Muench E, Bauhuf C, Roth H, Horn P, Phillips M, Marquetant N, et al. Effects of positive end-expiratory pressure on regional cerebral blood flow, intracranial pressure, and brain tissue oxygenation. Crit Care Med. 2005;33(10):2367–72. https://doi.org/10.1097/01.ccm.0000181732.37319.df.
41. Nemer SN, Caldeira JB, Azeredo LM, Garcia JM, Silva RT, Prado D, et al. Alveolar recruitment maneuver in patients with subarachnoid hemorrhage and acute respiratory distress syndrome: a comparison of 2 approaches. J Crit Care. 2011;26(1):22–7. https://doi.org/10.1016/j.jcrc.2010.04.015.
42. Della Torre V, Badenes R, Corradi F, Racca F, Lavinio A, Matta B, et al. Acute respiratory distress syndrome in traumatic brain injury: how do we manage it? J Thorac Dis. 2017;9(12):5368–81. https://doi.org/10.21037/jtd.2017.11.03.
43. Acute Respiratory Distress Syndrome Network, Brower RG, Matthay MA, Morris A, Schoenfeld D, Thompson BT, et al. Ventilation with lower tidal volumes as compared with traditional tidal volumes for acute lung injury and the acute respiratory distress syndrome. N Engl J Med. 2000;342(18):1301–8. https://doi.org/10.1056/NEJM200005043421801.
44. Bouma GJ, Muizelaar JP. Cerebral blood flow in severe clinical head injury. New Horiz. 1995;3(3):384–94.
45. Williamson CA, Sheehan KM, Tipirneni R, Roark CD, Pandey AS, Thompson BG, et al. The association between spontaneous hyperventilation, delayed cerebral ischemia, and poor neurological outcome in patients with subarachnoid hemorrhage. Neurocrit Care. 2015;23(3):330–8. https://doi.org/10.1007/s12028-015-0138-5.
46. Esnault P, Roubin J, Cardinale M, D'Aranda E, Montcriol A, Cungi PJ, et al. Spontaneous hyperventilation in severe traumatic brain injury: incidence and association with poor neurological outcome. Neurocrit Care. 2019;30(2):405–13. https://doi.org/10.1007/s12028-018-0639-0.
47. Chesnut R, Aguilera S, Buki A, Bulger E, Citerio G, Cooper DJ, et al. A management algorithm for adult patients with both brain oxygen and intracranial pressure monitoring: the Seattle International Severe Traumatic Brain Injury Consensus Conference (SIBICC). Intensive Care Med. 2020;46(5):919–29. https://doi.org/10.1007/s00134-019-05900-x.
48. Muizelaar JP, Marmarou A, Ward JD, Kontos HA, Choi SC, Becker DP, et al. Adverse effects of prolonged hyperventilation in patients with severe head injury: a randomized clinical trial. J Neurosurg. 1991;75(5):731–9. https://doi.org/10.3171/jns.1991.75.5.0731.
49. Carrera E, Schmidt JM, Fernandez L, Kurtz P, Merkow M, Stuart M, et al. Spontaneous hyperventilation and brain tissue hypoxia in patients with severe brain injury. J Neurol Neurosurg Psychiatry. 2010;81(7):793–7. https://doi.org/10.1136/jnnp.2009.174425.
50. Dastur CK, Yu W. Current management of spontaneous intracerebral haemorrhage. Stroke Vasc Neurol. 2017;2(1):21–9. https://doi.org/10.1136/svn-2016-000047.
51. Ni YN, Wang YM, Liang BM, Liang ZA. The effect of hyperoxia on mortality in critically ill patients: a systematic review and meta analysis. BMC Pulm Med. 2019;19(1):53. https://doi.org/10.1186/s12890-019-0810-1.
52. Brucken A, Kaab AB, Kottmann K, Rossaint R, Nolte KW, Weis J, et al. Reducing the duration of 100% oxygen ventilation in the early reperfusion period after cardiopulmonary resuscitation decreases striatal brain damage. Resuscitation. 2010;81(12):1698–703. https://doi.org/10.1016/j.resuscitation.2010.06.027.

53. Fallenius M, Raj R, Reinikainen M, Bendel S, Skrifvars MB. Association between high arterial oxygen tension and long-term survival after spontaneous intracerebral hemorrhage. Crit Care Med. 2016;44(1):180–7. https://doi.org/10.1097/CCM.0000000000001281.
54. Rincon F, Kang J, Maltenfort M, Vibbert M, Urtecho J, Athar MK, et al. Association between hyperoxia and mortality after stroke: a multicenter cohort study. Crit Care Med. 2014;42(2):387–96. https://doi.org/10.1097/CCM.0b013e3182a27732.
55. Lopez HV, Vivas MF, Ruiz RN, Martinez JR, Navaridas BG, Villa MG, et al. Association between post-procedural hyperoxia and poor functional outcome after mechanical thrombectomy for ischemic stroke: an observational study. Ann Intensive Care. 2019;9(1):59. https://doi.org/10.1186/s13613-019-0533-8.
56. Balan IS, Fiskum G, Hazelton J, Cotto-Cumba C, Rosenthal RE. Oximetry-guided reoxygenation improves neurological outcome after experimental cardiac arrest. Stroke. 2006;37(12):3008–13. https://doi.org/10.1161/01.STR.0000248455.73785.b1.
57. Steyerberg EW, Wiegers E, Sewalt C, Buki A, Citerio G, De Keyser V, et al. Case-mix, care pathways, and outcomes in patients with traumatic brain injury in CENTER-TBI: a European prospective, multicentre, longitudinal, cohort study. Lancet Neurol. 2019;18(10):923–34. https://doi.org/10.1016/S1474-4422(19)30232-7.
58. Coplin WM, Pierson DJ, Cooley KD, Newell DW, Rubenfeld GD. Implications of extubation delay in brain-injured patients meeting standard weaning criteria. Am J Respir Crit Care Med. 2000;161(5):1530–6. https://doi.org/10.1164/ajrccm.161.5.9905102.
59. Mayer SA, Copeland D, Bernardini GL, Boden-Albala B, Lennihan L, Kossoff S, et al. Cost and outcome of mechanical ventilation for life-threatening stroke. Stroke. 2000;31(10):2346–53. https://doi.org/10.1161/01.str.31.10.2346.
60. Karanjia N, Nordquist D, Stevens R, Nyquist P. A clinical description of extubation failure in patients with primary brain injury. Neurocrit Care. 2011;15(1):4–12. https://doi.org/10.1007/s12028-011-9528-5.
61. Wang S, Zhang L, Huang K, Lin Z, Qiao W, Pan S. Predictors of extubation failure in neurocritical patients identified by a systematic review and meta-analysis. PLoS ONE. 2014;9(12):e112198. https://doi.org/10.1371/journal.pone.0112198.
62. Scheinhorn DJ, Chao DC, Stearn-Hassenpflug M. Liberation from prolonged mechanical ventilation. Crit Care Clin. 2002;18(3):569–95. https://doi.org/10.1016/s0749-0704(02)00016-7.
63. Liu Y, Wei LQ, Li GQ, Lv FY, Wang H, Zhang YH, et al. A decision-tree model for predicting extubation outcome in elderly patients after a successful spontaneous breathing trial. Anesth Analg. 2010;111(5):1211–8. https://doi.org/10.1213/ANE.0b013e3181f4e82e.
64. Ko R, Ramos L, Chalela JA. Conventional weaning parameters do not predict extubation failure in neurocritical care patients. Neurocrit Care. 2009;10(3):269–73. https://doi.org/10.1007/s12028-008-9181-9.
65. Kayambu G, Boots R, Paratz J. Physical therapy for the critically ill in the ICU: a systematic review and meta-analysis. Crit Care Med. 2013;41(6):1543–54. https://doi.org/10.1097/CCM.0b013e31827ca637.
66. Villwock JA, Villwock MR, Deshaies EM. Tracheostomy timing affects stroke recovery. J Stroke Cerebrovasc Dis. 2014;23(5):1069–72. https://doi.org/10.1016/j.jstrokecerebrovasdis.2013.09.008.
67. Bosel J, Schiller P, Hook Y, Andes M, Neumann JO, Poli S, et al. Stroke-related Early Tracheostomy versus Prolonged Orotracheal Intubation in Neurocritical Care Trial (SETPOINT): a randomized pilot trial. Stroke. 2013;44(1):21–8. https://doi.org/10.1161/STROKEAHA.112.669895.
68. Schonenberger S, Niesen WD, Fuhrer H, Bauza C, Klose C, Kieser M, et al. Early tracheostomy in ventilated stroke patients: Study protocol of the international multicentre randomized trial SETPOINT2 (Stroke-related Early Tracheostomy vs. Prolonged Orotracheal Intubation in Neurocritical care Trial 2). Int J Stroke. 2016;11(3):368–79. https://doi.org/10.1177/1747493015616638.
69. Godet T, Chabanne R, Marin J, Kauffmann S, Futier E, Pereira B, et al. Extubation failure in brain-injured patients: risk factors and development of a prediction score in a prelimi-

nary prospective cohort study. Anesthesiology. 2017;126(1):104–14. https://doi.org/10.1097/ALN.0000000000001379.
70. Szeder V, Ortega-Gutierrez S, Ziai W, Torbey MT. The TRACH score: clinical and radiological predictors of tracheostomy in supratentorial spontaneous intracerebral hemorrhage. Neurocrit Care. 2010;13(1):40–6. https://doi.org/10.1007/s12028-010-9346-1.
71. Guerin C, Reignier J, Richard JC, Beuret P, Gacouin A, Boulain T, et al. Prone positioning in severe acute respiratory distress syndrome. N Engl J Med. 2013;368(23):2159–68. https://doi.org/10.1056/NEJMoa1214103.
72. Papazian L, Forel JM, Gacouin A, Penot-Ragon C, Perrin G, Loundou A, et al. Neuromuscular blockers in early acute respiratory distress syndrome. N Engl J Med. 2010;363(12):1107–16. https://doi.org/10.1056/NEJMoa1005372.
73. Young NH, Andrews PJ. High-frequency oscillation as a rescue strategy for brain-injured adult patients with acute lung injury and acute respiratory distress syndrome. Neurocrit Care. 2011;15(3):623–33. https://doi.org/10.1007/s12028-011-9550-7.
74. Roth C, Ferbert A, Deinsberger W, Kleffmann J, Kastner S, Godau J, et al. Does prone positioning increase intracranial pressure? A retrospective analysis of patients with acute brain injury and acute respiratory failure. Neurocrit Care. 2014;21(2):186–91. https://doi.org/10.1007/s12028-014-0004-x.
75. Le Roux P, Menon DK, Citerio G, Vespa P, Bader MK, Brophy GM, et al. Consensus summary statement of the International Multidisciplinary Consensus Conference on Multimodality Monitoring in Neurocritical Care: a statement for healthcare professionals from the Neurocritical Care Society and the European Society of Intensive Care Medicine. Neurocrit Care. 2014;21(Suppl 2):S1–26. https://doi.org/10.1007/s12028-014-0041-5.
76. Force ADT, Ranieri VM, Rubenfeld GD, Thompson BT, Ferguson ND, Caldwell E, et al. Acute respiratory distress syndrome: the Berlin Definition. JAMA. 2012;307(23):2526–33. https://doi.org/10.1001/jama.2012.5669.
77. Busl KM, Bleck TP. Neurogenic pulmonary edema. Crit Care Med. 2015;43(8):1710–5. https://doi.org/10.1097/CCM.0000000000001101.
78. Aljishi M, Jayathissa S. Neurogenic pulmonary oedema secondary to vertebral artery dissection while playing tennis. BMJ Case Rep. 2018;2018 https://doi.org/10.1136/bcr-2017-221753.
79. Raha A, Wadehra A, Sandhu K, Dasgupta A. Acute subdural hematoma causing neurogenic pulmonary edema following lumbar spine surgery. J Neurosurg Anesthesiol. 2017;29(1):63–4. https://doi.org/10.1097/ANA.0000000000000254.
80. Kondo R, Sugita Y, Arakawa K, Nakashima S, Umeno Y, Todoroki K, et al. Neurogenic pulmonary edema following Cryptococcal meningoencephalitis associated with HIV infection. Neuropathology. 2015;35(4):343–7. https://doi.org/10.1111/neup.12193.
81. Simon RP, Gean-Marton AD, Sander JE. Medullary lesion inducing pulmonary edema: a magnetic resonance imaging study. Ann Neurol. 1991;30(5):727–30. https://doi.org/10.1002/ana.410300515.
82. Lee DS, Kobrine A. Neurogenic pulmonary edema associated with ruptured spinal cord arteriovenous malformation. Neurosurgery. 1983;12(6):691–3. https://doi.org/10.1227/00006123-198306000-00019.
83. Baumann A, Audibert G, McDonnell J, Mertes PM. Neurogenic pulmonary edema. Acta Anaesthesiol Scand. 2007;51(4):447–55. https://doi.org/10.1111/j.1399-6576.2007.01276.x.
84. Sacher DC, Yoo EJ. Recurrent acute neurogenic pulmonary edema after uncontrolled seizures. Case Rep Pulmonol. 2018;2018:3483282. https://doi.org/10.1155/2018/3483282.
85. Ishiwata Y, Fujitsu K, Sekino T, Fujino H, Kubokura T, Tsubone K, et al. Subdural tension pneumocephalus following surgery for chronic subdural hematoma. J Neurosurg. 1988;68(1):58–61. https://doi.org/10.3171/jns.1988.68.1.0058.
86. Siegel JL, Hampton K, Rabinstein AA, McLaughlin D, Diaz-Gomez JL. Oxygen therapy with high-flow nasal cannula as an effective treatment for perioperative pneumocephalus: case illustrations and pathophysiological review. Neurocrit Care. 2018;29(3):366–73. https://doi.org/10.1007/s12028-017-0464-x.

Common Troubleshooting in Daily Practice

Ahmed Ibrahim Eissa

The aim of mechanical ventilation is to ensure adequate ventilation and oxygenation, reduce the work of breathing, and ensure patient comfort and synchrony with the ventilator while minimizing the risk of adverse effects.

A patient fighting (or bucking) the ventilator is an emergent situation. If the clinician cannot find the source of the problem and fix it, the patient may die in minutes.

Sometimes, the problem is easy to spot and solve, such as disconnected ventilator tubing. If the cause is not immediately obvious, primary responsibility is **to ensure adequate ventilation**. This is a priority over diagnosis.

Most troubleshooting are diagnosed by rapid clinical examination. Radiology and bedside lung ultrasound are helpful. But if the patient is dying, do not wait for radiology, just ACT.

Equally, most troubleshooting are manageable with simple clinical maneuvers.

Ventilator alarms provide safety for critically ill patients who are often unable to speak or communicate effectively. These audible or visual alarms are triggered when the ventilator/patient condition exceeds the preset alarm limits. This alert system prompts the clinicians to attend to the patient without delay.

Ventilator alarms have different classifications.

The European Committee for Standardization established the priority systems (high priority, medium priority, and low priority) to alert clinicians with patient safety concerns. The American Association for Respiratory Care published a consensus statement recommending three levels of alerts (level 1: immediately life threatening, level 2: potentially life threatening, level 3: non-ventilator events not likely to be life threatening).

In addition to these ventilator alarms, external alerts are also available to monitor the patient's changing physiologic status (SpO_2, heart rate, etc.) [1] (Table 1).

A. I. Eissa (✉)
Lecturer of Critical Care Medicine, Faculty of Medicine- Cairo University, Cairo, Egypt

J. Hidalgo et al. (eds.), *Personalized Mechanical Ventilation*,
https://doi.org/10.1007/978-3-031-14138-6_26

Table 1 Initial ventilator alarm settings

Ventilator alarm	Initial sittings
Peak pressure—High/low	10–15 cm above or below the peak inspiratory pressure
Minute ventilation—High/low	50% above or below the set volume
Low exhaled tidal volume	50% of the delivered tidal volume
High respiratory (frequency) rate	10–20% above the current total frequency Then, adjusted according to the clinical status
Low frequency/apnea	2–6 breaths/min below the current total
The high PEEP	2 cm H_2O above the current PEEP
The low PEEP alarm	2 cm H_2O below the current PEEP

1 High Airway Pressure Alarm

Excessive alveolar pressure may damage the lung, causing acute lung injury (or in more severe cases ARDS) and air leaks (e.g., pneumothorax, pneumomediastinum). In addition, the pressure that is transmitted from the alveoli to the pleural space will also have hemodynamic effects [2].

High airway pressure is not only important because of the risk of adverse effects, but because it also leads to inadequate ventilation. With most ventilators, inspiration is terminated if the airway pressure reaches the set upper pressure limit, and it results in the patient receiving a much lower tidal volume [3].

High airway pressure alarm in volume-preset modes has the same significance of low tidal volume alarm in pressure-preset modes.

1.1 Causes of High Airway Pressure [4, 5]

- Ventilator:
  - Inappropriate settings.
  - Ventilator malfunction.
- Circuit:
  - Kinking in the circuit.
  - Fluid/condensed water vapor in the inspiratory limb of the ventilator circuit.
  - Wet/obstructed filters causing resistance rise.
- Endotracheal tube:
  - Kinking of the tubing.
  - Obstructed with secretions, blood, etc.
  - Patient bites the tube.
  - Endobronchial intubation.
  - Herniation of the cuff of the endotracheal tube over its distal tip.

- Patient:
  - Airway narrowing *(increase in peak airway pressure* ***without*** *a proportional increase in plateau pressure).*

    Major obstruction of the airway.
    Bronchoconstriction.
    Acute exacerbation of asthma or chronic obstructive pulmonary disease.
    Retained secretions.

  - Decrease in lung compliance *(increase in peak airway pressure* ***with*** *a proportional increase in plateau pressure).*

    Pulmonary edema.
    Fluid overload.
    Consolidation.
    Acute respiratory distress syndrome.
    Dynamic hyperinflation associated with intrinsic positive end-expiratory pressure (PEEPi).
    Atelectasis/collapse.

  - Extrinsic compression *(increase in peak airway pressure* ***with*** *a proportional increase in plateau pressure).*

    Collection of pleural fluid (hemothorax, parapneumonic effusion, or transudative effusion).
    Pneumothorax.
    Abdominal distension (gastric distension, ileus, or ascites).
    Extensive eschar formation.
    Surgical emphysema.

  - Patient-ventilator dyssynchrony, coughing.

1.2 Initial Assessment and Management

1.2.1 Step One: Start Manual Bag-Mask Ventilation

The first response is to disconnect the patient from the ventilator, and start manual bag-mask ventilation with the bag connected to 100% oxygen. This step is both therapeutic and diagnostic [6]. If the distress resolves and the patient is easy to ventilate, it indicates that the problem is ventilator/circuit problem. If the distress continues and the patient is difficult to ventilate, it indicates patient/artificial airway problem.

Check pulse oximeter reading as hypoxia can be life threatening, although several factors can affect readings [7].

1.2.2 Step Two: Assess for Life-Threatening Major Airway Obstruction

If a major airway obstruction is suspected, it will commonly cause oxygen desaturation and an increase in peak airway pressure. The clinician should attempt to pass a suction catheter through the airway to determine if the airway is patent and to remove secretions or other materials that can cause obstruction. Failure to pass a suction catheter through the airway indicates obstruction and necessitates urgent changing of the tube, unless you were able to relieve the obstruction.

The endotracheal tube can become occluded with a variety of foreign bodies, including dried lubricant [4], surgical tape [4], a broken stylet sheath [5], plastic debris retained from the time of manufacturing the Murphy eye in the tube (Fig. 1) [6], and nasal turbinates avulsed during nasotracheal intubation [8].

External compression of an endotracheal tube as a result of an inflated cuff is a rare cause of airway obstruction (Fig. 2) [9].

Herniation of the cuff of an endotracheal tube over its distal tip can cause complete airway obstruction [10]. Most commonly, it occurs after changes in position of the tube or changes in the posture of the head and neck. Clues to diagnose include an increase in peak airway pressure, resistance during manual ventilation, a decrease in VT, difficulty in passing a suction catheter, and an abnormal musical sound during inspiration [11]. Deflation of the cuff produces immediate relief.

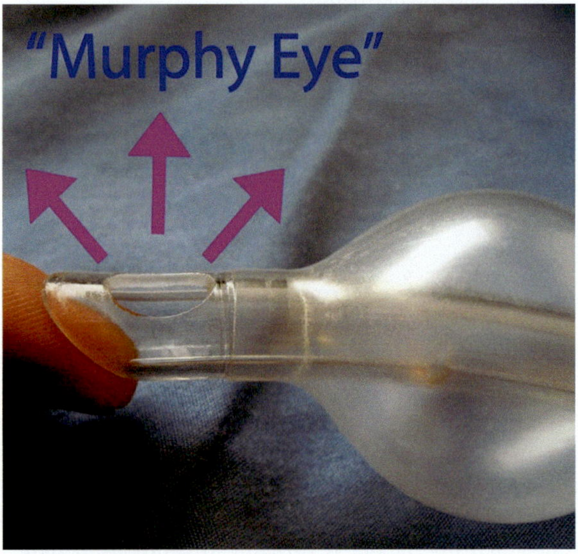

Fig. 1 Murphy eye of the endotracheal tube

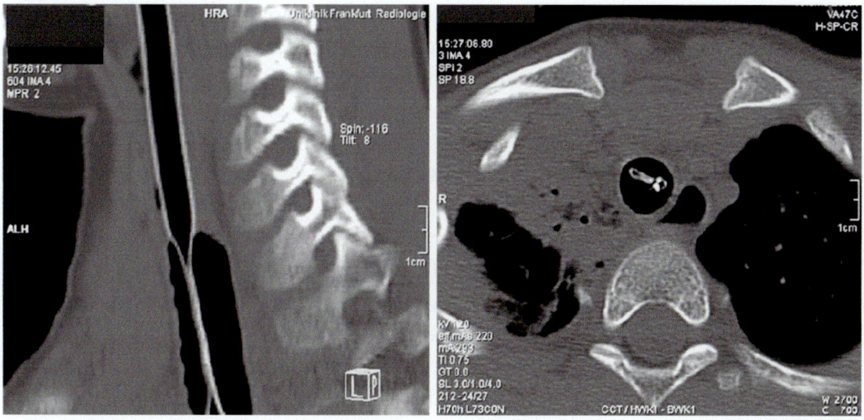

Fig. 2 External compression of endotracheal tube. Computed tomography images of the sagittal plane of the cervical spine and trachea (*left panel*) and transversal plane at the level of the first thoracic vertebra (*right panel*)

Fig. 3 Inspiratory pause pressure

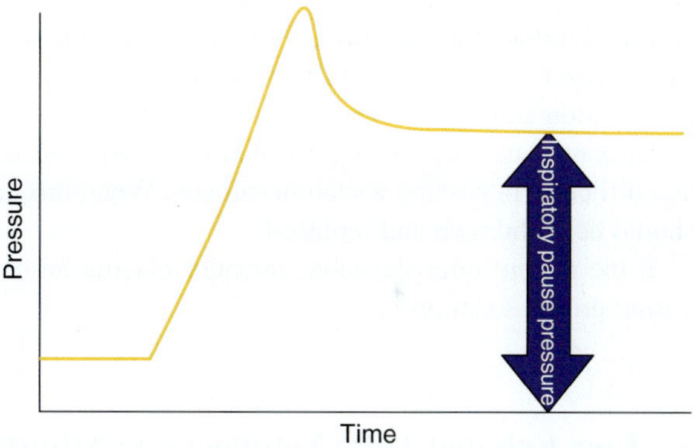

1.2.3 Step Three: Perform Inspiratory Pause Hold

Perform end-inspiratory occlusion maneuver "inspiratory pause hold" to measure the plateau pressure if possible (Fig. 3).

This pressure is measured at the end of inspiration when there is no flow.

Airway pressure = Flow × Resistance + Alveolar pressure.

If there is no flow, airway pressure = 0 × Resistance + Alveolar pressure and therefore.

Airway pressure = Alveolar pressure.

An increase in peak airway pressure **without** a proportional increase in plateau pressure indicates narrowing of the airway [3, 12].

However, an increase in peak airway pressure accompanied **with** a proportional increase in plateau pressure indicates a decrease in thoracic compliance, which may arise within the lung or from extrinsic compression.

1.2.4 Step Four: Urgent Cause Management

Pneumothorax is suspected if there is evidence of asymmetric expansion of each hemithorax, diminished air entry on the affected side with signs of hyperexpansion, and hyperresonance. Bedside lung ultrasound is a very useful diagnostic tool. Radiology should not be done for unstable patients [13].

Tension pneumothorax is suspected if there is evidence of hypotension and circulatory shock, congested neck veins, and tracheal deviation. In this case, immediate needle decompression should be performed. If a gush of air is heard, a thoracostomy tube is inserted.

Clues to diagnose endobronchial intubation include an increase in peak airway pressure with a proportional increase in plateau pressure, asymmetric expansion of each hemithorax, and a decrease in breath sounds over the contralateral lung.

If endobronchial intubation is suspected, the endotracheal tube should be pulled back a few centimeters, and the position of the tube should be confirmed by chest auscultation and by radiography.

Kinking is usually visible; it will also lead to an increase in peak airway pressure and difficulty in passing a suction catheter. When this occurs, the endotracheal tube should be withdrawn and replaced.

If the patient bites the tube, consider placing an oral airway or bite block and ensure proper sedation.

2 Low Exhaled Tidal Volume (VT)/Minute Ventilation Alarm

Inadequate tidal volume will result in inadequate ventilation and respiratory acidosis.

Monitoring the tidal volume is particularly important in patients who are being ventilated using pressure-control or pressure-support modes. For a change in system resistance or compliance, it will result in a change in tidal volume. In patients who are being ventilated in volume-preset modes, the tidal volume is unlikely to vary significantly unless the ventilator is malfunctioning [3].

Many ventilators do not incorporate an alarm for low or high tidal volume but do incorporate alarms for minute ventilation [3].

Exhaled tidal volume is a more accurate indicator of the tidal volume. A significant discrepancy between the inspiratory and expiratory tidal volume usually indicates a leak in the system.

2.1 *Causes of Low Exhaled Tidal Volume [4–6, 8]*

- Ventilator :
  - Inappropriate settings.
  - Ventilator malfunction.
- Circuit:
  - Disconnection in the circuit *(patient-disconnected alarm will be triggered if disconnected for more than 1 min).*
- Endotracheal tube:
  - Displacement of the endotracheal tube into the hypopharynx or esophagus.
  - Endotracheal tube cuff leak or deflation.
- Patient:
  - Patient-ventilator dyssynchrony.
  - Tracheoesophageal fistula.

2.2 *Initial Assessment and Management*

2.2.1 Step One: Start Manual Bag-Mask Ventilation

The first response is to disconnect the patient from the ventilator, and start manual bag-mask ventilation with the bag connected to 100% oxygen. Check pulse oximeter reading as hypoxia can be life threatening, although several factors can affect readings [7]. Check the ventilator and circuit for visible disconnection or leakage.

2.2.2 Step Two: Check Endotracheal Tube Position

A previous properly positioned endotracheal/tracheostomy tube may subsequently move up or down in a patient's airway. Downward or upward movement of an endotracheal tube is usually caused by inadequate external fixation of the endotracheal tube, excessive movement of the neck, or both [14].

An endotracheal tube may also migrate above the vocal cords or get dislodged into the esophagus [10]. Esophageal intubation may arise as a result of attempts to blindly reposition an endotracheal tube.

Clues to diagnose movement of the tube into the hypopharynx or esophagus are respiratory distress accompanied by phonation, audible escape of air through the nose and mouth, absence of tube condensation, decrease in tidal volume (VT), decrease (or increase) in peak airway pressure, and abdominal distension.

Chest radiography is not recommended and can be misleading because the trachea overlays the esophagus, making it difficult to tell whether the tube is located in the esophagus or trachea in the anteroposterior view obtained at bedside. Meanwhile, end-tidal CO2 of zero helps in detecting esophageal intubation.

The tip of endotracheal tube should be secured at least 3–4 cm above the carina, and a chest radiograph should be obtained at the time of intubation [14]. In addition, centimeter markings on an endotracheal tube should be documented and help as a reference, although not completely reliable [15]. In general, an endotracheal tube should be secured at reference markings of 23 cm in men and 21 cm in women [15]. On the chest radiograph, the tip of the endotracheal tube should be located at a level corresponding to the top of the aortic knob when the head is in a neutral position [16]. Auscultation of equal breath sounds is less reliable [15].

2.2.3 Step Three: Check for Cuff Leak

Clues to diagnose are low peak airway pressure, low exhaled VT, phonation, audible escape of air through the nose and mouth, frothy secretions in the patient's mouth, a discrepancy between expired and inspired VT, and failure to maintain a set level of PEEP [10].

It is most commonly caused by endotracheal tube malposition. Consequently, the development of a cuff leak should alert the clinician to reevaluate tube position.

Leak is not necessary in the cuff itself, but can also be in the pilot balloon or in the external valve assembly [16]. A temporal correction of this problem (without having to immediately replace the endotracheal tube) is to clamp the cuff inflation tubing proximal to the valve and pilot balloon.

Meanwhile, complete rupture of a cuff can lead to aspiration of saliva, vomit, or food; the entire endotracheal tube needs to be replaced.

2.2.4 Step Four: Assess the Patient

Patient-ventilator dyssynchrony is discussed in a separate chapter.

Tracheoesophageal fistula is a rare complication that is primarily caused by ischemia of the tracheal wall secondary to pressure from an overinflated cuff or by movement of a tracheal tube or its tip [17].

Patients with this complication typically have had both a tracheal tube and a nasogastric tube in place for a long time [10, 18].

Clues to diagnose include the inability to deliver a preset VT despite a functional cuff, gastric distension, audible leak of air through the mouth, copious airway secretions, suctioning of gastric contents from the lower respiratory tract, and clinical deterioration and coughing on deflation of the cuff [16].

Definitive diagnosis can be made by bronchoscopy with direct visualization or by imaging, i.e., esophagography or tracheography [16]. Treatment is surgical or bronchoscopic closure [16].

3 Low-Pressure Alarm

Low-pressure alarm will serve the same function of low exhaled tidal volume (VT)/minute ventilation alarms. Sometimes, the alarm limits are breached as a result of changing patient condition. For example, the low-pressure alarm during volume-preset modes may be triggered when the patient's compliance has improved significantly. Likewise, during pressure-preset modes, the low-volume alarm may be triggered when the patient's compliance has decreased significantly [1].

4 High-Frequency Alarm

Rapid shallow breathing is a clinical sign of respiratory distress as it increases dead-space ventilation, metabolism, and CO_2 production [19].

High-frequency alarm is triggered when the total frequency (mandatory and spontaneous) exceeds the preset high-frequency limit.

The high-frequency alarm limit should be lowered accordingly during the weaning process.

4.1 Common Causes of High-Frequency Alarm [19]

- Ventilator:
  - Inappropriate settings.
- Circuit:
  - Fluid/condensed water vapor in the ventilator circuit that increases the work of breathing.
- Endotracheal tube:
  - Secretions, blood, etc.
- Patient:
  - Experiencing pain, discomfort, or anxiety.
  - Delirium, hallucination.
  - Hypoxia.
  - Pulmonary edema.
  - Fluid overload.
  - Lung pathology.
  - Metabolic acidosis.
  - New sepsis.

4.2 Management

Check the ventilator, circuit, and endotracheal tube.

Ensure that the patient is comfortable, not in pain, and well sedated.

Treat the undelaying cause.

5 Low-Frequency and Apnea Alarms

Low-frequency and apnea alarms are triggered when the total frequency falls below the preset frequency limit. They are also triggered in circuit leak.

The low-frequency limit should be adjusted accordingly with the patient's spontaneous frequency. For patients with a high spontaneous breathing (e.g., awakening from anesthesia, hypoxia, anxiety), alarm limit is increased. For patients with a low spontaneous breathing (e.g., sleeping, under sedation, during weaning), alarm limit is decreased [1].

5.1 Common Causes of Low-Frequency Alarm

- Inappropriate ventilator setting.
- Circuit disconnection or similar conditions.

5.2 Common Causes of Apnea Alarm

- Inappropriate ventilator setting.
- Circuit disconnection or similar conditions.
- True apnea in patients who are ventilated in a pure support mode (e.g., pressure support).
- In patients with periodic respiration when the time between two consecutive inspiratory efforts exceeds the set alarm limit [3].

6 High Positive End-Expiratory Pressure (PEEP) Alarm

High PEEP alarm is used to alert the presence of auto-PEEP or intrinsic PEEP (PEEPi) that may occur as a result of air trapping in the lung (dynamic hyperinflation) [4–6].

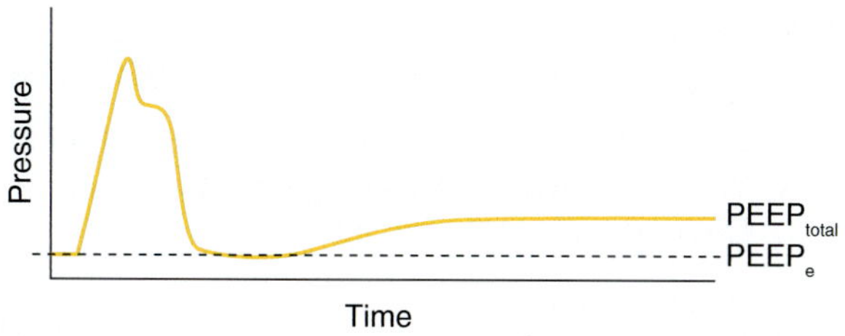

Fig. 4 Measuring total PEEP *(PEEPtotal)*

The high PEEP alarm may be set at 2 cm H_2O above the current PEEP.

Total PEEP can be estimated in apneic patients by activating the "expiratory pause hold" and noting the end-expiratory pressure when it plateaus (Fig. 4).

7 Low Positive End-Expiratory Pressure (PEEP) Alarm

Low PEEP alarm is triggered in conditions of losing airway pressure (e.g., cuff leak, circuit leak).

Low PEEP alarm may also be triggered when the inspiratory flow delivered by the ventilator is insufficient to meet the patient's inspiratory demand. The patient may show signs of air hunger, chest retraction, tachypnea, and tachycardia. On the flow-time waveform, the peak inspiratory flow may drop slightly because the positive inspiratory flow by the ventilator is partially overcome by the negative inspiratory flow by the patient.

The low PEEP alarm may be set at 2 cm H_2O below the current PEEP.

8 Desaturation and Hypoxia

If a patient desaturates while on a mechanical ventilator, the same principle is applied; consider both patient causes and equipment causes.

8.1 Causes of Desaturation and Hypoxia on Mechanical Ventilation [6, 20–22]

- Ventilator:
  - Inappropriate settings.
  - Ventilator malfunction.
  - Oxygen failure *(gas supply and oxygen concentration alarms will be triggered).*

- Circuit:
  - Kinking in the circuit.
  - Fluid/condensed water vapor in the inspiratory limb of the ventilator circuit.
  - Wet/obstructed filters causing resistance rise.
  - Disconnection in the circuit.
- Endotracheal tube:
  - Kinking of the tubing.
  - Obstructed with secretions, blood, etc.
  - Endobronchial intubation.
  - Displacement of the endotracheal tube into the hypopharynx or esophagus.
  - Endotracheal tube cuff leak or deflation.
- Patient:
  - Airway narrowing.

    Major obstruction of the airway.
    Bronchoconstriction.
    Acute exacerbation of asthma or chronic obstructive pulmonary disease.
    Retained secretions.
  - Decrease in lung compliance.

    Pulmonary edema.
    Fluid overload.
    Consolidation.
    Acute respiratory distress syndrome.
    Dynamic hyperinflation associated with intrinsic positive end-expiratory pressure (PEEPi).
    Atelectasis/collapse.
  - Extrinsic compression.

    Collection of pleural fluid (hemothorax, parapneumonic effusion, or transudative effusion).
    Pneumothorax.
    Abdominal distension (gastric distension, ileus, or ascites).
    Extensive eschar formation.
    Surgical emphysema.
  - Patient-ventilator dyssynchrony.
  - Aspiration (gastric or oropharyngeal) [6].
  - Pulmonary thromboembolism.
  - Systemic—nonpulmonary—problem affecting oxygenation, e.g., sepsis, shock, and seizure [6].

- Effects of interventions and procedures [6]:
  - Endotracheal suctioning.
  - Changes in body position.
  - Chest physiotherapy.
  - Bronchoscopy.
  - Thoracentesis.
  - Peritoneal dialysis.
  - Hemodialysis ventilator malfunction.
- Medications [6]:
  - Bronchodilators (cause ventilation/perfusion mismatch).
  - Vasodilators (cause ventilation/perfusion mismatch).
  - β-Blockers (cause bronchospasm).

8.2 *Initial Assessment and Management*

8.2.1 Step One: Check the Pulse Oximeter and Set the Fraction of Inspired Oxygen to 1

Quickly check the integrity of pulse oximeter waveform, and check if the heart rate measured by oximeter corresponds to the ECG heart rate. Set the fraction of inspired oxygen to 1. If hypoxemia is corrected, the cause of hypoxemia is likely ventilation/perfusion mismatch [1].

8.2.2 Step Two: Check Chest Movement: "Is the Patient Ventilating?"

Check that the patient's chest is still moving before going on to a more detailed examination. Assess for chest movement and its synergy, visually and manually, while looking at the ventilator for low tidal volumes or high-pressure alarm.

8.2.3 Step Three: Start Manual Bag-Mask Ventilation

Disconnect the patient from the ventilator, and start manual bag-mask ventilation with the bag connected to 100% oxygen.

If the patient is easy to ventilate and it is easy to squeeze the bag, but the chest is not moving, there is a leak in the circuit (e.g., cuff leak or disconnection) or the endotracheal tube has been dislodged and is no longer in the trachea. Refer to the causes of low exhaled tidal volume.

If the patient is easy to ventilate and it is easy to squeeze the bag, resulting in proper chest movement and improvement of saturation, this indicates that the problem is ventilator/circuit related.

If the patient is difficult to ventilate and it is difficult to squeeze the bag, it indicates patient/artificial airway problem.

8.2.4 Step Four: Urgent Cause Management

Special consideration should be given to the possibility of endobronchial intubation, pneumothorax, collapse of part of the lung, pulmonary edema, and bronchospasm as these are all easily treatable.

Also consider the possibility of pulmonary embolus as this is more common in critically ill patients and the clinical features are subtle [20–22].

Increasing PEEP will improve hypoxemia secondary to intrapulmonary shunting. PEEP increases the functional residual capacity (FRC) and residual volume (RV). Since normal gas exchange occurs at the FRC level, PEEP improves ventilation by overcoming the shunt-producing conditions (e.g., atelectasis, pulmonary edema) that reduce FRC. Another advantage of PEEP is its ability to reverse shunt and refractory hypoxemia when applied with a lung recruitment maneuver [1, 20–22].

9 Hypotension

Patients with good systolic cardiac function, normal sympathetic reflexes, and normal or increased intravascular volume tolerate mechanical ventilation well, especially if spontaneous triggering efforts continue.

Venous return is largely determined by intravascular volume and venous tone. Intrathoracic pressure rises during positive-pressure ventilation, especially when positive end-expiratory pressure (PEEP) is used or auto-PEEP is generated.

Profound deterioration may occur in patients developing auto-PEEP immediately after the institution of positive-pressure ventilation. Unlike hemorrhage and other states of hypovolemia, compensatory heart rate responses to the low cardiac output and blood pressure are often blunted [1].

9.1 Common Causes of Hypotension Occurring Immediately after the Initiation of Positive-Pressure Ventilation [1, 3]

- Hypovolemia is exacerbated by reduced venous return due to positive intrathoracic pressure.
- Drugs used for induction of anesthesia for intubation. Almost all anesthetic induction agents cause vasodilatation and myocardial depression.

- Loss of sympathetic tone as a result of the use of hypnotic/sedative agents.
- Gas trapping due to overventilation.
- Although far less common, being life threatening, tension pneumothorax should always be considered.

9.2 *Initial Assessment and Management*

9.2.1 Step One: Fluid Administration

The appropriate initial response is usually to give fluids as hypovolemia and drug-induced hypotension are by far the most common causes of hypotension occurring immediately after the initiation of positive-pressure ventilation.

9.2.2 Step Two: Temporarily Disconnect the Patient from the Ventilator

If this fails to correct the hypotension, temporarily disconnect the patient from the ventilator. If the cause is gas trapping, the blood pressure will rise within about 10–30 seconds as the trapped gas is released.

9.2.3 Step Three: Vasopressor Infusion

In severely ill patients, the use of vasopressor infusion may be required, and consideration should be given to preparing a vasopressor infusion prior to intubation/MV in selected high-risk patients.

9.2.4 Step Four: Assess for Tension Pneumothorax

If tension pneumothorax is suspected—especially if there is no response to fluids—immediate needle decompression should be performed. If a gush of air is heard, a thoracostomy tube is inserted.

References

1. Chang DW. Management of mechanical ventilation. In: Chang DW, et al., editors. Respiratory critical care. 1st ed. Burlington, MA: Jones & Bartlett Learning/MTP; 2020. p. 416–78.
2. Doelken P, Sahn SA. Pleural disease in the critically ill patient. In: Irwin RS, Rippe JM, editors. Intensive care medicine. 6th ed. Philadelphia, PA: Lippincott, Williams, and Wilkins; 2008. p. 636.
3. Gomersall C, Joynt G, Tang S, et al. Troubleshooting. In: Gomersall C, Joynt G, Tang S, et al., editors. Mechanical ventilation: beyond BASIC. Shatin, Hong Kong: The Department of Anaesthesia & Intensive Care, The Chinese University of Hong Kong; 2014. p. 91–9.

4. Tobin MJ. What should a clinician do when a patient "fights the ventilator"? Respir Care. 1991;36:395–406.
5. Tobin MJ. Mechanical ventilation. N Engl J Med. 1994;330:1056.
6. Tobin MJ, Jubran A, Laghi F. Fighting the ventilator. In: Tobin MJ, editor. Principles and practice of mechanical ventilation. 3rd ed. New York, NY: Mcgraw Hill; 2013. p. 1237–59.
7. Jubran A. Pulse oximetry. In: Tobin MJ, editor. Principles and practice of intensive care monitoring. New York, NY: McGraw-Hill; 1998. p. 261–87.
8. Tobin MJ. Nobel prize symposium physiologic basis of mechanical ventilation. Ann Am Thorac Soc. 2018;15(Suppl 1):S49–52.
9. Hofstetter C, Scheller B, Hoegl S, et al. Cuff overinflation and endotracheal tube obstruction: case report and experimental study. Scand J Trauma Resusc Emerg Med. 2010;18:18.
10. Stauffer J. Monitoring the use of tracheal tubes. In: Tobin MJ, editor. Principles and practice of intensive care monitoring. New York, NY: McGraw-Hill; 1998. p. 667–82.
11. Hudson LD. Diagnosis and management of acute respiratory distress in patients on mechanical ventilators. In: Moser K, Spragg R, editors. Respiratory emergencies. St. Louis, MO: Mosby; 1982. p. 201–13.
12. Rossi A. Monitoring respiratory mechanics in ventilator-dependent patients. In: Tobin MJ, editor. Principles and practice of intensive care monitoring. New York, NY: McGraw-Hill; 1998. p. 553–96.
13. Marini JJ, Dries DJ. Practical problems and complications of mechanical ventilation. In: Marini JJ, Dries DJ, editors. Critical care medicine—The Essentials and more. 5th ed. Philadelphia, PA: Lippincott Williams & Wilkins; 2018. p. 229–70.
14. Conrardy PA, Goodman LR, Lainge F, Singer MM. Alteration of endotracheal tube position. Flexion and extension of the neck. Crit Care Med. 1976;4(1):7–12.
15. Brunel W, Coleman DL, Schwartz DE, et al. Assessment of routine chest roentgenograms and the physical examination to confirm endotracheal tube position. Chest. 1989;96(5):1043–5.
16. Marcy TW, Marini JJ. Respiratory distress in the ventilated patient. Clin Chest Med. 1994;15(1):55–73.
17. Harley HR. Ulcerative tracheo-oesophageal fistula during treatment by tracheostomy and intermittent positive pressure ventilation. Thorax. 1972;27(3):338–52.
18. Wood DE, Mathisen DJ. Late complications of tracheotomy. Clin Chest Med. 1991;12(3):597–609.
19. Hill LL, Pearl RG. Flow triggering, pressure triggering, and autotriggering during mechanical ventilation. Crit Care Med. 2000;28:579.
20. Barbateskovic M, Schjørring OL, Russo Krauss S, et al. Higher versus lower fraction of inspired oxygen or targets of arterial oxygenation for adults admitted to the intensive care unit. Cochrane Database Syst Rev. 2019;2019(11):CD012631.
21. O'Driscoll BR, Howard LS, Earis J, et al. BTS guideline for oxygen use in adults in healthcare and emergency settings. Thorax. 2017;72:ii1.
22. Panwar R, Hardie M, Bellomo R, et al. Conservative versus Liberal oxygenation targets for mechanically ventilated patients. A pilot multicenter randomized controlled trial. Am J Respir Crit Care Med. 2016;193(43):43.

Correction to: Respiratory Physiology and Mechanics at the Bedside

Ahmed Mohamed Reda Taha and Prashant Nasa

Correction to:
Chapter 1 in: J. Hidalgo et al. (eds.), *Personalized Mechanical Ventilation*, https://doi.org/10.1007/978-3-031-14138-6_1

The affiliation of first author Ahmed Mohamed Reda Taha was incorrectly printed in Chapter 1 (Respiratory Physiology and Mechanics at the Bedside) as *Intensive Care and COVID 19 Unit, Belize Healthcare Partners, Belize, Belize*. It has now been corrected to "*Critical Care Institute, Cleveland Clinic, Abu Dhabi, UAE*" on pages iv and 1.

The updated original version of the chapter can be found at
https://doi.org/10.1007/978-3-031-14138-6_1

J. Hidalgo et al. (eds.), *Personalized Mechanical Ventilation*,
https://doi.org/10.1007/978-3-031-14138-6_27

Index

J. Hidalgo et al. (eds.), *Personalized Mechanical Ventilation*,
https://doi.org/10.1007/978-3-031-14138-6

N

Q

R

MIX
Papier aus verantwortungsvollen Quellen
Paper from responsible sources
FSC® C105338
FSC
www.fsc.org

If you have any concerns about our products,
you can contact us on
ProductSafety@springernature.com

In case Publisher is established outside the EU,
the EU authorized representative is:
Springer Nature Customer Service Center GmbH
Europaplatz 3, 69115 Heidelberg, Germany

Printed by Libri Plureos GmbH
in Hamburg, Germany